BAUER & BUSSE

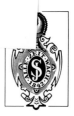

The Arterial System

Dynamics, Control Theory and Regulation

Edited by
R. D. Bauer and R. Busse

With 132 Figures

Springer-Verlag Berlin Heidelberg New York 1978

LQM K

International Symposium in Honor of Professor Dr. Erik Wetterer
"Dynamics and Regulation of the Arterial System"
Erlangen, Germany, October, 28-30, 1977

Privatdozent Dr. R. D. Bauer
Privatdozent Dr. R. Busse
Institut für Physiologie und Kardiologie
der Universität Erlangen-Nürnberg
D-8520 Erlangen, Waldstraße 6

ISBN 3-540-08897-0 Springer-Verlag Berlin Heidelberg New York
ISBN 0-387-08897-0 Springer-Verlag New York Heidelberg Berlin

Library of Congress Cataloging in Publication Data. Main entry under title: The Arterial System.
"Summarizes the papers presented at the symposium 'Dynamics and Regulation of the arterial system'
held at Erlangen on October 28-30, 1977, in honor of Prof. Erik Wetterer." Bibliography: p.
Includes index. 1. Arteries--Congresses. 2. Hemodynamics--Congresses. 3. Rheology (Biology)--Congresses.
4. Wetterer, Erik, 1909 - I. Bauer, Rudolf Dietrich - II. Busse, Rudi, 1943 - III. Wetterer, Erik, 1909 -
[DNLM: 1. Arteries--Physiology--Congresses. 2. Blood flow velocity--Congresses. 3. Coronary vessels--
Congresses. 4. Cardiovascular system--Congresses. WG510 A786   1977]   QP106.2.A77   612'.133
78-15945.

Offsetprinting and Binding: Julius Beltz, Hemsbach/Bergstr.   2127/3130-543210

Preface

This book summarizes the papers presented at the symposium "Dynamics and Regulation of the Arterial System" held at Erlangen on 28-30 October 1977 in honor of Professor Erik Wetterer. The aim of the symposium was an intensive exchange of ideas within a multidisciplinary group of scientists who are specialists in their fields of research. It is obvious that a two-day symposium covering such a wide range of topics could only highlight certain aspects of the latest research on the cardiovascular system.

The book is divided into three sections. The first part deals with arterial hemodynamics. Emphasized are the mechanical properties of the arterial wall, in particular the smooth muscle, fundamental parameters for the description of pulse wave propagation, such as attenuation, phase velocity, and reflection of pulse waves. Furthermore, new methods for recording arterial diameters and the latest results in determining pulsatile pressure and pulsatile diameter of arteries in vivo as well as from calculations based on models of the arterial system are presented.

The second part deals with applications of the control theory and the principles of optimality of the cardiovascular system in toto and of single regions of this system. Contributions to research in the field of regulation of blood volume and of regional hemodynamics are also presented.

The third part covers problems of interaction of the heart and the arterial system, including fluid mechanics of the aortic valves and the coronary blood flow under normal and pathologic conditions.

We hope that this book will contribute to a better understanding of the general physiologic principles underlying the various functions of the cardiovascular system.

We are deeply grateful for the friendly cooperation of all who were involved in preparing the manuscripts and acknowledge the valuable contributions of chairmen of various sessions of the symposium, in particular Professor Anliker, Professor Bretschneider, Professor Jacob, Professor Kenner, Professor Taylor, Professor Thurau, and Professor Reichel, who facilitated the fruitful exchange of ideas during the symposium.

The cost of the symposium and of this publication has been met by generous grants from the pharmaceutical and electromedical industries, which are herewith gratefully acknowledged.

Finally, we would like to thank Springer-Verlag for making it possible to publish this book quickly and without hitches.

Erlangen, May 1978   R.D. Bauer   R. Busse

Table of Contents

Control Theory and Regulation

Cardiovascular Dynamics and Coronary Arteries

Laudatio

Dynamics of the Arterial System

Mechanics of the Arterial Wall in Health and Disease

D. H. Bergel

University Laboratory of Physiology, Parks Road, Oxford OX1 3PT

Introduction

My purpose is to cover only parts of the literature on this large topic, paying special attention to studies concerned with or relevant to the human. There have been several comprehensive reviews dealing with this subject recently and reference should be made to these [18, 13, 66]. Taylor [70] and Roach [67] have discussed the whole area of cardiovascular fluid dynamics, while those who would like an introduction to this subject, with a distinctive personal and narrative style, are recommended to read McDonald [56].

The mechanics of arteries is an important topic in its own right. It involves the study of the deformation of a complex multiphase material containing active elements subjected to stresses occurring over a wide frequency range. At the present, we have very little knowledge of how the wall is put together and how its properties relate to the structure, and this seems to me to be a major deficiency. However, another reason to look at arteries has to do with understanding how their properties relate to their function within the circulation. They serve to distribute the blood to the tissues and appear to be put together in some optional way [69]. Arterial properties also influence the work of the heart; indeed, the hydraulic impedance presented to the heart by the arterial tree constitutes the load on the heart [57], and the manner in which the ventricle expels blood into a system of known hydraulic acceptance ought to tell us something important about the heart. We do not yet know how to extract this information and make use of it, although some progress has been made [37]. Nevertheless, we have learnt a great deal about the hydraulics of the arteries in the last 2 decades, and it is the arteries as components of the circulation that will be mainly considered here.

Methods

To be able to measure the mechanical properties of a blood vessel, it is necessary to know about its dimensions and the forces acting on it. In the physiological laboratory, it is now relatively simple to obtain high-fidelity records of pressure and other forces; this is not so easy to do with dimensions, even for rather simple geometries. Well – established methods exist for use on an exposed blood vessel;

3

these are discussed elsewhere [14]. But there are many situations in which it might be desirable to measure the dimensions of the undisturbed and unexposed vessel, and it is here that the real difficulties arise. One result of the measurement problems was the suggestion that the exposed artery is stiffer than when in its normal situation. This idea was based on angiographic [8] or ultrasonic [7, 50] measurements in humans. Others who have used x-rays [47] have found the vessel concerned, the ascending aorta, to be rather less compliant than Arndt and his colleagues, but both groups agree that the compliance is very much greater than that reported many years ago by Greenfield and Patel [43].

There seem to be two different problems behind this disagreement. Firstly, the early measurements by Patel and his associates were done with a caliper strain gauge, and it was later shown that they could have been in error [65]. Later determinations with this same device produced rather lower figures which agreed very well with the simultaneously recorded pulse wave velocity (PWV). Any discrepancies between the angiographic and caliper methods would appear to have disappeared, and both techniques result in predicted values for the PWV in the aorta which agree well with those directly recorded in animals and man [55, 56, 61].

The discrepancy between the ultrasonic methods and the mechanical ones arose from studies of human carotid artery distension [7] in which very large deformations were recorded, suggesting values for PWV much lower than those recorded in other species. A convincing explanation for the differences was put forward by Mozersky et al. [60] who showed how pressure on an underlying vessel from the transducer head could result in the recording of exaggerated diameter changes. It is encouraging to have a plausible explanation for these difficulties because the measurement of arterial distensibility by transcutaneous ultrasonic methods appears to be an ideal method for clinical use. Active development is now necessary, and some progress is being made [34, 62, 63].

There does not now appear to be convincing evidence that an exposed vessel is necessarily stiffer than an undisturbed one, quite apart from the fact that studies on the mechanical effect of smooth muscle activity on large arterial distensibility (and it is hard to see other ways in which vessel properties could alter significantly over short time intervals) show clear effects which are, however, very modest in magnitude [46].

Catheter tip instruments for the measurement of blood flow velocity and pressure are being increasingly used by clinicians and physiologists. Although arterial catheterization is a serious undertaking, the ability to include studies of arterial wall properties within a diagnostic catheterization would undoubtedly be valuable. Devices for animal use have been described [9, 51], but there are great technical problems to be overcome before human application could be contemplated.

There is an important indirect method of determining wall properties which is still relatively underemployed. The velocity of propagation of arterial pressure waves (PWV) is largely determined by the circumferential distensibility of the artery. Other waves also travel in the wall, such as the axial waves which provide information on longitudinal extensibility [6], but here I shall only discuss the

4

more familiar radial distension waves. The travel of these waves in viscoelastic thick-walled tubes has been the subject of much theoretic study and is well-discussed elsewhere [32, 56, 71]. There is considerable uncertainty concerning the behavior expected with small vessels (i.e., where Womersley's a-parameter is low, say < 3) but for major arteries the predictions of the various treatments all converge.

The relationship between wave velocity and wall properties is of the form set out in the familiar Moens-Korteweg equation:

$$c = \sqrt{E h / 2r\rho}$$

where c is the velocity, E the circumferential Young's modulus of elasticity, h/2r the ratio of wall thickness to tube diameter, and ρ the density of the contained fluid. Various modifications are required to cover the situation in anisotropic viscoelastic relatively thick-walled tubes, together with the fluid properties and any external wall restraints, but their combined effect on the high a-asymptote for c is only of the order of 20%.

In practice, the presence of the square root sign is a nuisance, measured velocities are a rather insensitive way to check distensibility data (but are nevertheless rightly used in this fashion), while the technical difficulties of determining PWV in vivo do lead to relatively great uncertainty in deduced values for the mechanical variables. But the method provides information on humans which would otherwise be very hard to come by and should, I believe, be more widely used clinically.

There have been surprisingly few experimental comparisons of actual wave velocity and simultaneously measured elasticity, but it has been reported for rubber tubes [25] dogs' aorta [65], and dogs' femoral artery [24] that agreement between measured and computed PWV is good.

Within the circulation, problems arise due to the presence of reflections, but for most purposes, the extraction of something like the foot-to-foot velocity is all that is necessary [55]. Other methods have been described by which the true propagation characteristics of the arterial wall can be determined in vivo [5, 33, 58], but they require highly invasive experimentation. However, it is relatively simple to measure propagation delays between accessible arteries in the human using external pulse detection devices [35, 44], and much useful data can be obtained, some of which will be discussed later. As is now well-known, the PWV is increased by raising the distending pressure, so its measurement also provides a useful way to estimate blood pressure on a beat-to-beat basis in the human without recourse to arterial puncture.

Observations on Normal Arteries

1. Structure and Composition

There have been relatively few new studies on blood vessel structure and little to add to the account given by Bergel [13]. The scanning electron microscope would seem to be an ideal instrument to explore the fibrous structure of blood vessels, but I can find few reports of its use. Carnes et al. [28] have described the elastin skeleton of the aorta. It appears that in addition to the dense lamellae, a fine felt of elastin pervades the intima and that the lamellae themselves are inter-linked and also bound to adventitial structures by sparse but coarse elastin fibers. Thus, the whole wall is bound into a whole. Earlier work had suggested that the collagen runs parallel, but not directly connected with, the elastin, while the aortic smooth muscle cells attach mainly to the elastic lamellae.

The changes seen in the growing rats' aorta have been much studied. Cliff [30] has showed that the growing aorta gets thicker while the number of cells per unit area falls, but this occurs without change in the number of elastic lamellae which form the basic structural unit [75]. The absolute amount of elastin and collagen increases as the animal grows, but the changes in relative amount of scleroprotein are slight and virtually absent after 20 weeks although increase in weight continues for a year [21]. There is significant remodelling of the wall in adult life, the scleroproteins becoming less concentrated into lamellae and forming a more diffuse network [30]. It is not sure how much of this represents formation of new material as opposed to mechanical splitting and redistribution, but since there is some increase in thickness in later life with no change in fibrous protein concentration, it seems that some new material is appearing. Later work by Berry et al. [22, 23] confirms this pattern and contains much data on chemical composition. Thus, the architecture of this vessel changes rather little in youth and middle age, but signs of wear and tear appear in later life. During this time there can be considerable changes in mechanical behavior as will be seen later.

2. Mechanical Properties

The form of the normal pressure radius relationship for an artery is too well-known to need much description. With increasing pressure, the wall becomes stiffer, but the changes are gradual with no point at which the low pressure, elastin dominated, region can be said to pass into a collagenous zone.

Fung [42] has observed that soft tissues can be characterized by a form of expression in which stiffness is linearly related to stress, and such behavior is also seen in as complex a material as the arterial wall [11, 41]; my own experience confirms this. The interrelationships between the various wall constituents have been examined by many authors. Minns et al. [59], looked at the stress-strain properties of ligmentum nuchae, tendon, and aorta and the way they altered following removal of the mucopolysaccharide matrix or the collagen. Removing the matrix affected predominately the stress relaxation, from which they have suggested that this material contributes to the viscous properties, and may also provide some cross-linkage between collagen fibres. They confirmed the observation that collagen protects a soft tissue against rupture and make the interesting point that its presence would protect against the effects of local weaknesses in an elastin network by limiting overextension and failure in those areas.

Because we know little about the mechanical arrangements of the wall elements, there appears to be a rather poor correlation between wall composition and elasticity, both between different types of vessels and the same one under differing conditions, e.g., age. However, Berry and Greenwald [21] have been able to relate the properties of the aortas of normal and hypertensive rats, at low strain, to the elastin concentration. Interestingly enough, an attempt to make a similar correlation for collagen failed, presumably because we don't know how one fiber attaches to the next, nor to what extent the collagen itself might have become altered.

The contribution of the third element, smooth muscle, to arterial wall mechanics is becoming clarified. Two recent volumes summarize recent advances concerning smooth muscle [26, 72]. It is generally accepted that the tensions generated by active muscle are large enough to have a noticeable effect even in large vessels without the need for any mechanical linkage to amplify it. Quite recently, studies of the mechanical properties of single isolated smooth muscle cells (admittedly from toad stomach) have shown that a force of up to 2 kg/cm^2 can be generated [38]. This is entirely consistent with what we know of the effects of muscle activation in whole vessels, and the figure agrees closely with that reported for active tension in strips of pigs' carotids [48]. In vivo, muscle activation produces constriction and a decrease in stiffness, when compared at similar pressures, but it increases elasticity when compared at constant dimensions [36, 46]. The latter authors have attempted to analyze their results in terms of the classic Hill model of striated muscle; the tissue has a relatively large 'series compliance' and the stiffness is proportional to the stress, as is the case in striated muscle [40].

Muscle also effects the time-dependent properties of the arterial wall. Early work (summarized in [13]) showed the dynamic elastic modulus to be higher than the static and that this increase was the more marked in relatively muscular vessels. Not unexpectedly, it has been shown that the size of the quasistatic hysteresis loop is greater when the muscle is active [11] and that stress relaxation phenomena are more prominent [68, 76]. There are rather few formal studies of the effect of muscle activity on wall viscoelasticity, but Bauer and Pasch [11] who looked at thick-walled muscular vessels from the rats' tail found them to be more 'viscous' than larger vessels, but this did not change after treatment with papaverine or noradrenalin. It would not appear that muscle effects influence arterial properties greatly apart, and it is an all important reservation, from the effects on luminal diameter. In this sense, it may be useful to think of vascular smooth muscle as a 'shortening machine.'

It has been known for centuries that arteries change with age; they become larger and have thicker walls. These changes are more marked in the central vessels [53]. In addition, the amount of longitudinal retraction seen when arteries are removed from the body diminishes steadily with age [10]; indeed, this is probably the most sensitive indicator of the ageing process. Studies on rats [20, 21] over the first 2 years of life showed rather small changes in dimensions after the end of growth, although Cliff [30], whose observations covered the full 3 years, found more marked changes in wall thickness.

In addition to the morphologic changes, the wall itself becomes less extensible [53]. The ageing process has been seen by Wolinsky [74] as a response to mechanical stress and different only in degree from that accompanying sustained hypertension. This is an attractive idea because it suggests a physical mechanism, but it is not possible at this time to test it closely for we really have a poor picture of what is going on to produce these changes; for example, are the fibrous proteins different in properties or are they differently interconnected?

There have been rather few studies of arterial ageing in humans in vivo. The study of arterial PWV is the most obvious one to perform, but there is little detailed work to show just what happens. O'Rourke et al. [64] found an age-related increase in transmission velocity in the distal aorta and iliac artery which did not appear to be correlated with clinical evidence of disease. No clear change was found for velocities in the proximal aorta. It is not clear whether the changes were independent of any age-related blood pressure changes. This is important because Gribbin [44] made a study of brachial transmission times and found no correlation, provided the comparison was made at a reference transmural pressure. It is possible, therefore, that at least a part of the changes previously related to subject age are a consequence of the arterial pressure at which the measurements were made. This, together with the undoubted fact that clear histologic changes can be found, stresses once again our poor understanding of the structural basis of vascular elasticity. A similar conclusion follows the demonstration by De Monchy and Van den Hoeven [35] that wave velocities change very little over the first 20 years of life. Finally, it is becoming clear that arterial reactivity changes significantly with age [31], and this will have to be taken account of in the future.

Arterial Wall in Disease

The whole arterial tree is affected in hypertension; indeed, Folkow [39] has argued persuasively that the primary defect is an increase in muscle mass in the systemic arterioles. He finds in spontaneously hypertensive rats no evidence of altered vascular reactivity. This is confirmed in more recent work by Holloway and Bohr [49] who do report altered reactivity in vessels from rats with experimental renal or DOCA implantation hypertension, a report which emphasizes the great problems in the use of animal models of disease. Further controversy surrounds the mechanism of microvascular damage in malignant hypertension: are the exudative lesions a consequence of raised pressure alone, or is also it necessary to postulate a humoral factor [12, 27]. All are agreed that a high pressure can damage small blood vessels, and it seems to be generally the case that blood vessels beyond a stenosis are protected from damage. The weight of evidence seems to suggest that no additional factor is generally present.

The large arteries are also affected, and Wolinsky [73, 74] has shown how the increase in wall thickness results in a wall of roughly normal gross composition in which the hydrostatic stress has been restored to normal. He suggests this is merely a more marked form of the ageing process, and he sees this as an adaptive response to increased wall stress. Rather similar changes were reported by Berry and Greenwald [21] in a very detailed study of aortic composition and properties in normal and hypertensive rats. They found a rather more marked increase in elastin (absolute and relative) and lesser collagen increase than did Wolinsky. The elasticity changes were complex, but the appropriate way to compare normal and hypertensive vessels is not obvious. A greater relative wall thickness means that less stress is produced by the same pressure; thus, thick vessels will expand less and, since wall strain is the primary determinant of elasticity (Bergel, 1972a), it will be more distensible at all pressures as Berry and Greenwald [21] found. It would be more appropriate to compare at some standard strain, but no easy way of matching strain suggests itself. Similar problems were faced by Aars [1] who was driven to make comparisons on the basis of inflexion points in the stress strain diagram. Such inflexions are often gentle and hard to locate unambiguously, so that this solution is not generally applicable.

Thus, it is not easy to predict the distensibility of hypertensive vessels and not too surprising that Gribben [44] could find no evidence that PWV was raised in hypertension, provided the comparison was made at the same distending pressure. The PWV is certainly higher in hypertensives and the distensibility of the arteries lower (viz., the effects on baroreceptor function), and this contributes to the increased cardiac workload but apparently no more so than in the normal vessel temporarily exposed to a high pressure. Clearly we need more delicate measures.

Other forms of arterial disease have received increasing study, particularly the hemodynamic factors possibly involved in the atheromatous process. The early phase in which various rather simple single etiologies were being proposed has now passed, and it is realized that the process is a very complex one in which subtle changes occurring over long time periods are involved. The field is developing fast, and a brief general account is given by Bergel et al. [17]. Berry et al. [19] have shown how prenatal flow disturbances leave detectable vascular alterations years later, while the fascinating problem of poststenotic dilation in arteries is still being investigated, especially the demonstrated effect of sonic-frequency vibrations on the arterial wall [67].

Arterial Baroreceptors

The specialized regions of the arterial tree, carotid sinus and aortic arch, which are provided with nerves which respond to pressure present a most interesting problem for those concerned with arterial mechanics. It is well-established that the nerves respond, as they must, to wall strain rather than stress, but there are few detailed studies of the relation between distensibility and baroreceptor function. Aars [1, 2, 3] has examined the aortic arch region in normal and hypertensive rabbits and shown how the change in baroreceptor properties in hypertension (resetting) appears to relate to the thickening and dilation of the aorta. His results are consistent with the idea that the resetting process has to do mainly with altered arterial mechanics rather than changes in the nerve endings. Studies on the human baroreflex [44, 45, 54] are also explicable in the same way on the assumption that what little is known of human arterial distensibility applies also to the baroreceptor regions. Further, Angell-James and Lumley [4] have showed a direct effect of surgical endarterectomy on both carotid sinus mechanics and nerve output.

In collaboration with Sleight's group, we have begun direct measurements of carotid sinus distensibility, using an ultrasonic transit time technique [25] together with conventional nerve recording techniques. Our results to date do not support the conclusion of Koushanpour and Kelso [52] that the saturation of the nerve output at high distending pressures is independent of the 'mechanical' saturation, whereby the distensibility of the sinus becomes much reduced at high pressures. Our results, [15] would indicate that the nerve firing is simply related to the diameter changes. We have also looked at the effect of altered smooth muscle activity, produced by noradrenaline [16]. The results confirm Aars' [3] findings that firing at constant vessel size is increased by muscle activation, suggesting that the nerve endings are mechanically in series with the smooth muscle. We have also constructed length-tension diagrams for the sinus (on the admittedly false assumption that the wall is a cylinder) and thereby related firing changes to tension changes. We find a pleasing linearity here and a relationship of the same slope when a similar analysis is done on the inflation and deflation limb of a slow pressure change. The suggestion that the hysteresis effects are predominantly due to changes in muscle stretch receives here a rather satisfying confirmation.

Acknowledgements: My grateful thanks to my collaborators C. Bertram, A. MacDermott, R. Peveler, and P. Sleight, and to B. Gribbin for permission to quote from his unpublished work.

References

1. Aars, H.: Relationship between blood pressure and diameter of ascending aorta in normal and hypertensive rabbits. Acta. Physiol. Scand. 75, 397-405 (1969)
2. Aars, H.: Relationship between aortic diameter and aortic baroreceptor activity in normal and hypertensive rabbits. Acta. Physiol. Scand. 75, 406-414 (1969)
3. Aars, H.: Effects of altered smooth muscle tone on aortic diameter and aortic baroreceptor activity in anaesthetised rabbits. Circ. Res. 28, 254-262 (1971)
4. Angell-James, J.E., Lumley, J.P.S.: The effects of carotid endarterectomy on the mechanical properties of the carotid sinus and carotid sinus nerve activity in atherosclerotic patients. Br. J. Surg. 61, 805-810 (1974)
5. Anliker, M., Histand, M.B., Ogden, E.: Dispersion and attenuation of small artificial pressure waves in the canine aorta. Circ. Res. 23, 539-551 (1968)

6. Anliker, M., Moritz, W.E., Ogden, E.: Transmission characteristics of axial waves in blood vessels. J. Biomech. 1, 235-246 (1968)
7. Arndt, J.O., Klauske, J., Mersch, F.: The diameter of the intact carotid artery in man and its change with pulse pressure. Pflügers Arch. 301, 230-240 (1968)
8. Arndt, J.O., Stegall, H.F., Wicke, H.J.: Mechanics of the aorta in vivo. A radiographic approach. Circ. Res. 28, 693-704 (1971)
9. Baan, J., Szidon, J.P., Noordergraaf, A.: Dynamic local distensibility of living arteries and its relation to wave transmission. Biophys. J. 14, 343-362 (1974)
10. Band, W., Goedhard, W.J.A., Knopp, A.A.: Effects of ageing on dynamic visco-elastic properties of the rats thoracic aorta. Pflügers Arch. 331, 357-364 (1972)
11. Bauer, R.D., Pasch, Th.: The quasistatic and dynamic circumferential elastic modulus of the rat tail artery studied at various wall stresses and tones of the vascular smooth muscle. Pflügers Arch. 330, 335-346 (1971)
12. Beilin, L.E., Goldby, F.S., Möhring, J.: High arterial pressure versus humoral factors in the pathogenesis of the vascular lesion of malignant hypertension. Clin. Sci. Mol. Med. 52, 111-117 (1977)
13. Bergel, D.H.: The properties of blood vessels. In: Biomechanics. Fung, Y.C.B. et al. (eds.), New Jersey: Prentice Hall (1972)
14. Bergel, D.H.: The measurement of lengths and dimensions. In: Cardio-vascular Fluid Dynamics. Bergel, D.H. (ed.). London: Acad. Pr. (1972)
15. Bergel, D.H., Brookes, D.E., MacDermott, A.J., Robinson, J.L., Sleight, P.: The relation between carotid sinus dimension, nerve activity and pressure in the anaesthetised greyhound. J. Physiol. (London) 263, 156-157 P (1976)
16. Bergel, D.H., Brooks, D.E., MacDermott, A.J., Robinson, J.L., Sleight, P.: Baroreceptor firing frequency and activation of carotid sinus smooth muscle. J. Physiol. 266, 27 P (1977)
17. Bergel, D.H., Nerem, R.M., Schwartz, C.J.: Fluid dynamic aspects of arterial disease. Atherosclerosis 23, 253-261 (1976)
18. Bergel, D.H., Schultz, D.L.: Arterial elasticity and fluid dynamics. Prog. Biophys. Mol. Biol. 22, 1-36 (1971)
19. Berry, C.L., Gosling, R.G., Laogun, A.A., Brian, E.: Anomalous iliac compliance in children with a single umbilical artery. Br. Heart. J. 38, 510-515 (1976)
20. Berry, C.L., Greenwald, S.E., Rivett, J.F.: Static mechanical properties of the developing and mature rat aorta. Cardiovasc. Res., 9, 669-678 (1975)
21. Berry, C.L., Greenwald, S.E., Effects of hypertension on the static mechanical properties and composition of the rat aorta. Cardiovasc. Res. 10, 437-451 (1976)
22. Berry, C.L., Looker, T., Germain, J.: The growth and development of the rat aorta. 1, morphological aspects. J. Anat. 113, 1-16 (1972)
23. Berry, C.L., Looker, T., Germain, J.: Changes in nucleic acid and sclero-protein content. J. Anat. 113, 17-34 (1972)
24. Bertram, C.D.: Studies in cardiovascular mechanics: ultrasonic measurement of femoral artery properties. D. Phil thesis, University of Oxford (1975)

25. Bertram, C.D.: Ultrasonic transit-time system for arterial diameter measurement. Med. Biol. Eng. 15, 489-499 (1977)
26. Bulbring, E., Shuba, M.F. (eds.): Physiology of Smooth Muscle. New York: Raven (1976)
27. Byrom, F.B.: Tension and the artery: the experimental elucidation of pseudo-uraemia and malignant nephrosclerosis. Clin. Sci. Mol. Med. 51, 3s–11s (1976)
28. Carnes, W.H., Hart, M.L., Hodgkin, N.: Conformation of aortic elastin revealed by scanning electron microscopy of dissected surfaces. Adv. Exp. Med. Biol. 79, 61-70 (1977)
29. Cleary, E.G., Mount, M.: Hypertension in weanling rabbits. Adv. Exp. Med. Biol. 79, 61-70 (1977)
30. Cliff, W.J.: The aortic tunica media in ageing rats. Exp. Mol. Pathol. 13, 172-180 (1970)
31. Cohen, M.L., Berkowitz, B.A.: Vascular contraction: effect of age and extravellular calcium. Blood Vessels. 13, 139-154 (1976)
32. Cox, R.H.: Blood flow and pressure propagation in the canine femoral artery. J. Biomech. 3, 131-149 (1970)
33. Cox, R.H.: Determination of the true phase velocity of arterial pressure waves in vivo. Circ. Res. 29, 407-418 (1971)
34. Daigle, R.E., Miller, C.W., Histand, M.B., McLeod, F.D., Hokanson, D.E.: Non traumatic aortic blood flow velocity sensing by use of an ultrasonic oesophageal probe. J. Appl. Physiol. 38, 1153-1160 (1975)
35. De Monchy, C., Van den Hoeven, G.M.A.: Pulse wave transmission time in central aorta and peripheral arteries in normal children. Blood Vessels 13, 129-138 (1976)
36. Dobrin, P.B., Canfield, T.R.: Series and contractile elements in vascular smooth muscle. Circ. Res. 33, 147-151 (1973)
37. Elzinga, G., Westerhof, N.: End-diastolic volume and source impedance of the heart. In: Ciba Symposium 24: The physiological basis of Starling's law of the heart. London: Elsevier (1974)
38. Fay, F.S., Cooke, P.H., Canaday, D.G.: Contractile properties of isolated smooth muscle cells. In: Physiology of Smooth Muscle. E. Bülbring, M.F. Shuga, (eds.). New York: Raven (1976)
39. Folkow, B.: The haemodynamic consequences of adaptive structural changes of the resistance vessels in hypertension. Clin. Sci. Mol. Med. 41, 1-12 (1971)
40. Ford, L.E., Huxley, A.F., Simmons, R.M.: Tension responses to sudden length change in stimulated frog muscle fibres near slack length. J. Physiol., (London) 269, 441-515 (1977)
41. Frank, O.: Die Elastizität der Blutgefäße. Z. Biol. 71, 255-272 (1920)
42. Fung, Y.C.B.: Elasticity of soft tissues in simple elongation. Am. J. Physiol. 213, 1532-1544 (1967)
43. Greenfield, J.C., Patel, D.J.: Relation between pressure and diameter in the ascending aorta of man. Circ. Res. 10, 778-781 (1962)
44. Gribbin, B.: A Study of baroreflex function and arterial distensibility in normal and hypertensive man. D.M. Thesis, University of Dundee (1974)

12

45. Gribbin, B., Pickering, T.G., Sleight, P., Peto, R.: Effect of age and high blood pressure on baroreflex sensitivity in man. Circ. Res. 29, 424-431 (1971)
46. Gow, B.S.: The influence of vascular smooth muscle on the visco-elastic properties of blood vessels. In: Cardiovascular Fluid Dynamics. Bergel, D.H. (ed.). London: Acad. Pr. (1972)
47. Gozna, E.R., Marble, E.A., Shaw, A.J., Winter, D.A.: Mechanical properties of the ascending thoracic aorta of man. Cardiovasc. Res. 7, 261-265 (1973)
48. Herlihy, J.T., Murphy, R.A.: Length-tension relationship of smooth muscle of the hog carotid artery. Circ. Res. 33, 275-283 (1973)
49. Holloway, E.T., Bohr, D.: Reactivity of vascular smooth muscle in hypertensive rats. Circ. Res. 33, 678-685 (1973)
50. Kober, G., Arndt, J.O.: Die Druck-Durchmesser-Beziehung der A. Carotis Communis des wachen Menschen. Pflugers Arch. 314, 27-39 (1970)
51. Kolin, A., MacAlpin, R.N.: Induction angiometer electromagnetic magnification of microscopic vascular diameter variations in vivo. Blood Vessels 14, 141-156 (1977)
52. Koushanpour, E., Kelso, D.M.: Partition of the carotid sinus baroreceptor response in dogs between the mechanical properties of the wall and the receptor elements. Circ. Res. 31, 831-845 (1972)
53. Learoyd, B.M., Taylor, M.G.: Alterations with age in the viscoelastic properties of human arterial walls. Circ. Res. 18, 278-292 (1966)
54. Lindblad, L.E.: Influence of age on sensitivity and effector mechanisms of the carotid sinus baroreflex. Acta. Physiol. Scand. 101, 43-49 (1977)
55. McDonald, D.A.: Regional pulse-wave velocity in the arterial tree. J. Appl. Physiol. 24, 73-78 (1968)
56. McDonald, D.A.: Blood Flow in Arteries. London: Arnolds (1974)
57. Milnor, W.R.: Arterial impedance as ventricular afterload. Circ. Res. 36, 565-570 (1975)
58. Milnor, W.R., Nichols, W.W.: A new method of measuring propagation coefficients and characteristic impedance of blood vessels. Circ. Res. 36, 631-639 (1975)
59. Minns, R.J., Soden, P.D., Jackson, D.S.: The role of the fibrous components and ground substance in mechanical properties of biological tissues. J. Biomech. 6, 153-165 (1973)
60. Mozersky, D.J., Sumner, D.S., Strandness, D.E.: Transcutaneous measurement of the elastic properties of the human femoral artery. Circulation 46, 948-955 (1972)
61. Nichols, W.W., McDonald, D.A.: Wave velocity in the proximal aorta. Med. Biol. Eng. 10, 327-335 (1972)
62. Olsen, R.M.: Human carotid artery wall thickness, diameter and blood flow by a non-invasive technique. J. Appl. Physiol. 37, 955-960 (1974)
63. Olsen, R.M., Shelton, D.K.: A nondestructive technique to measure wall displacement in the thoracic aorta. J. Appl. Physiol. 32, 147-151 (1972)
64. O'Rourke, M.F., Blazek, J.V., Morreels, C.L., Krovetz, L.J.: Pressure wave transmission along the Human aorta. Circ. Res. 23, 567-579 (1968)

65. Patel, D.J., Janicki, J.S., Carew, T.E.: Static anisotropic properties of the aorta in living dogs. Circ. Res. 25, 765-779 (1969)
66. Patel, D.J., Vaishnav, R.N.: The rheology of large blood vessels. In: Cardiovascular Fluid Dynamics. Bergel, D.H. (ed.). London: Academic Press (1972)
67. Roach, M.R.: Biophysical analyses of blood vessel walls and blood flow. Annu. Rev. Physiol. 39, 51-71 (1977)
68. Seidel, C.L. and Murphy, R.A.: Stress relaxation in hog carotid artery as relate to contractile activity. Blood Vessels, 13, 78-91 (1976)
69. Taylor, M.G.: Arterial impedance and distensibility. In: The Pulmonary Circulation and Interstitial Space. Fishman, A.P. (ed.). Chicago: Chicago U. Pr. (1969)
70. Taylor, M.G.: Haemodynamics. Annu. Rev. Physiol. 35, 87—118 (1973)
71. Wetterer, E., Kenner, T.: Grundlagen der Dynamik des Arterienpulses. Berlin-Heidelberg-New York: Springer (1968)
72. Wolf, S., Werthessen, N.T. (eds.): The smooth muscle of the artery. Adv. Exp. Med. Biol. 57, (1975)
73. Wolinsky, H.: Comparison of medial growth of human thoracic and abdominal aortas. Circ. Res. 27, 531-538 (1970)
74. Wolinsky, H.: Long term effects of hypertension on the rat aortic wall and their relation to concurrent aging changes. Circ. Res. 30, 301-309 (1972)
75. Wolinsky, H., Glagov, S.: A lamellar unit of aortic medial structure and function in mammals. Circ. Res. 20, 99-111 (1967)
76. Wurzel, W., Cowper, G.R., McCook, J.M.: Smooth muscle contraction and viscoelasticity of arterial wall. Can. J. Physiol. Pharm. 48, 510-523 (1970)

Prediction of Shape Changes of Propagating Flow and Pressure Pulses in Human Arteries

M. Anliker, J. C. Stettler, P. Niederer, and R. Holenstein

Institut für Biomedizinische Technik der Universität Zürich und der
ETHZ Moussonstraße 18, CH-8044 Zürich

Introduction

The ultimate utility of theoretical studies is judged by the understanding they provide of the phenomena which are modeled and by their ability to predict new features of this phenomena which had not yet been recognized. In our mathematical analysis of the cardiovascular system, we aim at identifying those properties of the heart and vessels which are responsible for the characteristic shapes of the pressure and flow pulses in the different parts of the arterial tree. In particular, we are interested in quantifying the modifications of these pulse shapes due to anatomic changes caused by disease and ageing. For a reliable interpretation of such changes, we need, however, a sufficiently accurate mathematical description of the phenomena and also the capability to experimentally verify the theoretical results.

Thanks to recent advances in ultrasound diagnostics, we can obtain progressively more data on the hemodynamics of the heart and larger blood vessels and on their geometric features without penetrating the skin. For example, a new 128-channel ultrasound Doppler velocity meter [1, 10] permits the determination of instantaneous velocity profiles and the flow patterns in vessels within a range of about 10 cm. With this device, it should be possible to clinically quantify the flow through the four major arteries in the neck which supply blood to the brain. Likewise, it is expected to allow an evaluation of flow patterns in the larger arteries in the abdomen, in particular the abdominal aorta and the renal arteries. Besides this, by superposing the Doppler or velocity signal onto the echogram, one would arrive at an ultrasonic angiogram which displays anatomic as well as functional information.

In our early mathematical models of the arterial system, we considered an arterial conduit from the heart to the foot of the hindleg of a dog [3, 13]. This conduit was assumed to behave like a straight elastic tube with a circular cross-section and a radius which diminishes continuously with distance from the heart. The various branches were simulated by leakage of the wall which appropriately varies with distance from the heart. The elastic behavior of the conduit with regard to distension was given in terms of the wave speed as a function of distance from the heart and as a function of pressure. At the proximal end, the ejection pattern of the heart was prescribed in the fashion described by Wetterer and Kenner [16] and at the distal end the capillary pressure was assumed as

15

constant. With the aid of the method of characteristics, which takes nonlinear effects into account, we computed the pressure and flow patterns and their variations along the conduit for various physiologic conditions.

The results of these studies have shown that the familiar features of the natural pressure and flow pulses in arteries can be reproduced mathematically if the physical and geometric cardiovascular parameters are properly specified. However, the theoretical model does not predict backflow during the early diastolic phase in the abdominal aorta, the iliac, and the femoral arteries when the outflow through the porous wall is assumed to be proportional to the difference between the local arterial pressure and the capillary pressure [3]. By modifying this outflow law in such a way that the seepage through the wall is also proportional to the local flow rate in the arterial conduit, one arrives at the familiar backflow pattern which one observes in these vessels under normal conditions [4, 8]. A detailed examination of the computed pressure and flow pulses also verified some facts regarding the attenuation mechanisms. The effects of viscosity of the blood alone cannot account for a realistic damping of the propagating pulses, especially when they reach the more distal part of the conduit. The numerical procedure associated with the method of characteristics itself produces a certain damping which can be predicted and related to the size of the temporal and spatial increments utilized in the computations. The taper of the conduit measurably influences the damping pattern through its effects on the energy density. The three traditional simple models for viscoelasticity do not characterize the damping mechanism provided by the arterial wall as they do not yield a logarithmic decrement which is independent of frequency [9].

Arterial Conduits With Discrete Branches

The simulation of all branches, irrespective of their size, by a leaking wall constitutes an unsatisfactory approximation in earlier theoretical studies [3, 13] utilizing the method of characteristics. A new approach has, therefore, been devised by subdividing the conduit into tapered segments in accordance with the location of major discrete branches as illustrated in Figure 1. Between two successive segments, one or more — depending on the diameter of the branch artery — axial computing intervals (Δz) are declared as an outflow region. At the lateral sides of this region, the boundary conditions for the adjoining segments must be compatible with the laws governing the outflow into the branch. The loss of blood through smaller branches which may be located within each segment is still simulated by a continuously distributed and appropriately chosen seepage through the wall. In this study, the tapered vessel segments are first considered as being purely elastic; the effects of a viscoelastic wall behavior are later examined in a preliminary fashion.

16

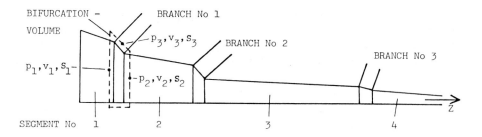

Fig. 1. Schematic drawing of model of arterial conduit with discrete segments. The conduit is subdivided into tapered segments and bifurcation volumes, i. e., discrete outflow regions of major branches. In the segments between successive branches, the pressure p, the velocity v, and the cross-sectional area S are determined with the aid of the method of characteristics and the expression for the wave speed c as a function of S, p, and the axial coordinate z. The six unknowns p_j, v_j and the cross-sectional areas S_j of each bifurcation volume are evaluated as described in the text

Assumptions and Basic Equations

The blood is treated as an incompressible fluid, and the effects of viscosity are taken into account in an approximate manner. As a further approximation, we postulate the flow to be one-dimensional at all times (t) which implies that only spatial averages of the pressure [p (z, t)] and the flow velocity [v (z, t)] are considered at each cross-section. The interaction of the blood with the elastic wall is defined by the cross-sectional area S_0 (z) at reference pressure p_0 and the speed c (p, z) of small distension waves [2] as a function of p and z.
This speed [c (p, z)] and the cross-sectional area [S (p, z)] are interrelated through

$$c^2 = \frac{S}{\rho \cdot \frac{\partial S}{\partial p}} \tag{1}$$

where ρ denotes the density of the blood. By integrating Eq. 1, we obtain

$$S(p, z) = S_0 (z) \cdot \exp \left(\frac{p - p_0}{\rho \cdot c(p_0, z) \cdot c (p, z)} \right) \tag{2}$$

With the assumptions stated, the Navier-Stokes equation for the z direction reduces to

$$\rho \cdot S \cdot \left(\frac{\partial v}{\partial t} + v \cdot \frac{\partial v}{\partial z} \right) + S \cdot \frac{\partial p}{\partial z} = f \tag{3}$$

where f represents the general expression for the friction force due to the viscosity of the blood. For a Hagen-Poiseuille-type flow, we would have the relation

17

$$f = -8 \cdot \pi \cdot \mu \cdot v \qquad (4)$$

in which μ is the viscosity coefficient. In formulating conservation of mass for the segments of the arterial conduit, the outflow per unit length in terms of a pressure- and flow-dependent leakage [ψ (p, v, z)] which also varies with the distance z must be taken into account

$$\frac{\partial S}{\partial p} \cdot \frac{\partial p}{\partial t} + S \cdot \frac{\partial v}{\partial z} + \frac{\partial S}{\partial p} \cdot v \cdot \frac{\partial p}{\partial z} + v \cdot \frac{\partial S}{\partial z} + \psi = 0 \qquad (5)$$

For ψ we postulate

$$\psi = \phi_B(z) \cdot (p - p_c) + \phi_Q(z) \cdot v \cdot S \qquad (6)$$

where p_c is the capillary pressure and $\phi_B(z)$ and $\phi_Q(z)$ are the local parameters which characterize the partial dependence of the leakage on pressure and flow, respectively.

Boundary Conditions

As boundary condition at the root of the aorta (z = 0), we give the ejection pattern of the left ventricle in terms of the volume flow rate [q_0 (t)], whereby the basic shape of the curve q_0 (t) is assumed to be identical with that given by Wetterer and Kenner [16]. At the distal end of the conduit, a constant capillary pressure or a peripheral resistance is prescribed. To derive the boundary conditions for the segments adjoining an outflow region (Fig. 1), we enforce conservation of mass

$$v_1 \cdot S_1 = v_2 \cdot S_2 + v_3 \cdot S_3 + \frac{d}{dt} \int_1^2 S(z) \cdot dz \qquad (7)$$

In addition, we disregard the energy dissipation due to viscosity as well as the energy required to distend the arterial wall in the outflow region. Consequently, we have according to Bernoulli

$$p_1 + \frac{1}{2} \cdot \rho \cdot v_1{}^2 = p_3 + \frac{1}{2} \cdot \rho \cdot v_3{}^2 + \rho \cdot \int_1^3 \frac{\partial v}{\partial t} dz \qquad (8)$$

Furthermore, we assume that the outflow through the branch is, in analogy to Eq. 6, defined by

$$v_3 \cdot S_3 = R_B \cdot (p_1 - p_c) \cdot S_3{}^2 + R_Q \cdot v_1 \cdot S_1 \qquad (9)$$

18

where R_B and R_Q characterize the partial dependence of the outflow on the pressure and the local flux in the arterial conduit, respectively. The factor $S_3{}^2$ is introduced to account for the fact that in case of Hagen-Poiseuille flow the flux is proportional to the square of the lumen area.

Computational Aspects

The system of Eqs. 3 and 5 which governs the pulse propagation between two branch points is solved numerically by the method of characteristics [6]. If ψ and f are algebraic functions of v and p, one obtains for the characteristic directions

$$\frac{dz}{dt} = v \pm c \ \text{ with } \ c^2 = \frac{S}{\rho \cdot \frac{\partial S}{\partial p}} \tag{10}$$

and, after transformation, in lieu of Eqs. 3 and 5

$$dv \pm \frac{dp}{\rho c} = [\ f \mp \frac{v \cdot c}{S}(\frac{\partial S}{\partial z}) \mp \frac{c}{S} \cdot \psi\ ] \cdot dt \tag{11}$$

In order to solve the system (11) numerically, we choose as specified time and space intervals $\Delta t = 0.002$ s and $\Delta z = 2.5$ cm. For numerical stability, the relation $\frac{\Delta z}{\Delta t} > c$ has to be fulfilled for all points. An initial condition is prescribed along the line t = 0. Such a procedure is feasible because this line does not coincide with a characteristic in the (z, t) plane. As the calculation proceeds in fixed time steps (Δt), we compute the values of v and p at the time t_1 from the solution known in equally spaced points along the line $t = t_1 - \Delta t$. Because of the non-linear terms in the analysis, the characteristic lines (10) are not straight. Therefore, the lines a_1 and a_2 (Fig. 2) which determine the solution in point A do not in general intersect the line $t = t_1 - \Delta t$ in points like B, C, D, in which the solution is known. As a consequence of introducing discrete branches where the cross-sectional area in the arterial conduit exhibits a jump, the outflow function ψ and the cross-section S show only small variations along the segment between successive branch sites. Because of the relatively small changes of ψ and S along the integration path, we arrive at a satisfactory numerical accuracy for the solution if we choose as coefficients in Eq. 11 the values in point C and if for the computation of increments Δp and Δv the linearly interpolated p and v values for points E and F, respectively, are utilized.
At the branch sites, the solutions given by Eq. 11 for the two adjoining segments have to be combined with Eqs. 7 through 9 which hold for the bifurcation volume. The six unknowns, i. e., (Fig. 1) the pressures p_1, p_2, and p_3 and the velocities v_1, v_2, and v_3, are determined from the three equations 7, 8, and 9 as well as the upstream and downstream characteristic equations in point 1 and the upstream characteristic equation in point 2. The values for S_j follow from Eq. 2.

19

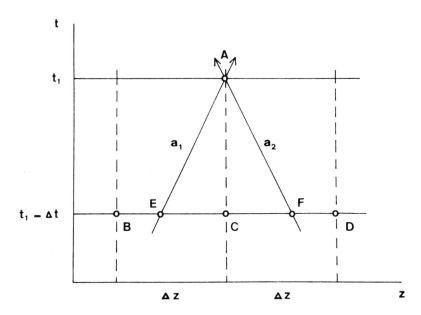

Fig. 2. Method of characteristics as implemented on the computer. The values of the two unknowns p and v at time t_1 in point A are determined by proceeding along the two characteristic curves a_1 and a_2. At this time instant, the solutions are known in equally spaced points along $t = t_1 - \Delta t$, i. e., in points like B, C, and D. The values of p and v in the points E and F are obtained by linear interpolation. With $t = 0.002$ s and $z = 2.5$ cm, the numerical errors are insignificant in relation to some of the inadequacies of the model

As initial condition at time $t = 0$, we select $v = 0$ and $p = $ const. The calculation has to be allowed to proceed through successive heart beats until the differences of the solution between the last two beats is negligible, which is usually the case after six to ten beats.

Model Parameters for Arterial Conduit

We considered a human arterial conduit which extends from the root of the aorta to the foot as illustrated in Figure 3. It is modeled as a straight tube with a progressively diminishing cross-section. Eight discrete outflow regions simulate major branches while the loss of blood through the smaller branches is approximated by a continuously distributed seepage through the wall. In the sense of

Fig. 3. Model of human arterial conduit from the heart to the foot (standard case). Eight major branches are defined which subdivide the conduit into nine segments. The areas listed are those corresponding to the reference pressure $p_0 = 100$ mm Hg

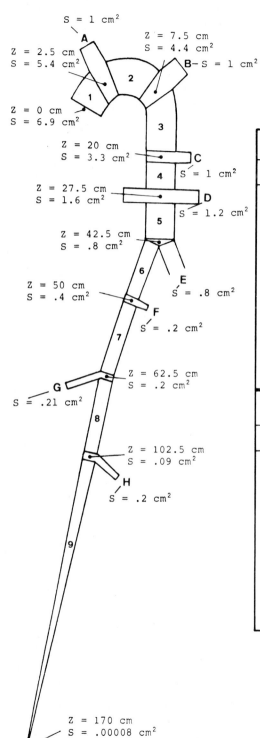

S = 1 cm²

A

Z = 7.5 cm
S = 4.4 cm²

B— S = 1 cm²

Z = 2.5 cm
S = 5.4 cm²

2

1

Z = 0 cm
S = 6.9 cm²

3

Z = 20 cm
S = 3.3 cm²

C

4

S = 1 cm²

Z = 27.5 cm
S = 1.6 cm²

D

5

S = 1.2 cm²

Z = 42.5 cm
S = .8 cm²

6

E

S = .8 cm²

Z = 50 cm
S = .4 cm²

F

S = .2 cm²

7

Z = 62.5 cm
S = .2 cm²

G

S = .21 cm²

8

Z = 102.5 cm
S = .09 cm²

H

S = .2 cm²

9

Z = 170 cm
S = .00008 cm²

SEGMENT DESCRIPTION	
NO	SEGMENT
1	ASCENDING AORTA
2	AORTIC ARCH
3	THORACIC AORTA
4	UPPER ABDOMINAL A.
5	LOWER ABDOMINAL A.
6	COMMON ILIAC
7	EXTERNAL ILIAC AND COMMON FEMORAL
8	SUPERFICIAL FEMORAL AND POPLITEAL
9	A. TIBIALIS, A. DORSALIS PEDIS

BRANCH DESCRIPTION	
	BRANCH
A	CORONARY, R. SUBCLAVIAN, R. CAROTID
B	L. CAROTID, L. SUBCLAVIAN
C	HEPATIC, GASTRIC AND SPLENIC
D	A. RENALIS
E	ILIAC BIFURCATION
F	HYPOGASTRIC
G	A. PROFUNDA FEMORALIS
H	A. TIBIALIS POSTERIOR, A. PERONAEA

defining a standard case, we choose a set of parameter values within the range of normal healthy adults in a supine position:

Density of blood:	ρ	= 1.06 g/cm³
Viscosity of blood:	μ	= 0.049 poise
Capillary pressure:	p_c	= 25 mm Hg
Reference pressure:	p_0	= 100 mm Hg
Cardiac period:	T	= 0.8 s
Stroke volume:		70 cm³

1. Cross-section of Arterial Conduit

The values of S at the reference pressure p_0 indicated in Figure 3 denote the cross-sectional areas immediately after the depicted branch. They are selected on the basis of references 14 and 15. The difference between two successive values for S is divided equally into a cross-sectional change due to taper along the corresponding segment and a jump in cross-section at the discrete downstream branch site. Along the segment, the variation of the vessel radius is assumed to be linear.

2. Wave speed

Based on references 3 and 13, we choose for the functional form of the wave speed the expression

$$c\,(p, z) = (30 + 3.2 \cdot p) \cdot g\,(z) \tag{12}$$

in which p is defined in mm Hg. The function g (z) describing the dependence of c on z is piecewise linear and defined by the three values

$$c(p_0, 0) = 350 \text{ cm/s}; \quad c(p_0, 102.5 \text{ cm}) = 800 \text{ cm/s};$$
$$c(p_0, 170 \text{ cm}) = 1000 \text{ cm/s}$$

3. Outflow Parameters for Discrete Branches R_B, R_Q

In order to determine the outflow parameters R_{Bj} and R_{Qj} (j = 1, ..., N) (N = number of branches) we integrate Eq. 9 for every branch over one period

$$\int_0^T v_3\, S_3\, dt = R_B \int_0^T (p_1 - p_c) \cdot S_3{}^2\, dt + R_Q \int_0^T v_1\, S_1\, dt \tag{13}$$

Published data on the physiologic outflow patterns in the aorta and in the leg [5] provide values for the following expressions

$\begin{matrix} T \\ \int \\ 0 \end{matrix} v_3 \cdot S_3 \, dt$ Total flow through the side branch at the branch point under consideration

$\begin{matrix} T \\ \int \\ 0 \end{matrix} v_1 S_1 \, dt$ Total flux in the main branch immediately in front of the bifurcation

The integral $\int_0^T (p_1 - p_c) S_3^2 \, dt$ is approximated by $(\bar{p}_1 - p_c) \cdot S_3^2 (\bar{p}_2) \cdot T$, whereby $\bar{p}_1$ is known for the standard case (Table 1). Therefore, Eq. 13 establishes a linear relation for each pair of parameters R_{Bj} and R_{Qj}. To determine these values, a second condition is required for each branch site. These second conditions are chosen empirically in such a manner as to ascertain realistic pressure and flow patterns for the standard case. Even though this procedure is unsatisfactory insofar as the values for R_{Bj} and R_{Qj} are not derived directly from measured physiological quantities, it can be justified by the fact that realistic results are also obtained with the same parameter values when a stenosis is introduced or when the heart rate is increased.

Table 1. Outflow parameters and mean pressures for discrete branches

Branch No. j	R_Q	$R_B \cdot 10^4$ $(\dfrac{cm}{dyn \cdot s})$	$\bar{p}_1$ mm Hg
1	0.1	1.0	95
2	0.094	0.74	95
3	0.277	0.19	95
4	0.54	0.17	94
5	0.25	7.5	93
6	0.25	5.0	93
7	0.25	2.2	92
8	0.25	1.2	90

4. Parameters for Seepage Through Wall of Conduit

In view of the fact that the predicted pressure and flow pulses are not noticeably affected by a small seepage through the walls of the first eight segments, the corresponding ϕ values in Eq. 6 are chosen to be zero. For the last segment from the knee to the foot, we select $\phi_B = 4 \cdot 10^{-7} \dfrac{cm^4}{dyn \cdot s}$, $\phi_Q = 0$.

Results for Standard Case

The characteristic features of the arterial pressure and flow pulses in man as well as their changes with propagation from the heart to the foot are also exhibited by the model (Fig. 4a, b). In particular, we recognize the presence of the in-

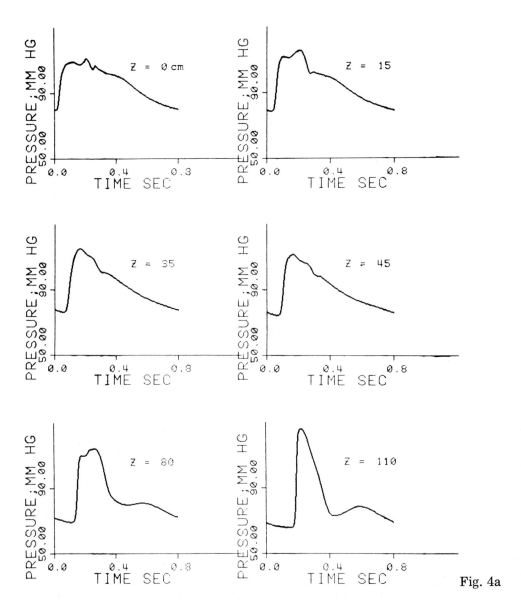

Fig. 4a

Fig. 4. Pressure and flow pulses at different sites z for the standard case. The pressure pulses (a) and flow pulses (b) are plotted for representative locations along the conduit (see also Fig. 3)

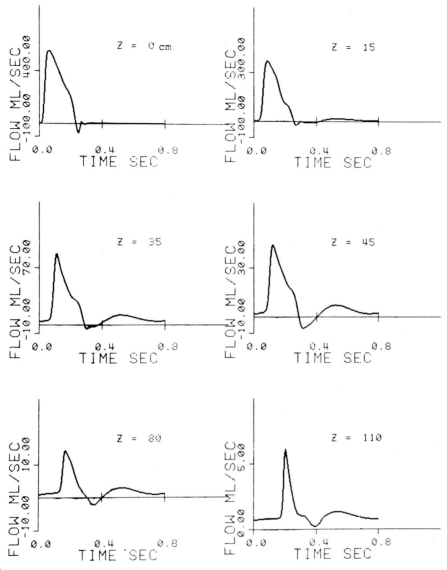

Fig. 4b

cisura within the first 50 cm from the root of the aorta, the gradual decrease of the diastolic pressure with distance from the heart, the continuous increase in the systolic pressure, and the associated steepening of the wave front up to a distance of about 140 cm, as well as the development of a well-defined dicrotic wave in the conduit section beyond the bifurcation. Besides this, the flow pulse shows a progressively pronounced backflow during diastole with increasing distance from the heart until the diameter is reduced to approximately 0.3 cm. All of these features are preserved when the heart rate is raised from 75 to 100 beats per minute and each of the other parameters is left unchanged. This fact can be interpreted as supporting evidence for the realistic behavior of the mathematical model used in this analysis. Yet, it should also be mentioned that the peaks of the computed flow and pressure pulses are somewhat sharper than those recorded from man. From this, we infer the need to take into account the viscoelasticity of the arterial wall. With regard to the distal boundary condition, the results do not seem to change noticeably when a constant peripheral resistance is prescribed at z = L in lieu of a constant capillary pressure.

Verification of Computational Accuracy Through Energy and Mass Balance Tests

1. Energy Balance Test

At any time instant (t) of the cardiac cycle, the pressure and flow patterns predicted for the arterial conduit considered should be in agreement with the energy theorem. Accordingly, the energy input between the beginning of the cardiac cycle at t = 0 and any time instant (t) is equal to the energy transferred to the surrounding, plus the energy dissipated during this time interval, plus the internally stored energy. With the time and space intervals chosen, we find for the standard case with eight discrete branches that the energy balance has a deficiency of about 3.9% of the input energy. This discrepancy must be attributed to the numerical damping described by Rockwell et al [13].

2. Mass Balance Test

By considering a complete cardiac cycle and terminating the arterial conduit at various lengths, we find that on the average the mass balance has an offset of approximately 2.8% of the stroke volume. The conservation of mass test is, therefore, better satisfied than the energy theorem. This may be a consequence of the fact that only v and S enter the conservation of mass theorem in contrast to the energy test which also includes the pressure.

Model of a Stenosis

As a further test of the realistic behavior of the mathematical model, we analyzed the pressure and flow pulses in a conduit with a short stenosis which begins and ends abruptly, as illustrated in Figure 5. Its length is assumed to be one integration step Δz, i.e., 2.5 cm. Also for convenience and because of its frequent occurrence, the stenosis is chosen to be located immediately after a branch site.

The pressure drop (Δp) across the stenosis is separated into three parts, one due to changes in the flow velocity (instationary Bernoulli term), one due to flow separation (Borda-Carnot term), and one due to the Hagen-Poiseuille-type flow. For Δp, we therefore have the expression

26

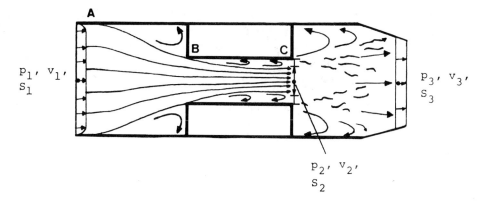

Fig. 5. Model of a short stenosis. Across an abrupt constriction in a vessel, a major part of the pressure drop is caused by flow separation at the locations A, B, and C. The contribution to this pressure drop from A and B is taken into account by defining an effective cross-section S_2 at C for the actual lumen with the aid of an empiric relation for stationary flow [11]. This additional narrowing can be as high as 40% of the stenosis lumen. In our case, we have included this flow contraction effect in the value of S_2 which is 20% of the cross-sectional area of the unobliterated conduit. Flow separation in C is responsible for the Borda-Carnot term in the expression (14) [see also 12]

$$\Delta p = p_1 - p_3 = \underbrace{\frac{\rho}{2} \cdot (v_3{}^2 - v_1{}^2) + \rho \cdot \int_1^3 \frac{\partial v}{\partial t} dz}_{\text{I}} + \underbrace{\frac{\rho}{2} \cdot v_1{}^2 \cdot \left(\frac{S_1}{S_2} - 1\right)^2}_{\text{II}} +$$

$$+ \underbrace{\frac{8 \cdot \pi \cdot \mu \cdot L \cdot Q_1}{S_2{}^2}}_{\text{III}} \qquad (14)$$

in which the indices refer to the various sections shown in Figure 5, and S_2 denotes the effective cross-section of the stenosis. In the arterial conduit designated as our standard case, we consider and 80% stenosis of this type at $z = 42.5$ cm. All other properties of the standard case are left unchanged. The quantities p_1, p_3, v_1, and v_3 are computed by making use of one characteristic equation at each end of the stenosis, by satisfying Eq. 14 for Δp, and by enforcing the conservation of mass theorem for the stenosis segment, which for this purpose is assumed to be rigid.

The pressure and flow pulses one obtains in presence of such a stenosis are plotted in Figure 6. They clearly differ from those of the standard case insofar as we now have a marked reduction of blood flow into the arterial conduit below the stenosis, an elevation of the pressure in the proximal region, a pressure drop of about 40 mm Hg across the stenosis (note the change in scale at $z = 45$

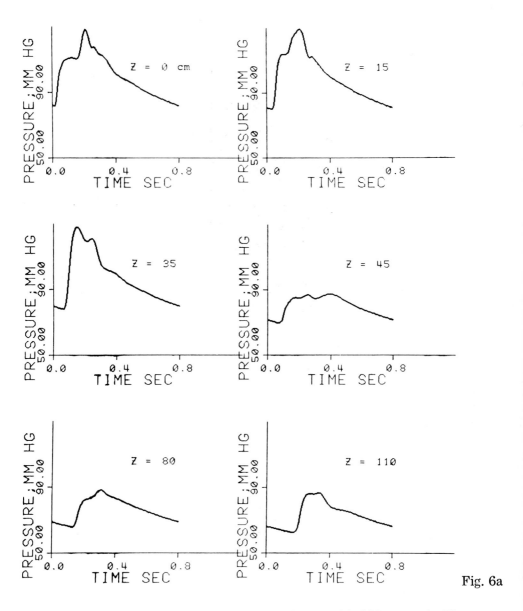

Fig. 6a

Fig. 6. Pressure and flow patterns in standard case with 80% stenosis. The curves correspond to the situation where a stenosis of the type illustrated in Figure 5 is introduced immediately distal to the branch at z = 42.5 cm

cm), and a clear manifestation of a reflection of the pulse at the stenosis. In addition, we no longer have backflow during diastole, except near the root of the aorta. Also, the flow pulses show a broadening below the stenosis, and during diastole, the flow rate is higher in relation to the peak flow than that in the flow pulse of the standard case.

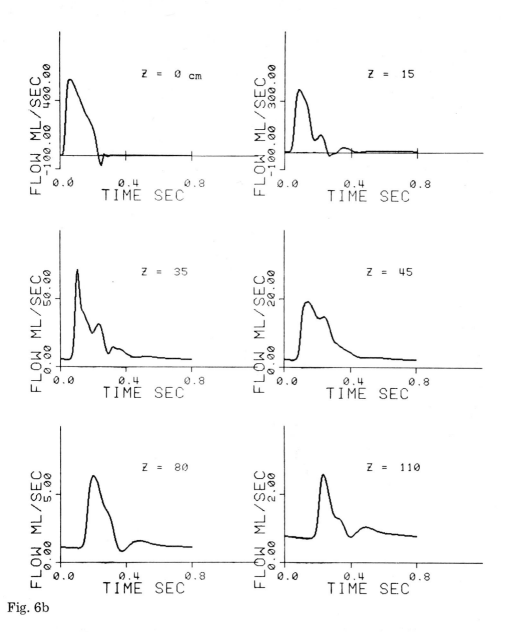

Fig. 6b

Model for Wall Viscoelasticity

To ascertain realistic pulse shapes, the mathematical model has to include the damping due to the viscoelasticity of the vessel wall as well as that due to the blood viscosity. In Eq. 3, the friction force associated with blood viscosity is approximated by the term $- 8 \pi \cdot \mu \cdot v$. Besides this, only a small damping due to the numerical procedure is present. For large arteries, the effect of wall viscoelasticity is more prominent than the damping due to the blood viscosity.

Several experimental studies have shown that the logarithmic decrement caused by the wall viscoelasticity of sinusoidal arterial pressure changes is independent of the frequency in the range of 20-200 Hz [2]. This type of damping, which in aeroelasticity is known as "structural damping," can be described in a straight-forward way by replacing the Young's modulus E by a complex quantity $E_1 + i E_2$ with constant E_1 and E_2. Such a procedure is, however, not amenable in our nonlinear analysis using the method of characteristics. Other models, e.g., Kelvin, Voigt, or more complicated concepts [13] do not exhibit a logarithmic decrement which is independent of frequency. Therefore, a different approach had to be utilized.

We have chosen one which originally was applied in computerized traffic accident simulation [7]. Accordingly, a pressure-area relationship of the vessel is prescribed in such a manner that only the sign and the magnitude of the pressure change but not its time rate define the response. In other words, the pressure-area relationship is "static" but different for loading and unloading. Departing from the elastic curve "a" in Figure 7, which is defined by Eqs. 2 and 12, a master hysteresis cycle is established between the systolic and the diastolic pres-

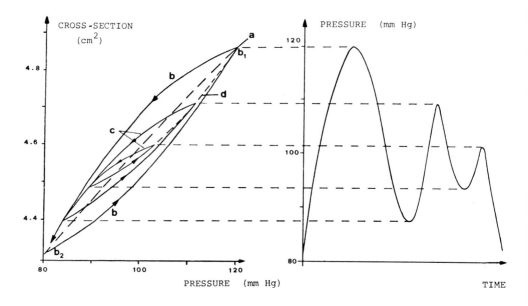

Fig. 7. Hysteresis cycles of cross-section — pressure relationship in case of visco-elastic wall behavior.
a: Original elastic curve.
b: Master hysteresis cycle between systolic (b_1) and diastolic (b_2) pressures.
c: Higher order cycles.
d: Path leading back to master cycle.
The depicted situation results from the hypothetic pressure pulse shown which generates one master cycle and two higher order cycles

sures labeled b_1 and b_2, respectively. While choosing an appropriate hysteresis cycle, care has to be taken that the tangent is always directed such that the pressure rises with increasing cross-sectional area. Therefore, maximal dissipation is achieved when the cycle approaches a rectangular shape between the two extreme pressures (Fig. 7).

In the present version of the computer program, the shape of the hysteresis loop is fixed. However, the user may choose the width of the loop according to the desired level of energy dissipation. Loops involving loading and unloading cycles within the master loop like those denoted by "c" in Figure 7 are defined in a similar way. Such higher order loops may occur as part of a regular heart beat. They are bounded by those whose minimum pressures are smaller and whose maximum pressures are higher. Whenever the pressure continues to increase beyond the maximum pressure of the just completed cycle, it follows a curve which passes through the culmination points of those cycles whose maximum pressures are higher as indicated by the dashed line "d" in Figure 7. This model automatically provides for an energy dissipation which is independent of the frequency because it does not depend on the speed at which a cycle is executed.

The introduction of this new viscoelasticity model requires a modification of the computational procedure used so far. Now the wave speed has to be determined from Eq. 1, whereby the derivative of S with respect to the pressure is defined analytically by the shapes of the hysteresis loops. The fact that this derivative is discontinuous in the inversion points of the loops proved to be of no consequence for the computation process because the discrepancies shown by the energy and mass balance tests are of the same order as in the case of a purely elastic wall behavior. A preliminary evaluation of this model was made by applying it to the standard case. The flow patterns at z = 90 cm plotted in Figure 8 for the elastic and viscoelastic wall demonstrate a blunting of the

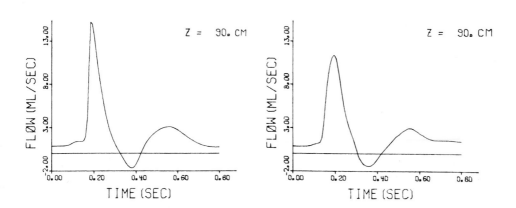

Fig. 8. Influence of viscoelasticity of vessel wall on flow pulse shape. The effect of introducing the viscoelasticity model in the standard case is demonstrated for the flow pulse at z = 90 cm

peaks and a substantial reduction in the amplitude of the systolic pulse as a result of the viscoelastic wall behavior.

Discussion

A new mathematical model has been devised which is expected to provide a more realistic simulation of human arterial conduits than previous models. It was designed to fulfil requirements which were not met in a satisfactory way in earlier mathematical studies such as:

1. Capability to model arbitrary networks
2. Possibility to accomodate pathological features (e.g., stenosis) without essential changes in the model
3. Inclusion of viscoelasticity of the vessel wall
4. Systematic tests of numerical accuracy

A segmented model in which individual pieces with different properties can be arranged to form any desired network is believed to facilitate the achievement of some of these goals. Three types of elements which could be used to build up a network of arbitrary arterial conduits are for example:

1. Single tapered tube segments with a small continuous outflow
2. Bifurcations or branch elements
3. Segments exhibiting pathological properties

In the present analysis, the major branches are still lumped rather than modeled in terms of segments and branches of their own. Associated with the lumped treatment of a major branch is the stipulation that the blood flow into the branch depends on the flow rate in the conduit and on the difference between the local and the capillary pressures. This dependence is characterized in terms of two constant parameters which implies that possible reflections from the distal regions of the branch artery are lumped with those generated at the beginning of the branch. Accordingly, the model simulates the actual branch behavior in a relatively coarse manner. In a more refined study, the method of characteristics should be utilized to predict the propagation of flow and pressure pulses in the branch arteries as well. Nevertheless, the present model provides not only physiologically realistic results in the standard case but also when a severe stenosis is added or when the heart rate is increased and no other parameter value is changed including those for the branch flow.

Experience has shown that the systematic application of the energy and mass balance tests can be a valuable warranty for the reliability and accuracy of the results. They not only reveal errors in programming but also provide information on regional blood and energy flow. A preliminary evaluation of the new viscoelasticity model for the vessel wall indicates that it produces reasonable damping and shape changes of the pulses in the standard case. However, a more detailed study of the properties of this model has to be performed in conjunction with a comprehensive network analysis of the arterial tree.

Summary

A human arterial conduit from the heart to the foot is modeled as a straight
tube with a progressively diminishing cross-section. Eight major branch arteries
are simulated by discrete outflow regions, whereas the loss of blood through
smaller branches is approximated by a continuously distributed and appropriately chosen seepage through the wall. The blood is treated as an incompressible
fluid and the flow as one-dimensional. Besides this, a standard conduit is defined
whose distensibility is given by the speed of small pressure waves as a function
of pressure and distance from the heart and whose axial variation of the lumen
is prescribed at a reference pressure. Furthermore, the stroke volume, heart rate,
and outflow through the branches are chosen within the corresponding ranges
for normal healthy adults.

With the aid of the method of characteristics, the pressure and flow patterns are
predicted numerically and plotted for various sites along the conduit. The computed pulse shapes and their changes with propagation exhibit the characteristic
features observed in man, as do those determined for the standard conduit with
a short 80% stenosis at the beginning of the iliac artery. However, in both cases,
the systolic peaks are somewhat too sharp and the wave front too steep at the
larger distances from the heart when the blood viscosity is the only source of
damping. By way of an example, it is shown that a new model for the viscoelastic behavior of the vessel wall promises better agreement between predicted
and measured pressure and flow pulses.

References

1. Anliker, M.: Current and future aspects of biomedical engineering. Triangle
   16, 129-140 (1977)
2. Anliker, M., Histand, M.B., Ogden, E.: Dispersion and attenuation of small
   artificial pressure waves in the canine aorta. Circ. Res. 23 539-551 (1968)
3. Anliker, M., Rockwell, R.L., Ogden, E.: Nonlinear analysis of flow pulses
   and shock waves in arteries. Part I: Derivation and properties of mathematical model. Part II: Parametric study related to clinical problems. J. Appl.
   Math. Phys. (ZAMP) 22, 217-246 (Part I), 563-581 (Part II) (1971)
4. Bollinger, A., Fromm, U., Brunner, H.H., Mahler, F., Casty, M., Anliker, M.,
   Siegenthaler, W.: Die Wirkung von Isosorbid-Dinitrat (ISD) auf den peripheren Kreislauf: Eine Studie mit kontinuierlicher perkutaner Flußmessung
   in der A. Femoralis. In: Nitrate, Wirkung auf Herz und Kreislauf. Hrsg.:
   W. Rudolph, W. Siegenthaler, München: Urban und Schwarzenberg 1976
5. Bühlmann, A.A., Froesch, E.R.: Pathophysiologie. Berlin-Heidelberg-New
   York: Springer 1974
6. Courant, R., Hilbert, D.: Methods of Mathematical Physics. New York:
   Interscience 1962, Vol. II
7. Danforth, J.P., Randall, C.D.: Modified ROS Occupant Dynamics Simulation User Manual. Gen. Mot. Res. Warren, Mi. Res. Publ. 1254, (1973)

8. Doriot, P.A., Casty, M., Milakara, B., Anliker, M., Bollinger, A., Siegen-thaler, W.: Quantitative analysis of flow conditions in simulated vessels and large human arteries and veins by means of ultrasound. Proc. 2nd Europ. congress on ultrasonics in medicine. Munich: Excerpta Medica Int. Congress Ser. 363 (May 1975)

9. Elsner, J.: Mathematische Modellstudien der Druck- und Flußpulse in menschlichen Arterien. Diss. ETH 5582, Zürich 1975

10. Hübscher, W., Anliker, M.: Instantane Flußmessungen in großen Blutge-fäßen mittels 128-kanaligem Ultraschall-Doppler-Gerät und Mikroprozes-sor. medita 9a, 135-138 (1977)

11. Prandtl, L., Oswatitsch, K., Wieghardt, K.: Führer durch die Strömungs-lehre. Braunschweig: Vieweg 1969

12. Raines, J.K., Darling, R.C., Jaffrin, J.Y.: Detection and simulation of peripheral occlusive disease. 4th Annual Meeting, Biomed. Eng. Soc. p. 2.4 (1973)

13. Rockwell, R.L., Anliker, M., Elsner, J.: Model studies of the pressure and flow pulses in a viscoelastic arterial conduit. J. Franklin Institute 297, 405-427 (1974)

14. Snyder, M.F., Rideout, V.C., Hillestad, R.J.: Computer modeling of the human systemic arterial tree, J. Biomech. 1, 341 (1968)

15. Westerhof, N., Bosmann, F., DeVries, C.J., Noordergraaf, A.: Analog studies of the human systemic arterial tree. J. Biomech. 2, 121-143 (1969)

16. Wetterer, E., Kenner, Th.: Dynamik des Arterienpulses. Berlin - Heidelberg - New York: Springer 1968

New Ways of Determining the Propagation Coefficient and the Visco-Elastic Behaviour of Arteries in situ

E. Wetterer, R. D. Bauer, and R. Busse

Institut für Physiologie und Kardiologie der Universität Erlangen-Nürnberg, D-8520 Erlangen

In the theoretic treatment of the pulse waves generated by the left ventricle in the arterial system, two basic equations are important, the equation of motion and that of continuity. The first equation contains the longitudinal impedance (z_l) as the relation between the longitudinal pressure gradient and the local flow, while in the second, the transverse impedance (z_t) represents the relation between the local pressure and the longitudinal flow gradient. Each of the two impedances is related to the unit of vessel length. Pressure (p) and flow (i) are functions of the point (x) on the longitudinal axis of the vessel and of the time (t) [for literature, see 2, 9, 12, 13, 18, 20].

Regular arterial pulses can be treated as rhythmic events in a steady state and Fourier analysis can be used. The sinusoidal harmonic components are independent of one another if the system is linear. For a given harmonic, we have

$$p(x, t) = P(x) \cdot \exp(j\omega t) \tag{1}$$

$$i(x, t) = I(x) \cdot \exp(j\omega t) \tag{2}$$

$P(x)$ and $I(x)$ are the complex amplitudes of pressure and flow at point x, ω is the angular frequency, and j is $\sqrt{-1}$. The pulses are propagated along the system due to the combined effects of mass inertia of the blood and compliance of the vessel wall. Energy dissipation and thus attenuation are due to fluid and wall viscosity. While the longitudinal impedance takes into account mass inertia and the friction of fluid, the compliance and friction of the wall are considered in the transverse impedance. Thus, the two impedances are relevant to propagation and damping of the waves. The complex propagation coefficent (γ), which comprises the damping constant (a) and the phase constant (β), can be obtained from the two impedances

$$\gamma = a + j\beta = \sqrt{z_l/z_t} \tag{3}$$

Due to wave reflections, any recorded pulsatile pressure or flow is the sum of that of a forward running wave (f) and that of a backward running wave (b). In contrast to the pressure, the flow of a backward running wave is always opposite in phase to the flow that the wave would exhibit while running in the forward direction. If P_f and P_b are the pressure of a forward and a backward running wave at point x = 0, we have

$$P(x) = P_f \cdot \exp(-\gamma x) + P_b \cdot \exp(\gamma x) \tag{4}$$

$$I(x) = [P_f \cdot \exp(-\gamma x) - P_b \cdot \exp(\gamma x)]/Z \tag{5}$$

The phase velocity of forward waves is

$$c_{ph} = \omega/\beta \tag{6}$$

and is also called true phase velocity, in contrast to the apparent phase velocity which is related to the sum of forward and backward waves. Eq. 5 contains a further important quantity, the characteristic impedance Z, which is defined as the local pressure-to-flow ratio of forward waves

$$Z = P_f(x)/I_f(x) = \sqrt{z_l \cdot z_t} \tag{7}$$

It is obvious that there is an interrelationship between γ, Z, z_l, and z_t so that from two of these quantities the other two can be calculated. The transverse impedance z_t of an arterial segment which is tethered in longitudinal direction and has no side branches depends on the complex compliance per unit of length and on the frequency

$$z_t = \frac{1}{j\omega} \cdot P(x)/A(x) \tag{8}$$

where P(x) and A(x) are the complex amplitudes of pressure and internal cross-sectional area at point x, respectively. Thus z_t can be determined experimentally from the recorded pressure and, for example, the recorded external diameter if the wall thickness is known. If the wall viscosity is zero, there is no phase difference between P(x) and A(x) and the phase angle of Z_t is $-90°$, as seen from Eq. 8. In reality, A(x) lags behind P(x) so that the phase angle of z_t is somewhat less negative than $-90°$. Another more complicated way of determining z_t experimentally might be the direct application of the equation of continuity by measuring the flow gradient from simultaneous flow recordings at two points and the pressure at the intermediate point.

The experimental determination of the longitudinal impedance z_l may be based directly on the equation of motion. In this case, the pressure gradient is measured by pressure recordings at two points or by recording the differential pressure between them. The flow is recorded at the intermediate point. A method based on this procedure is described below. If the fluid viscosity is zero, the phase angle of z_l is $+90°$ (pressure leads flow) while in the case of a viscous fluid it is less than $90°$ [cf. 13, 20, 21]. It is obvious that the phase angle of the propagation coefficient γ is $+90°$ if the viscosities of the fluid and wall are zero. This means that the damping constant a is zero. The phase angle of the characteristic impedance Z is also zero in this case. If the fluid or the wall viscosity or both are greater than zero, the phase angle of γ must always be less than $+90°$, while the sign of the phase angle of the characteristic impedance Z depends on how much each of the phase angles of z_l and z_t deviates from $+90°$ and $-90°$, respectively.

36

The direct in vivo determination of the propagation coefficient γ is not difficult, if only forward waves are concerned. For this purpose, simultaneous recordings of pressure have to be carried out at two points of an artery. However, these simple conditions are present only in the case of artificially induced waves of such high frequencies that the short wave lengths and the strong damping virtually prevent any interference between forward and backward waves. Anliker and his co-workers [1] performed experimental studies of this kind. By means of an electrically driven impactor, they induced, in the thoracic aorta of dogs, trains of sine waves between 40 and 200 Hz which were superimposed on the natural pressure pulses. The pressure was recorded at two points 4-8 cm apart. In this way, true phase velocity and damping were determined for each of the frequencies applied; from these, the propagation coefficient can be derived. In the frequency range used, the phase velocity changed only moderately, while damping increased markedly with frequency in such a way that the attenuation per wave length was almost constant, corresponding to a logarithmic decrement of 0.7-1 per wave length.

If the propagation coefficient γ is to be determined experimentally in vivo in the frequency range of the natural arterial pulses, which does not exceed 10-20 Hz, the natural pulses themselves must be used. These pulses are the result of a superimposition of forward and backward waves which are not related to one another in any known way. Therefore, the number of unknowns is augmented by one and an additional measurement is required. As Milnor and Nichols [15] have pointed out, the experimental determination of γ is based only on the following conditions: γ must be constant along the length of the vessel segment examined and must have the same value for forward and backward waves; the attenuation of the propagated wave must be exponential; the Fourier components must be independent of one another, which is the case in a linear system.

Following a suggestion made by Taylor [17], McDonald and Gessner [14] determined γ in the canine carotid artery from three simultaneous pressure recordings (P_1, P_2, P_3) at equidistant points (Fig. 1, top). It follows from Eq. 4 that

$$\cosh \gamma L = \frac{P_1 + P_3}{2P_2} \tag{9}$$

where L = distance between two adjacent measuring points. The determination of Z would require an additional recording of flow or diameter so that, altogether, four simultaneous recordings would be necessary.

In the approach employed by Cox [6] in the canine femoral artery (Fig. 1, middle), z_l and z_t were determined separately. (Instead of z_t, its reciprocal value, the transverse admittance was used). According to the equation of motion, the longitudinal impedance was determined by recording the differential pressure between two points and the flow at the intermediate point. The transverse admittance was obtained by recording the arterial pressure and diameter at the first of the measuring points and calculating the internal cross-sectional area (A in Eq. 8) from the diameter and the wall thickness. Thus, again, four recordings were needed. γ and Z could be calculated from z_l and z_t according to Eqs. 3

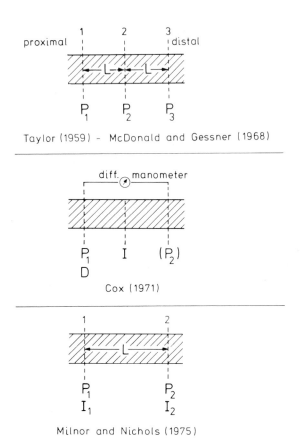

Milnor and Nichols (1975)

Fig. 1. Three different principles of the determination of the propagation coefficient γ and the characteristic impedance Z in homogeneous arterial segments in situ using natural pulses. Top: "three-point method" suggested by Taylor [17] and used by McDonald and Gessner [14] for the determination of γ. For the determination of Z, an additional measurement of flow or diameter would be needed. Middle: determination of γ and Z by means of z_l and z_t according to Cox [6]. Bottom: determination of γ and Z by Milnor and Nichols [15] from recordings of pressure and flow at each of two points of the arterial segment. For further explanation see text

and 7. In the case of γ, the author was mainly interested in the true phase velocity and its dependence on frequency and mean arterial pressure, while the damping constant, although contained in his numeric results, was not discussed.

The procedure suggested by Milnor and Nichols [15] and applied to the canine femoral artery is based on simultaneous recordings of pressure and flow at each of two points (1 and 2) at a distance (L) apart (Fig. 1, bottom). It permits γ and Z to be determined from the four measured values according to the formula

$$\cosh \gamma L = \frac{1 + (P_1/P_2)(I_1/I_2)}{(P_1/P_2) + (I_1/I_2)} \tag{10}$$

where P_1, I_1, P_2, and I_2 are the complex amplitudes of pressure and flow at points 1 and 2, respectively. The characteristic impedance Z was calculated by the authors from a formula containing the quotients P_2/P_1 (or I_2/I_1) and P_1/I_1 and hyperbolic functions of γL. It is possible to use another formula which can be derived by expressing z_l and z_t by means of the differential equations of motion and continuity and then making $Z^2 = z_l \cdot z_t$. The final integration yields

$$Z^2 = \frac{P_2^2 - P_1^2}{I_2^2 - I_1^2} \tag{11}$$

The main difficulty inherent in all determinations of γ using natural pulses is the fact that the superimposition of waves of opposite directions of propagation leads to the loss of the linear term (and also the higher odd terms) contained in the series of the exponential functions. This is a property of the hyperbolic cosine but is also effective if the determination of γ is carried out in such a way that the hyperbolic cosine does not appear. Thus, γ is determined virtually by the relatively small quadratic term alone. This makes very high demands on the accuracy of the measuring systems. The determination of the damping constant is more affected than that of the phase constant because the former is smaller. Since the loss of the linear term can on no account be circumvented when forward and backward waves are involved, the only possible way to obtain an improvement is to reduce the number of simultaneous measurements. Therefore, we tried to modify the three-point method (Eq. 9) and to determine γ from only two simultaneous pressure recordings [5]. This is possible if a well-defined relationship between forward and backward waves exists. This can be achieved by temporarily clamping the artery at the distal measuring point (point 2 in Fig. 2)

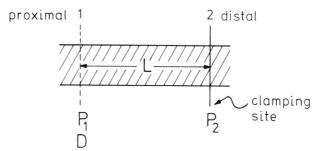

Fig. 2. Determination of the propagation coefficient γ from pressure recordings at only two points of an arterial segment. Artery clamped at distal measuring point. Additional diameter recording at proximal measuring point to derive the characteristic impedance Z. Modified from Busse [5]

so that total positive reflection occurs. The other pressure measurement is carried out at point 1 at a distance (L) proximal to point 2. If, in Eq. 4, we make x = 0 for point 1, the pressure of the incident wave entering the arterial segment is P_f, and, due to the total positive reflection at the clamped end, the backward pressure is $P_b = P_f \cdot \exp(-2\gamma L)$. We then have

$$P_1 = P_f [1 + \exp(-2\gamma L)] \tag{12}$$

The wave arriving at point 2 exhibits the pressure $P_f \cdot \exp(-\gamma L)$ which is doubled due to the total positive reflection

$$P_2 = 2P_f \cdot \exp(-\gamma L) \tag{13}$$

It follows from Eqs. 12 and 13 that

$$\cosh \gamma L = P_1/P_2 . \tag{14}$$

The most crucial conditions of this method are that the closed end of the arterial segment be kept as rigid as possible and the pressure P_2 be measured at the most distal point. To obtain a rigid closure, we initially used a special compound cylinder surrounding the artery and the catheter of the intravascular pressure transducer at the closed end. In the mean time, this cylinder has been replaced by another clamping device which consists, in principle, of a special snare of thick flexible plastic material and provides the closed end of the arterial segment with a firmer support.

To determine the transverse impedance z_t (and hence the characteristic impedance Z from z_t and γ), the arterial diameter is recorded at point 1. In this respect, we follow the principle applied by Cox [6]. We use a contact-free photoelectric device which was developed at our laboratory [19]. A method based on a similar principle, and applicable to elastic tubes contained in technical devices, was used by Flaud and his co-workers [7]. Our device is shown in Figure 3. Its func-

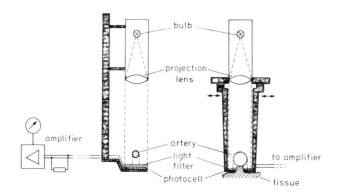

Fig. 3. Photoelectric device for contact-free recording of the outer diameter of an artery in situ. For explanation see text. Modified from Wetterer et al [19]

tion is, in principle, as follows. The light emitted by an electric bulb is collimated by a projection lens and directed to a flat silicone photocell covered by a light filter. The area of the shadow cast by the artery on the photocell is proportional to the artery's outer diameter. The intensity of the collimated light, the density of the filter, and the value of the load resistor of the photocell are chosen in such a way that there is a rectilinear relationship between the signal voltage of the photocell and the arterial diameter. The combined frequency response of photocell and amplifier is flat up to 200 Hz. The time lag of the signal is about 0.2 ms. The device shown on the left of Figure 3 is suitable for arteries of diameters up to 7 mm. For larger arteries, the double arrangement seen on the right is used.

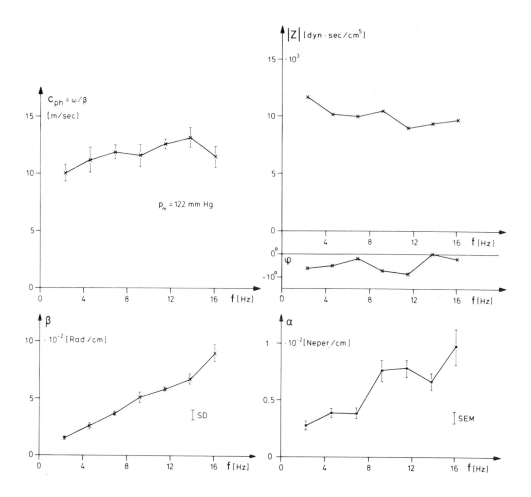

Fig. 4. Results obtained with the method of Figure 2 in the canine carotid artery of a dog. Mean blood pressure was 122 mm Hg. Pressures were recorded with two catheter-tip transducers (Millar PC 350 A) at a distance of about 10 cm apart. The other instruments are mentioned in the text. Left side: phase constant β (bottom) and phase velocity c_{ph} (top). Bars indicate standard deviation. Right side: damping constant a (bottom, bars indicate standard error of the mean) and modulus and phase of the characteristic impedance Z (top)

Figure 4 shows the results obtained in the carotid artery of a dog. The phase constant β increases with frequency in such a way that the phase velocity, which is in the range of 10-13 m/s, also increases. This increase, however, is not significant above 6 Hz. Bars indicate standard deviation. The damping constant increases with frequency; this corresponds, in principle, to the known results of previous authors. The bars which now indicate the standard error of the mean reveal a relatively large scatter, which can be explained by the previously mentioned peculiarity of the hyperbolic cosine. It is surprising that the values of the damping constant a are much lower than those reported by other workers. For example, they are only about one-quarter of those obtained by McDonald and Gessner [14] in the dog carotid with the three-point method. At the present stage of investigation, we will not try to explain this discrepancy. A comparison of our damping values with those of Moritz and Anliker [16] obtained with the impactor method reveals much smaller differences. These authors found, in the range of 25-40 Hz, a logarithmic decrement per wave length of 1.1 in the carotids of six dogs. From our a value, a logarithmic decrement per wave length of between 0.8 and 0.9 can be calculated; this is not much smaller than that found by Moritz and Anliker. The values of McDonald and Gessner would give a logarithmic decrement per wave length of 2 to more than 3. The modulus of the characteristic impedance Z is about 11,000 CGS units and decreases slightly when the frequency increases. There is a fair agreement with results reported in the literature. The same is true with respect to the phase angles of the characteristic impedance, which are negative and small. Similar results were obtained in three other dogs. These initial findings must be confirmed by further experiments.

Our second main topic is related to the viscoelastic properties of the arterial wall. As mentioned above, the application of Fourier analysis in the determination of wall parameters relevant to wave propagation presupposes a linear system. It is, however, well-known that the elastic behavior of arteries deviates from linearity. The question arises as to whether, in the range of the usual pulsatile blood pressure changes, the extent of this deviation is great enough to give rise to noticeable errors. Some workers believe this to be a point of serious concern [1, 11].

Our approach to this problem is as follows. Due to the combined effects of wall elasticity and wall viscosity, the pressure-diameter diagram of pulsating arteries shows the well-known hysteresis loop in which pressure leads diameter. Figure 5 shows a record of pressure and external diameter of a canine carotid artery. The diameter was recorded with the previously mentioned photoelectric device and the pressure with a catheter-tip transducer at the same point. On the right, the pressure-diameter loop is plotted. For the evaluation of the purely elastic

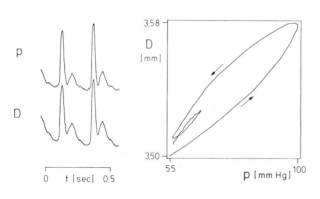

Fig. 5. Left: time course of pressure (p) and external diameter (D) of the common carotid artery of a dog. Pressure was recorded with a catheter-tip transducer (Millar PC 350 A), diameter with a contact-free photoelectric device [19]. Right: pressure-diameter loop of the first pulse of left side. From Bauer [3].

42

and the purely viscous wall properties, we try to separate the two in the following way. By definition, the purely elastic pressure-diameter relationship is independent of the strain rate and must, of necessity, yield the same curve for lengthening and shortening of the circumference or diameter so that there is no loop at all. The viscous effect, however, depends on the rate of strain, whose sign is positive during lengthening and negative during shortening. Therefore, we subdivide the recorded pulsatile pressure (p) into an "elastic pressure" component (p_{el}), related to the circumference or diameter (D) itself, and a "viscous pressure" component (p_{vis}), related to the rate of change of circumference or diameter (dD/dt)

$$p = p_{el} + p_{vis} \tag{15}$$

As first approximation, we use a linear relationship between p_{vis} and dD/dt

$$p_{vis} = F \cdot dD/dt \tag{16}$$

where F is a factor, so that we obtain from the two equations

$$p_{el} = p - F \cdot dD/dt \tag{17}$$

This formula corresponds to the classic Voigt model. Since, as will be seen below, Eq. 17 did not yield fully satisfactory results, we developed, quite empirically, the following modification

$$p_{vis} = (F_1 + F_2|dD/dt|)dD/dt \tag{18}$$

from which another expression of p_{el} is obtained

$$p_{el} = p - (F_1 + F_2|dD/dt|)dD/dt \tag{19}$$

The factor F_1 behaves in the same way as the previous factor F, while the factor F_2 is multiplied by the absolute value of dD/dt so that the square of the differential quotient also influences the result.

To begin with the simpler one-factor calculation, the optimal value of the factor F is found by trial and error using the criterion of elimination of the loop. This can be performed by means of an appropriate computer program. The result is seen in Figure 6. In Figure 6a we see the same, unchanged loop as in Figure 5. In Figure 6b, Eq. 17 is applied using a factor F of 0.75, which is obviously too small. The loop area is reduced, but not eliminated. In Figure 6c, the factor is 1.69; this reduces the loop to the minimum obtainable by means of Eq. 17. However, the loop has not completely disappeared but has been converted to a flat double loop. Only in Figure 6d where Eq. 19 with $F_1 = 2.5$ and $F_2 = -0.15$ has been applied, is the loop virtually eliminated.

In all cases examined so far, the factor F_2 proved to be negative. Similar results were obtained in the abdominal and thoracic aorta and femoral artery of the dog. A further example is shown in Figure 7, where a dog abdominal aorta is

43

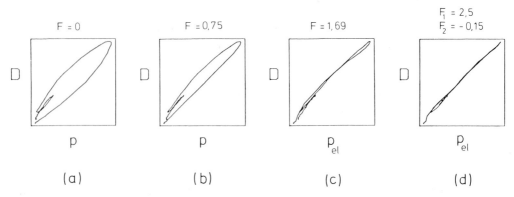

Fig. 6. Carotid pulse taken from Figure 5. a: p-D loop unchanged; b: loop area somewhat reduced by using Eq. 17 with F = 0.75; c: loop almost completely eliminated by using Eq. 17 with F = 1.69; d: optimal elimination of the loop by using Eq. 19 with F_1 = 2.5 and F_2 = –0.15. Units used for the calculations: p[mm Hg], D[mm], time [s]. From Bauer [3]

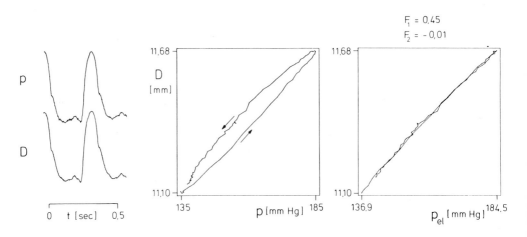

Fig. 7. Pressure (p) and diameter (D) of a canine abdominal aorta. Methods as in Figure 5. From left to right: time course of pressure and diameter. Original p-D loop. p_{el}-D curve calculated by means of Eq. 19 using F_1 = 0.45 and F_2 = –0.01. From Bauer [3]

examined. The original unchanged loop and the purely elastic pressure-diameter curve are seen. In the latter, the loop is completely eliminated by the two-factor method of Eq. 19.

The most obvious characteristic of these purely elastic pressure-diameter relationships of canine arteries is the very small curvature so that considerable errors in Fourier analysis due to elastic nonlinearity can be excluded. It should be emphasized, however, that in cases of abnormally high pulse pressure, marked curvatures can be observed so that the objections made by various authors, for example by Gow and Taylor [11], are undoubtedly justified in these cases.

A small number of pressure and diameter recordings have also been made in human carotid arteries exposed during operations. As far as can be judged from the few examples examined so far, the curvature of the elastic pressure-diameter diagram of the human carotid is stronger than that of the canine carotid. This will be shown in the contributions by Schabert and Summa presented at these proceedings.

For many purposes of hemodynamic interest, the arterial stress-strain (σ – ϵ) relationship is more relevant than the p-D relationship. Since σ must always be in phase with p and ϵ in phase with D, the criterion of loop elimination also applies to the σ – ϵ curve in which σ comprises a pure elastic part σ_{el} and a pure viscous part σ_{vis}. The σ_{el}–ϵ curve and the σ_{vis}–$d\epsilon/dt$ curves can be calculated directly from the respective p-D curves if the wall thickness is known and the arterial wall is regarded as incompressible. Theoretically, the σ_{el}–ϵ curve must be concave to the ϵ-coordinate if the p_{el}-D curve is linear.

For the transverse impedance z_t (Eq. 8), the relationship between pressure and internal cross-sectional area (A) is relevant and can also be calculated from the p-D curve. If the p_{el}-D curve is linear, the p_{el}-A curve must be concave to the A coordinate. The curvature is very small in the range of normal pulse pressures. If, at greater pulse pressure, the p_{el}-D curve is nonlinear, its curvature counteracts that of the p_{el}-A curve.

Figure 8 shows a p_{vis}-dD/dt plot of a carotid pulse calculated with the aid of Eq. 18. In the course of the pulse, both variables run through positive values in the first quadrant and negative values in the third quadrant. If the factor F_2 were zero, a rectilinear relationship would result. Since, however, F_2 is negative and multiplied by $|dD/dt|$, the p_{vis}-dD/dt relationship is represented by an S-shaped curve, which is convex to the p_{vis} coordinate and deviates the more from linearity the greater the value of dD/dt is. The result is that the two limbs in the first and third quadrants differ in length and curvature. In spite of the

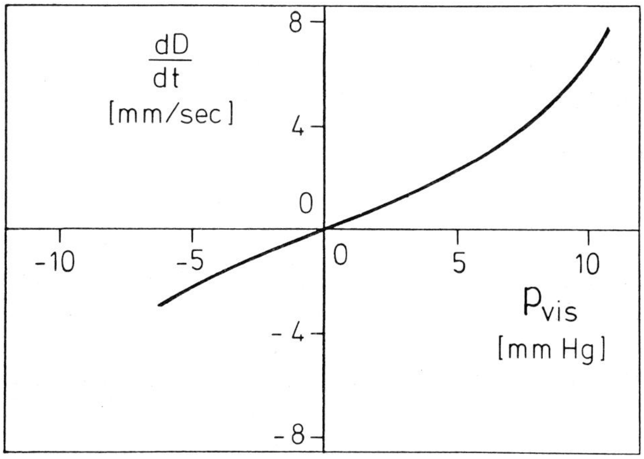

Fig. 8. p_{vis}-dD/dt curve calculated from the canine carotid pulse of Figure 5 using Eq. 18 with $F_1 = 2.5$ and $F_2 =$ –0.15. From Bauer [3]

curvature seen in Figure 8, the viscous nonlinearity cannot be expected to induce major errors in Fourier analysis since the viscous part is usually small as compared with the elastic part of arterial viscoelasticity.

Numerous models have been suggested in the literature to describe the viscoelastic behavior of arteries [for surveys, see 4, 8, 10, 13]. To interpret our results obtained in pulsating arteries in vivo under steady-state conditions, a modified Voigt model seems to be suitable. The classic Voigt model consists of the parallel arrangement of a purely elastic spring and a purely viscous dashpot. The latter is assumed to possess a linear relationship between frictional force and velocity of distension. In contrast, the dashpot of the modified Voigt model we would like to suggest exhibits a nonlinear force-velocity curve whose steepness decreases when the velocity of distension increases. Such behavior is known from thixotropic materials. It should be emphasized that the nonlinearity of the viscous behavior of the arterial wall as described here is no single, isolated finding. The literature contains several pointers to the fact that the coefficient of wall viscosity decreases when the frequency or velocity of stretching increases. We would like to refer to a few results, discussions, and surveys [4, 10, 11].

For a description of the manifold manifestations of arterial viscoelasticity, some authors have suggested very intricate models comprising several or many elastic and viscous elements arranged in parallel and/or in series. The relatively simple modified Voigt model that we suggest is limited to pulsating arteries under steady-state oscillatory conditions.

References

1. Anliker, M., Histand, M.B., Ogden, E.: Dispersion and attenuation of small artificial pressure waves in the canine aorta. Circ. Res. 23, 539-551 (1968)
2. Attinger, E.O. (ed.): Pulsatile Blood Flow. New York: McGraw 1964
3. Bauer, R.D.: Die quantitative Bestimmung der nichtlinearen Visko-Elastizität von Arterien in vivo — ein bisher ungelöstes Problem. Habilitationsschrift, Erlangen 1977
4. Bergel, D.H. (ed.): Cardiovascular Fluid Dynamics. London-New York: Acad. Pr. 1972, Vol. I and II
5. Busse, R.: Ein neuer theoretischer und experimenteller Weg zur Bestimmung des Übertragungsmaßes und des Wellenwiderstandes an Arterien in situ. Habilitationsschrift, Erlangen 1976
6. Cox, R.H.: Determination of the true phase velocity of arterial pressure waves in vivo. Circ. Res. 29, 407-418 (1971)
7. Flaud, P., Geiger, D., Oddou, C., Quemada, D.: Experimental study of wave propagation through viscous fluid contained in viscoelastic cylindrical tube under static stresses. Biorheology 12, 347-354 (1975)
8. Flügge, W.: Viscoelasticity. 2nd ed., Berlin-Heidelberg-New York: Springer 1975
9. Frank, O.: Die Theorie der Pulswellen. Z. Biol. 85, 91-130 (1926)

10. Fung, Y.C.: Stess-strain history relations of soft tissues in simple elongation. In: Biomechanics — its Foundations and Objectives. Fung, Y.C., Perrone, N., Anliker, M. (eds.). New Jersey: Prentice Hall 1972, pp. 181-208
11. Gow, B.S., Taylor, M.G.: Measurement of viscoelastic properties of arteries in the living dog. Circ. Res. $\underline{23}$, 111-122 (1968)
12. Kenner, Th.: Flow and pressure in the arteries. In: Biomechanics — its Foundations and Objectives. Fung, Y.C., Perrone, N., Anliker, M. (eds.). New Jersey: Prentice Hall 1972, pp. 381-434
13. McDonald, D.A.: Blood flow in arteries. 2nd ed. London: Arnold 1974
14. McDonald, D.A., Gessner, U.: Wave attenuation in viscoelastic arteries. In: Hemorheology. Copley, A.L. (ed.). Oxford: Pergamon Pr. 1968, pp. 113-125
15. Milnor, W.R., Nichols, W.W.: A new method of measuring propagation coefficients and characteristic impedance in blood vessels. Circ. Res. $\underline{36}$, 631-639 (1975)
16. Moritz, W.E., Anliker, M.: Wave transmission characteristics and anisotropy of canine carotid arteries. J. Biomech. $\underline{7}$, 151-154 (1974)
17. Taylor, M.G.: Wave travel in arteries. Ph. D. Thesis, London 1959
18. Taylor, M.G.: Hemodynamics. Annu. Rev. Physiol. $\underline{35}$, 87-116 (1973)
19. Wetterer, E., Busse, R., Bauer, R.D., Schabert, A., Summa, Y.: Photoelectric device for contact-free recording of the diameters of exposed arteries in situ. Pflügers Arch. $\underline{368}$, 149-152 (1977)
20. Wetterer, E., Kenner, Th.: Grundlagen der Dynamik des Arterienpulses. Berlin-Heidelberg-New York: Springer 1968
21. Womersley, J.R.: An Elastic Tube Theory of Pulse Transmission and Oscillatory Flow in Mammalian Arteries. WADC Technical Report TR 56-614. Wright Air Development Center 1957

Arterial Reflection

N. Westerhof, G. C. van den Bos, and S. Laxminarayan.
With technical assistance of A. van der Vos and F. O. M. Pot

Laboratorium voor Fysiologie, Vrije Universiteit, Amsterdam/Holland

Introduction

To study wave reflection in the arterial system, we can choose either of two
approaches. In the first place, we can look at pressure or flow as a function of
location: amplitudes of pressure or flow harmonics are computed as function
of place; the maxima and minima of these harmonics give information about
the main site and magnitude of reflection [5]. Secondly, we can look at reflection at a single site, i.e., pressure and flow are measured at one location only and
the overall reflections from points distal to this location are calculated. If we opt
for this approach, several ways are open. All give basically the same information,
but each method stresses a particular aspect. We can obtain the input impedance
of the vascular bed under study from measurement of pressure and flow through
Fourier analysis. This input impedance can give information about reflection
directly [10]. We can further calculate the reflection coefficient (the relation
between the wave running into the system and the reflected wave) [16]. These
methods use the frequency domain: pressure-flow relations as a function of
frequency (input impedance), pressure-pressure relations as function of frequency
(reflection coefficient). We can also use the time domain: impulse response function and the breakdown of measured pressure and flow into forward and reflected
waves [16, 4]. For both techniques, pressure and flow are measured at one location only. The impulse response function is the pressure measured when a δ-
function of flow is applied to the system. Like input impedance and reflection
coefficient, the impulse response function characterizes the system. This is not
the case with the method that calculates forward and backward waves.

We will review the methods based on analysis of pressure and flow measured at
a single site only. The techniques will be applied to two models of the arterial
system and to some experimental situations in anesthetized dogs. We have studied the systemic arterial system and two peripheral beds (brachiocephalic and
femoral).

Theory and Calculations

1. Input Impedance

Location and amount of reflection can be found from the input impedance as follows: at the lowest frequency where the modulus of the impedance is minimal, one-quarter of the wave length is equal to the length of the system [6, 19]. From the pulse wave velocity and this first minimum we find

$$l = c/4f_{min} \tag{1}$$

where l is the effective length, c the phase velocity, and f_{min} the lowest frequency where the modulus is a minimum or the phase crosses zero [12]. Similar relations hold for the other minima and maxima of the modulus of the impedance and also for the phase crossings.

When reflections are negligible, the input impedance is equal to the characteristic impedance of the section of artery where pressure and flow are measured. Inversely, if the input impedance deviates strongly from the characteristic impedance, reflections are large. The input impedance is calculated from the pressure and flow harmonics obtained through Fourier analysis of the measured pressure and flow signals.

2. Reflection Coefficient

The reflection coefficient relates harmonics of the reflected pressure wave with the harmonics of the centrifugal (forward) pressure wave. Flow waves are reflected with the same magnitude as pressure waves but the phase differs by 180 degrees [16]. The reflection coefficient gives direct information about the reflections in the arterial tree but not about its effective length. Waves reflected from different parts of the arterial system cannot be studied: the summated reflected wave is determined and we must speak of the global reflection coefficient.

The measured pressure and flow waves are the sum of their forward and reflected components. To perform the separation, we make use of the fact that the ratio of the forward pressure and flow harmonics is the characteristic impedance of the artery of measurement [16]. The reflected pressure and flow harmonics are also related through the characteristic impedance but 180 degrees out of phase. For large arteries, the characteristic impedance is approximately a real quantity and can be found from the value of the modulus of the input impedance between 3 and 10 Hz [1]. In this case, the ratio of the whole forward pressure and flow waves as a function of time is equal to the characteristic impedance. The reflected pressure and flow waves also have the characteristic impedance as their ratio but they are inversed. For the case of a real characteristic impedance, we can calculate the forward and reflected waves directly

$$P_m(t) = P_f(t) + P_b(t) \tag{2}$$

$$F_m(t) = F_f(t) + F_b(t) \tag{3}$$

$$P_f(t)/F_f(t) = Z_c = -P_b(t)/F_b(t) \tag{4}$$

where P and F are pressure and flow, Z_c the characteristic impedance, and the indices m, f, and b indicate measured, forward and reflected, respectively. We can, after rearrangement, write

$$P_f(t) = \frac{1}{2}[P_m(t) + Z_c F_m(t)] = +F_f(t) Z_c \tag{5}$$

$$P_b(t) = \frac{1}{2}[P_m(t) - Z_c F_m(t)] = -F_f(t) Z_c \tag{6}$$

Eq. 5 and 6 can be used to study forward and reflected waves in the arterial system [16, 2]. Fourier analysis of the reflected and forward waves and computation of the amplitude ratios (and phase differences) of the harmonics give the reflection coefficient as a function of frequency.

The reflection coefficient can also be calculated from the input impedance. The reflection coefficient written as an impedance relation is given by

$$\Gamma(\omega) = [Z_l(\omega) - Z_c(\omega)]/[Z_l(\omega) + Z_c(\omega)] \tag{7}$$

where Γ and Z_l are the reflection coefficient and the impedance distal to the location where Γ is to be determined. Since we assume that the characteristic impedance is a real, frequency-independent constant, it can be obtained from the modulus of the input impedance [1]. The $Z_l(\omega)$ is the input impedance of the entire arterial system if the location of measurement is the ascending aorta. For other locations, Z_l is the input impedance of the bed distal to the site of measurement.

3. Impulse Response Function

Reflections in the arterial system can also be studied if an impulse of flow is delivered to the system and the response signal (pressure) is studied. This response is called the impulse response function. The impulse of flow (δ-function) must be much shorter than all time constants in the arterial system, while the area should be unity (area is volume). The time delay (ΔT) between the given impulse and the impulses returning from the system is related to the effective length

$$l = \Delta T c/2 \tag{8}$$

The impulse response function (z(t)) can be calculated from the so-called convolution integral

$$P(t) = \int_{-\infty}^{t} F(t - \tau)\, z(\tau)\, d\tau \tag{9}$$

where τ is a running variable representing time. Since we have not been able to solve z(t) by direct deconvolution, we have used inverse transforms. The input impedance is the Fourier transform of the impulse response function. Inverse transformation of the input impedance gives the impulse response function. However, the values of the high harmonics of the impedance modulus cannot be determined accurately. The amplitudes of the higher harmonics do not vanish like the amplitudes of the higher harmonics of pressure and flow. The impedance moduli must, therefore, be filtered so that they decrease smoothly to negligible amplitudes [4]. The filtered moduli and the original phase angles of the impedance are then transformed to the time domain (inverse Fourier) to obtain the impulse response function. Since we start from pressures and flows with repetition frequency of the heart rate, the impulse response function is not the result of a single impulse of flow but is repeated with the heart rate.

Methods

Dogs (mean weight 34.3 kg, range 24-54 kg) were anesthetized with nembutal (30 mg/kg) and ventilated with positive pressure (O_2 and N_2O). We did a right thoracotomy in the third interspace to put electromagnetic blood flow transducers on the ascending aorta and brachiocephalic artery. Pacing electrodes were sutured on the right atrium and right ventricle. We put snares around the common carotid arteries. The femoral arteries were dissected to obtain the main vessel and a small branch. Via the left femoral, we passed a catheter tip manometer (Microtip Millar Instr.) and a balloon catheter into the aorta. The tip of the former was positioned in the ascending aorta on the cardiac side of the flow transducer and the balloon catheter was placed in the aorta where it curves away from the vertebral column. On the main right femoral artery, we put a flow transducer and the side branch was used to measure femoral blood pressure (Microtip Millar Instr.). Sites where we measured femoral pressure and flow were never more than 10 mm apart. We used snares on brachiocephalic and femoral arteries for occlusive zeros. The flow transducers were calibrated in vitro.
We recorded ECG lead 2, aortic pressure and flow (Skalar TM 503), brachiocephalic artery flow (Skalar TM 503), and femoral pressure and flow (Skalar TM 503 or SE Medic Flowmeter SEM 275) on analogue tape (SE 7000) and paper (Elema-Schönander). To study reflections in the systemic circulation in general and in two specific beds in particular (femoral and brachiocephalic), we used the following interventions:
1. Pacing of the heart. To reduce the basic heart rate we injected up to 0.3 ml of formalin into the atrioventricular conduction system [13] to produce heart

block. Complete AV dissociation caused irregular ventricular filling and thus considerable fluctuation in output. To prevent this, we caused atrial fibrillation (stimulation of the right atrium with 5 V, 50 Hz).

2. Aortic occlusion.

3. Occlusion of both common carotid arteries.

We began the experiments with the occlusions. Interventions lasted 2 min and were preceded by 5 min control periods. We then produced AV block to study the system at different heart rates. Pressure and flow recordings were digitized (sample rate 200/s) after they had been passed through identical analogue filters to avoid aliasing (80 Hz, roll off 48 dB/oct). All moduli and phases are the average values calculated from ten consecutive beats in a steady state. Since we did not measure brachiocephalic pressure separately, we used ascending aortic pressure for the calculations in this bed. To correct for flow meter phase lag and for the fact that pressure and flow could not always be measured at the same location, we superimposed pressure incisura and backflow of the aortic tracings and the upstrokes of the femoral and brachiocephalic pressure and flow recordings. The impulse response function was calculated after applying a Dolph-Chebychev filter [4] to the modulus of the input impedance. We calculated the characteristic impedance as the average of the impedance moduli between 3 and 10 Hz.

Results

1. Windkessel and Uniform Tube

The above discussed characterizations are applied to two models of the arterial system: the modified windkessel [15] and the uniform tube model [14]. The results are given in Figure 1. The modified windkessel was chosen with a peripheral resistance and characteristic resistance of 7230 and 240 g cm^{-4} s^{-1}, respectively. Total arterial compliance was set at 0.0005 g^{-1} cm^4 s^2. In the windkessel model, wave travel does not exist. Nevertheless, the reflection coefficient was calculated to make all comparisons with the real system possible.

The input impedance of the modified windkessel is similar to the input impedance of the entire arterial system of animal and man [15]. The modulus of the apparent reflection coefficient of the modified windkessel model decreases smoothly to very low values with increasing frequency (Fig. 1). The impulse response function is a δ-function followed by an exponential decay. Due to the limited number of harmonics used in the calculation (up to 20 Hz) and the use of the filter, the δ-function in the impulse response function is lowered and widened. The exponential decay time is equal to the decay time of the pressure wave during diastole and is the product of total arterial compliance and peripheral resistance.

The uniform tube was chosen 30 cm long and had a characteristic impedance and a phase velocity of 500 g cm^{-4} s^{-1} and 430 cm s^{-1}, respectively; both were slightly frequency dependent. The tube contained a viscous liquid and the wall material was viscoelastic. The tube is terminated with a resistance of

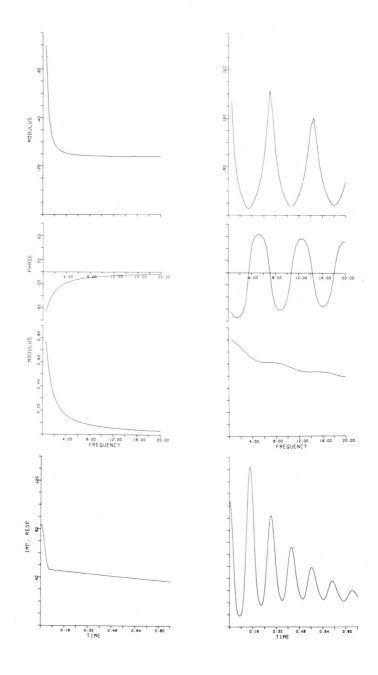

Fig. 1. The windkessel (left) and uniform tube (right). From top to bottom: modulus (in 10^3 g cm^{-4} s^{-1}) and phase (in degrees) of the input impedance; the modulus (dimensionless) of the reflection coefficient; the impulse response function (in 10^3 g cm^{-4} s^{-2}). Frequencies are given in Hz, time in seconds. For details on model parameters, see text

5500 g cm^{-4} s^{-1} in series with a small inertia term. The input impedance shows the well-known behavior [14]; modulus and delete phase both oscillate strongly with frequency. The modulus of the reflection coefficient at the entrance of the tube decreases slightly with frequency due to losses in the tube, but it remains large for the entire frequency range studied.

The impulse response function consists of a series of peaks that decrease in amplitude due to damping. The peaks widen as a result of dispersion [6, 19]. The second peak is larger than the first because the once reflected peak is immediately and completely reflected again at the "pump." The distance between the peaks gives the length of the tube when Eq. 8 is applied.

2. Dog

For dog 1640 we present the input impedance, the reflection coefficient, and the impulse response function at a series of heart rates, during occlusion of the aorta and during occlusion of the carotid arteries. We have done this for the systemic, the femoral (not during aortic occlusion), and the brachiocephalic beds. Figure 2 shows the input impedance of these three arterial beds. The line has been drawn by hand and is not a mathematic description of the data points. We have included beats during AV block and pacing at different rates to obtain a wide range of frequencies. Each rate has been indicated with a different symbol. The plots suggest that the system behaves reasonably linear since there is little difference between points calculated at various heart rates. Mean pressure in the aorta ranged from 73 mm Hg (HR 32 bpm) to 108 mm Hg (HR 129 bpm) (Table 1). The impedance plots compare well with data from the literature [8, 9, 10]. Occlusion of the aorta creates a circumscribed reflection site. Occlusion of the carotids increases peripheral resistance and thus probably increases reflection from all points where this normally occurs. In Figure 3, we have drawn the

Table 1. Mean pressure in aorta ($\overline{P}_{ao}$, in mm Hg); peripheral resistance (R_p, in 10^3 g cm^{-4} s^{-1}), and characteristic impedance (Z_c, in 10^3 g cm^{-4} s^{-1}) of the three arterial beds

	$\overline{P}_{ao}$	R_p			Z_c		
		Aorta	Brach. ceph.	Fem.	Aorta	Brach. ceph.	Fem.
Control	73-108[a]	7.47	13.0	150.	0.24	0.40	3.50
Aort. occl.	142	8.73	10.2	—	0.24	0.40	3.50
Occl. both car. A.	177	9.88	48.7	251.	0.24	0.40	3.50

[a] Lowest value at heart rate 32 bpm; highest value at heart rate 129 bpm.

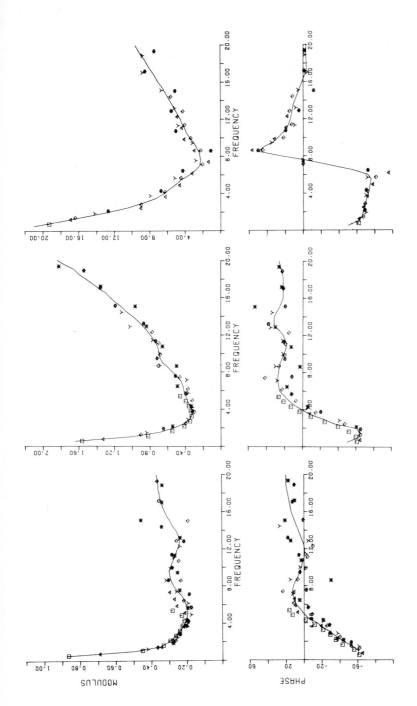

Fig. 2. Input impedance (modulus in 10^3 g cm^{-4} s^{-1} and phase in degrees) as a function of frequency (in Hz) for the whole arterial tree (left), brachiocephalic bed (middle), and femoral bed (right). Each symbol pertains to one heart rate

55

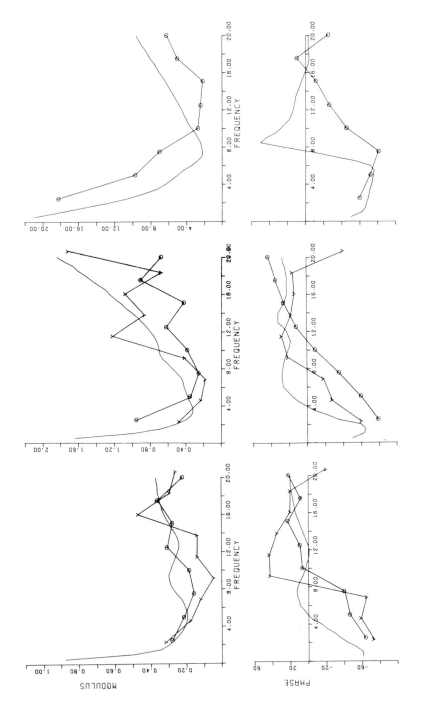

Fig. 3. Input impedance (modulus in 10^3 g cm^{-4} s^{-1} and phase in degrees) as a function of frequency (in Hz). Control situation: solid line (see Fig. 2). Aortic occlusion: y; occlusion of both carotid arteries: 0. Left: whole arterial tree; middle: brachiocephalic bed; right: femoral bed

results during the occlusions. The line represents control while both occlusions are indicated with different symbols. With aortic occlusion, the impedance of the entire arterial system has a more definite minimum [17]. After occlusion of the carotids, the minimum is slightly more pronounced, and has also moved to the right indicating an increased pulse wave velocity but constant effective reflection site. The input impedance of the brachiocephalic artery shows a somewhat more pronounced minimum of the modulus. The frequencies of the minimum and the zero crossing of the phase are shifted to higher frequencies. This shift to higher frequencies is also observed for the input impedance of the femoral bed.

The reflection coefficient as a function of frequency has been plotted in Figure 4 for control and both occlusions. For the entire arterial tree, we see that total reflection is increased most when the aorta occluded. In the brachiocephalic bed, aortic occlusion does not change reflection greatly; occlusion of both carotid arteries not only increases peripheral resistance but also introduces an extra reflection site; the reflection coefficient increases for all lower frequencies. In the femoral artery, the pattern of the reflection coefficient as a function of frequency is retained during occlusion of both carotid arteries but is shifted to higher frequencies. In Figure 5, the impulse response function for the three beds during control and the two interventions is given. All control situations clearly show one returning δ-function. In the femoral bed, the first returning δ-function is large. The differences in level are a result of the increase in peripheral resistance during the interventions.

The aortic occlusion shows for the two beds studied an increase in the first returning δ-function with respect to the original δ-function (at time zero). The occlusion of both carotid arteries shows a decrease of the first returning δ-function in the femoral bed. Occlusion of both carotid arteries results in a very complex picture of the impulse response function of the entire arterial system.

Discussion

The three descriptions of the arterial system, i.e., input impedance, reflection coefficient, and impulse response function, are characterizations of the system. They contain the same information since they are derived from the same signals: pressure and flow. However, each characterization emphasizes different aspects of the arterial tree or bed. Input impedance is the most widely used description. It does not seem very sensitive to alterations in the arterial bed (Fig. 3) [17].

Our impedance plots (Fig. 2). show that in the systemic circulation the impedance reaches the level of the characteristic impedance for higher frequencies. In the brachiocephalic and femoral beds, this is not the case. This indicates in the first place that the modified windkessel model is a good approximation of the total systemic bed but not of more peripheral beds. Those beds behave more like uniform tubes. Secondly, reflections in the total arterial system vanish for higher frequencies but are not negligible in the peripheral beds. We can calculate the effective length of the system with Eq. 1. However, this calculation is only per-

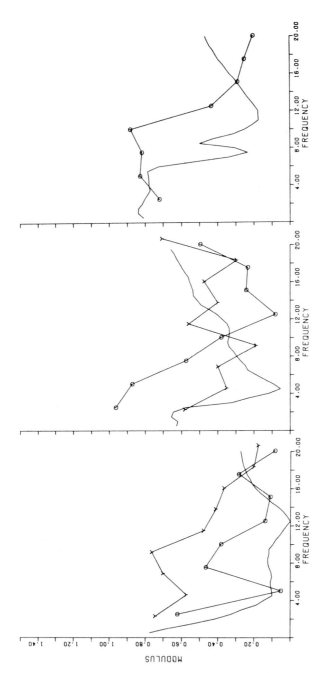

Fig. 4. Reflection coefficient modulus as a function of frequency (Hz). Control situation: solid line; aortic occlusion: y; occlusion of both carotid arteries: 0. Left: whole arterial tree; middle: brachiocephalic bed; right: femoral bed

58

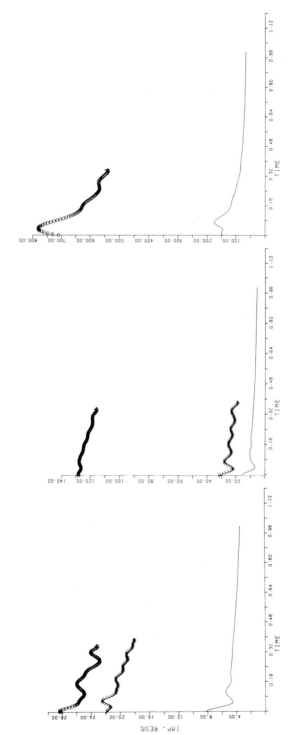

Fig. 5. Impulse response function (in 10^3 g cm^{-4} s^{-2}) as a function of time (in seconds). Control situation: solid line (bottom); aortic occlusion: y (top); occlusion of both carotid arteries: 0 (middle). Left: whole arterial tree; middle: brachiocephalic bed; right: femoral bed

mitted if the reflection coefficient at the effective reflection site is a real, frequency-independent constant. If this is not the case, errors may arise as is evidenced from the observation that minima and maxima of the impedance modulus and the zero crossings of the phase angle do not coincide and are not found at multiple frequencies [12]. During occlusions, both the mean pressure and the pulse wave velocity increase [11]. If the effective reflection site is assumed to be fixed, then the minimum of the impedance should shift to higher frequencies. This is indeed the case.

The reflection coefficient gives direct information on the amount of reflection in the arterial system. The reflection in the whole systemic arterial tree is small for higher frequencies. The brachiocephalic and femoral beds show more reflection than the total system. The calculation of the reflection coefficient is related to the calculation of forward and reflected waves in the arterial bed. The pressure and flow wave shapes (and their forward and reflected components) are the result of the interaction of the heart and the arterial system and are not as characterization of the arterial bed only. Moreover, the forward pressure and flow waves consist of the wave generated by the heart plus the wave that arises from reflection at the heart of the reflected wave. The reflection coefficient at the heart is not known and may vary during the cardiac cycle. Therefore, the separation of the forward wave into its subcomponents is impossible. Forward and reflected waves have recently been calculated by Van den Bos et al. [2] for the whole arterial tree during control and various interventions. They found that the introduction of a reflection site in the aorta by means of a liquid-filled balloon clearly affected the reflected wave and the forward wave. In the literature, measured pressure and flow waves have been superimposed to indicate that the differences are due to arterial reflection [3, 6, 19]. From Eq. 6, we can see that the difference between measured pressure and flow (assuming a constant characteristic impedance) is twice the reflected pressure wave.

The impulse response function describes the arterial bed as a function of time and is a third characterization of the arterial bed. It emphasizes the moments of return of the reflected wave. Eq. 8 shows how the effective length of the system can be calculated from the impulse response function. Although the impulse response function is a time function, the relation between pressure and flow is still very involved. The impulse response function does not show relations in shape between pressure and flow more clearly than input impedance. The advantage of the impulse response function is that the system is characterized with a single graph. One tends to pay more attention to the impedance modulus than to its phase but both are of equal importance.

In all calculations, we have assumed, when necessary, that the characteristic impedance is the average of the modulus between 3 and 10 Hz. It would be of interest to determine the characteristic impedance as a function of frequency more accurately in an independent way. Measurements of internal radius and wall thickness would be needed. The overall results presented will probably not be affected by an independent determination of the characteristic impedance, but details of the results might differ.

Characterizations of the arterial system and the study of reflections have contributed greatly to the understanding of arterial hemodynamics. They have not been used often in man, because measurement techniques are complicated, the mathematics are complex and, last but not least, because clinicians have seldom been trained to think in the frequency domain. Nevertheless, a quantitative description of the arterial system in patients would be most useful. These characterizations might help to separate cardiac from vascular abnormality. That application of the methods to man is indeed possible is illustrated by the work of Mills et al. [7] and Westerhof et al. [18].

Acknowledgments. The suggestions by and the discussions with Drs. G. Elzinga and P. Sipkema are gratefully acknowledged.

References

1. Bergel, D.H., Milnor, W.R.: Pulmonary vascular impedance in the dog. Circ. Res. 16, 401-415 (1965)
2. Bos, G.C. van den, Westerhof, N., Elzinga, G., Sipkema, P.: Reflection in the systemic arterial system: effects of aortic and carotid occlusion. Cardiovasc. Res. 10, 565-573 (1976)
3. Kouchoukos, N.T., Sheppard, L.C., McDonald, D.A.: Estimation of stroke volume in the dog by a pulse contour method. Circ. Res. 26, 611-623 (1970)
4. Laxminarayan, S., Sipkema, P., Westerhof, N.: Characterization of the arterial system in the time domain. IEEE Trans. Biomed. Eng. BME 25, 177-183 (1978)
5. Luchsinger, P.C., Snell, R.E., Patel, D.J., Fry, D.L.: Instantaneous pressure distribution along the human aorta. Circ. Res. 15, 503-510 (1964)
6. McDonald, D.A.: Blood flow in arteries. London: Arnold, 1974
7. Mills, C.J., Gabe, I.T., Gault, J.H., Mason, D.T., Ross, J. (Jr.), Braunwald, E., Shillingford, J.P.: Pressure flow relationships and vascular impedance in man. Cardiovasc. Res. 4, 405-417 (1970)
8. Noble, M.I.M., Gabe, I.T., Trenchard, D., Guz, A.: Blood pressure and flow in the ascending aorta of conscious dogs. Cardiovasc. Res. 1, 9-20 (1967)
9. O'Rourke, M.F., Taylor, M.G.: Vascular impedance of the femoral bed. Circ. Res. 18, 126-139 (1966)
10. O'Rourke, M.F., Taylor, M.G.: Input impedance of the systemic circulation. Circ. Res. 20, 365-380 (1967)
11. Schimmler, W.: Untersuchungen zu Elastizitätsproblemen der Aorta. Arch. Kreislaufforsch. 47, 189-233 (1965)
12. Sipkema, P., Westerhof, N.: Effective length of the arterial system. Ann. Biomed. Eng. 3, 296-307 (1975)
13. Steiner, C., Kovalik, A.T.W.: A simple technique for production of chronic complete heart block in dogs. J. Appl. Physiol. 25, 631-632 (1968)

14. Taylor, M.G.: An approach to the analysis of the arterial pulse wave. I., II. Phys. Med. Biol. 1, 258-269; 1, 321-329 (1957)
15. Westerhof, N., Elzinga, G., Sipkema, P.: An artificial arterial system for pumping hearts. J. Appl. Physiol. 31, 776-781 (1971)
16. Westerhof, N., Sipkema, P., Van den Bos, G.C., Elzinga, G.: Forward and backward waves in the arterial system. Cardiovasc. Res. 6, 648-656 (1972)
17. Westerhof, N., Elzinga, G., Van den Bos, G.C.: Influence of central and peripheral changes on the hydraulic input impedance of the systemic arterial tree. Med. Biol. Eng. 11, 710-723 (1973)
18. Westerhof, N., Murgo, J.P., Sipkema, P. Giolma,J.P., Elzinga, G.: Arterial impedance. In: Engineering Principles in Cardiovascular Research. Hwang, N.H.C., Gross, D.R. (eds.). Baltimore: U. Park Pr. 1978 (in press)
19. Wetterer, E., Kenner, Th.: Grundlagen der Dynamik des Arterienpulses. Berlin-Heidelberg-New York: Springer 1968

Arterial Smooth Muscle Mechanics

Robert H. Cox

Bockus Institute, Graduate Hospital and Department of Physiology
University of Pennsylvania Philadelphia, PA. 19146 USA

Introduction

Studies of the mechanics of arterial smooth muscle have been guided both con-
ceptually and methodologically by past work on striated muscle mechanics.
Studies using striated muscle are usually performed on small muscle fibers. The
contractile cells in such preparations are oriented in the direction of the long
axis of the fiber. Such a configuration greater simplifies the methods required
for mechanical testing and analysis, i.e., unidirectional.
Following the lead of work on striated muscle, most investigators of arterial
smooth muscle have sought one-dimensional preparations with which to study
mechanics. The most widely employed preparations include helical strips [19]
and narrow circumferential rings cut from intact arteries [1]. The strips or rings
are usually mounted by either ligatures, clamps, or pins between a force transducer and a loading device, e.g., a lever. Such methods yield essentially one-
dimensional length-tension or stress-strain relations. Following striated muscle
methods, the active length-tension curve for such arterial smooth muscle preparations is usually obtained from the ordinate difference between length-tension
curves determined under active and passive conditions at particular values of
muscle length.
This method of determining active mechanical properties of arterial smooth
muscle ignores the effects of passive tissue elements which are functionally connected both in series and in parallel with the contractile apparatus [22]. It has
been shown in striated muscle that such passive tissue elements "distort" the
intrinsic properties of the contractile apparatus in muscle when the latter are
measured in terms of the mechanical properties of whole muscle [4, 21, 28].
There is much more passive tissue and much less muscle in arterial preparations
than in striated muscle [7, 25, 30]. Therefore, the potential for such a distortion
of the properties of the contractile system by passive elements is much greater
in arterial smooth muscle. Such considerations are usually ignored in studies of
the active properties of arteries.
Preparations of arterial tissue in the form of strips and rings also suffer from
other limitations. The geometry of the preparation is obviously altered from
the normal, i.e., that of an intact cylindric arterial segment. End effects where
the tissue is coupled to the loading and the force measuring devices are difficult

to evaluate. The orientation of the cells and therefore contractile apparatus with respect to the axis of the sample is different from that of the intact artery.

As a result of these deficiencies, attempts have been made by a number of investigators to develop improved methods for studying arterial smooth muscle mechanics [3, 6, 13, 23, 29]. These methods involve both the preparations employed as well as the methods used in data analysis. The preparations are in the form of intact cylindric segments of arteries. The analytic methods involve the determination of both active stress-strain relations of segments as well as measures of the constriction capacity of the segment, i.e., its ability to reduce wall diameter. In addition, attempts are currently under way to develop methods whereby the properties of the contractile apparatus can be determined using digital computer simulation from measurements of active and passive muscle properties.

Active Smooth Muscle Responses

1. Methods

Samples of arteries are removed from animals either under anesthesia (pentobarbital, 30 mg/kg i.v.) or sacrificed with a captive bolt device. The segments are rapidly removed from the animals, placed in an aerated (95% O_2 5% CO_2) physiologic salt solution (PSS) maintained at 37 °C, and trimmed of loose connective tissue. The composition of the PSS in millimoles per liter is: 116.5 NaCl, 22.5 Na_2HCO_3, 1.2 NaH_2PO_4, 2.4 Na_2SO_4, 4.5 KCl, 1.2 $MgSO_4$, 2.5 $CaCl_2$, and 5.6 dextrose. The segments are cannulated at both ends with stainless steel adapters and mounted in the experimental apparatus shown in Figure 1 [6]. One end is attached to an isometric force transducer for the measurement of total axial wall force. The other end is connected to a manifold on a movable slide assembly used for positioning the segment in the bath and for the introduction of inflation pressure to the segment. Inflation pressure is measured through a side port in the manifold. The external diameter of the segment is measured near its midpoint using a cantilever transducer [27] pivoted from above the segment.

The recorded data are continuously displayed on a dual beam oscilloscope (Tektronix Model D-13) and on an X-Y plotter (Hewlett Packard Model 7046A) as plots of diameter and force versus inflation pressure. The analogue data are also recorded on an analogue tape recorder (Sangamo Model 3500). Transmural pressure within the segment is controlled either by means of an infusion pump apparatus or a regulated pressure supply. Continuous variations of transmural pressure are achieved by the infusion of water from the pump (Harvard Model 906) into a half-filled aspirator bottle. Constant values of transmural pressure are achieved through a regulated supply.

Following mounting in the experimental apparatus, the arterial segments are allowed to incubate for at least 1 h in normal PSS with internal pressure set to 150 mm Hg and axial length set at its in vivo value. Then slow continuous in-

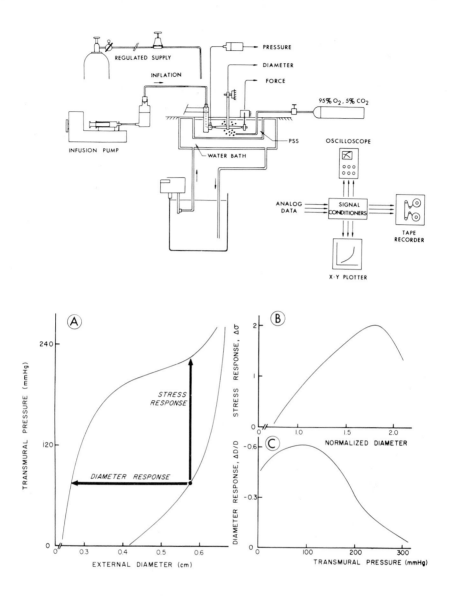

Fig. 1. Diagrammatic summary of the experimental apparatus and methods used for determination of vascular smooth muscle mechanics. A: pressure-diameter relations under active (upper curve) and passive (lower curve) conditions; isobaric diameter responses and isometric stress responses are also indicated. B: a typical variation of the isometric stress response with vessel diameter. C: a typical variation of the isobaric diameter response with transmural pressure

flation/deflation cycles at a rate of 1 mm Hg/s are performed between 0 and 250 mm Hg. After a variable number of such cycles (ca. 3-7) reproducible pressure/diameter/force curves are obtained. The purpose of this preliminary condition-

65

ing procedure is to minimize values of spontaneous vascular smooth muscle tone [6, 8, 29].

Transmural pressure is then usually set to about 75 mm Hg and diameter allowed to stabilize. Norepinephrine (NE) is added to the bath (5 μg/ml) and the artery allowed to constrict for 2 min at this pressure. The pressure is lowered to about 2-5 mm Hg and held constant until diameter stabilizes (5-10 min). Inflation at a constant rate is performed up to a maximum pressure of usually 250 mm Hg. The subsequent deflation response is usually not recorded. Continuous measurements of pressure, diameter, and external force are made. The bath is then drained, rinsed with fresh PSS, and refilled with a calcium-free PSS solution containing 2 mM EGTA. Pressure is again set at 150 mm Hg and the vessel allowed to incubate for a period of at least 30 min. At the end of this second incubation period, continuous pressure/diameter/force responses to continuous inflation/deflation cycles are recorded until reproducible closed loop curves have been obtained. These data are then recorded on magnetic tape and assumed to represent data for a condition of passive vascular smooth muscle [5].

At the end of each experiment on a particular artery segment, the vessel's length is measured in the apparatus and subsequently removed. The unstressed length is then measured and the vessel segment weighed in an ultrabalance (Mettler). Segment volume was obtained from its weight, assuming a density of 1.06g/cm^3.

Values of external diameter and axial wall force are obtained from the X-Y plotter records in steps of 10 mm Hg from 0 to 250 for the inflation responses only. Values of these data at 0 mm Hg are obtained by linear extrapolation of values at 5 and 10 mm Hg, respectively. These pressure, diameter, and force data along with values of segment volume and in vivo length are used to compute values of the three-dimensional wall stresses. The equations used for this purpose are given below [12]

$$\text{Tangential stress} \qquad \sigma_\theta = \frac{a}{b-a} P_i \qquad\qquad (1)$$

$$\text{Radial stress} \qquad \sigma_r = -\frac{a}{b+a} P_i \qquad\qquad (2)$$

$$\text{Axial stress} \qquad \sigma_x = \frac{a^2}{b^2-a^2} P_i + \frac{1}{\pi(b^2-a^2)} T_x \qquad\qquad (3)$$

where a and b are internal and external radii, respectively, P_i is transmural pressure, and T_x is total axial wall force. Values of external radius are obtained from values of external diameter. Values of internal radius are obtained from values of b, segment volume, and in vivo length. These values of three-dimensional wall stresses are computed for conditions of activated (NE) and passive smooth muscle (2 mM EGTA).

2. Results

The effects of activation of smooth muscle have been quantitated using two general approaches. The first approach treats the arterial wall in a manner similar to that applied to other muscles [8]. The second approach treats the arterial wall as an elastomer [9].

A schematic representation of the methods used to quantitate the effects of vascular smooth muscle activation using inflation responses is given at the bottom of Figure 1. Pressure-diameter data recorded under active and passive conditions (panel A) are used to determine values of wall stress and of diameter responses to activation. The active diameter response is quantitated as the difference in values of diameter under active and passive conditions at a given value of transmural pressure. These diameter differences are normalized by dividing by the initial passive diameter at each given pressure. An example of normalized diameter response as a function of transmural pressure is given in panel B of Figure 1. Active stress responses are quantitated from the difference in transmural pressure under active and passive conditions at a given value of blood vessel diameter. Values of wall stress are determined from the pressure differences using Eq. 1. An example of the active stress response to smooth muscle activation determined in this manner is given in panel C of Figure 1.

Responses to activation of vascular smooth muscle obtained from inflation responses as described above are similar to, but not identical with, isometric stress responses and isobaric diameter responses recorded directly on smooth muscle with either diameter or pressure held constant during the complete course of the vasoactive response [8, 14]. This continuous inflation method is based upon the assumption that the steady-state pressure-diameter curve with fully activated muscle is unique and independent of the manner in which it is determined. The relationship between pressure and diameter during continuous inflation under active conditions is determined by the true active pressure-diameter relation, the contribution from stretching as a result of the negative velocity of shortening (i.e., lengthening), and any influence on the degree of activation of vascular smooth muscle as a result of length changes of the contractile elements during the inflation response [8]. In order to establish the validity of this continuous inflation method, a series of experiments was performed [8], to compare the effects of variations in inflation rate on computed vascular smooth muscle responses with responses obtained by direct isometric and isobaric methods.

A summary of the results of these experiments is given in Figure 2. Inflation rate was varied between 0.2 and 5 mm Hg/s. The initial portion of the pressure diameter curve from about 0-100 mm Hg is essentially unaffected by inflation rate (top panel). At higher values of transmural pressure, pressure-diameter curves for slower inflation rates are shifted down and to the right in a nonuniform manner. Maximum values of diameter and of stress responses for various inflation rates are summarized in Table 1. The maximum value of diameter response is essentially independent of inflation rate as is the pressure at which the maximum response occurs, since this maximum occurs in the range where the pressure-diameter curve is little influenced by inflation rate. Values of maximum

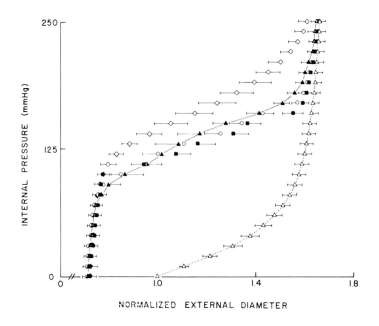

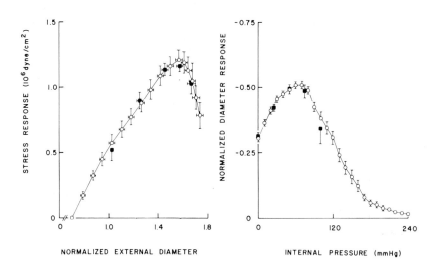

Fig. 2. Evaluation of the continuous inflation method of quantitating vascular smooth muscle mechanics. The panel at the top shows average pressure-diameter data for different inflation rates. Symbols are 5.0 (open diamonds), 1.0 (closed triangles), 0.5 (open circles), and 0.2 (closed squares) mm Hg/s after NE. Passive data are given by open triangles. The lower panels compare responses from continuous inflation at 0.2 mm Hg/s (open circles) with direct isometric or isobaric responses (closed squares). Left panel compares active stress responses while right panel compares active diameter responses. Bars represent ±1 SEM

68

Table 1. Effect of inflation rate on maximum diameter and stress responses to norepinephrine

Inflation rate mm Hg/s	Diameter response		Stress response	
	max $\Delta D/D$ %	P_i mm Hg	max $\Delta\sigma_\theta$ 10^3 dyn/cm^2	D/D_o
5.0	− 51.2 ± 0.8	88 ± 3	1605 ± 40[a]	1.56 ± 0.02[a]
2.0	− 50.9 ± 0.8	86 ± 4	1232 ± 32[a]	1.55 ± 0.03
1.0	− 50.5 ± 0.9	80 ± 9	932 ± 53	1.55 ± 0.03
0.5	− 50.9 ± 1.1	85 ± 10	914 ± 48	1.50 ± 0.02
0.2	− 51.2 ± 0.6	95 ± 3	866 ± 60	1.48 ± 0.03

[a] $P < 0.05$; comparing 0.2 data with other rates.

active stress response and the diameter (i.e., strain) at which the maximum occurs decreases as the inflation rate decreases. For inflation rates below 1 mm Hg/s, no significant differences were found in maximum values of active stress response or the value of strain at which this occurred.

A comparison of active stress responses obtained at an inflation rate of 0.2 mm Hg/s with direct isometric stress responses to NE obtained at initial strains corresponding to passive pressure levels of 5, 25, 50, 75, and 100 mm Hg is shown in Figure 2 (lower left panel). No significant difference was found between active stress response obtained using the slow continuous inflation method and those recorded from direct isometric responses. A summary of normalized diameter responses to NE is given in the lower right panel of Figure 2. Isobaric or constant pressure responses to NE were obtained in the same vessels using separate activations at transmural pressures of 0, 25, 50, 75, and 100 mm Hg. No significant difference existed in values of normalized diameter response obtained using the continuous inflation or the direct methods.

The data shown in the bottom of Figure 2 are representative of the active mechanical properties of arterial smooth muscle. The active stress response increases nearly linearly in magnitude from small values of diameter to a maximum at some optimum length (L_{max}). Further increases in length result in a decrease in the active stress response. Such a relation between active force development and muscle length is similar to that of other types of muscle and suggests a sliding filament-type arrangement of the contractile apparatus. The active diameter response exhibits a similar variation with transmural pressure, i.e., a maximum value for this quantity exists at pressures in the range of 50-100 mm Hg.

In the elastomer approach, the effects of smooth muscle activation are quantitated in terms of two variables: the incremental elastic modulus and the characteristic impedance. The incremental elastic modulus represents the slope of the tangential stress-strain curve and is computed using the following relation [9]

$$E_{inc} = \frac{2a^2b}{b^2 - a^2} \frac{\Delta P}{\Delta b} \qquad (4)$$

Values of theoretic characteristic impedance represent the high frequency asymptote about which values of vascular impedance oscillate [2] and represents the ratio of pulsatile pressure and flow. It is determined primarily by the elastic and geometric properties of the blood vessel segment close to the measurement site and determined from the following equation [9]

$$Z_0 = \frac{1}{\pi a^2} \sqrt{\frac{\rho E(b^2 - a^2)}{3b^2 + a^2}} \qquad (5)$$

where ρ is the density of blood.
The effects of smooth muscle activation on incremental elastic modulus of canine iliac arteries are summarized in the left panel of Figure 3. Activation produces a

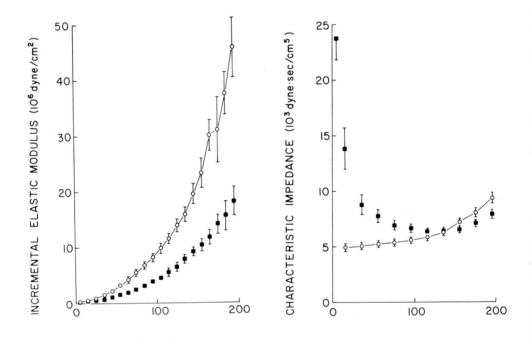

TRANSMURAL PRESSURE (mmHg)

Fig. 3. Comparison of the pressure dependence of the incremental elastic modulus (left panel) and the characteristic impedance (right panel) of iliac arteries. Data are for conditions of passive (open circles) and active smooth muscle (closed squares)

70

reduction in values of incremental elastic modulus at specific values of transmural pressure [9]. The magnitude of this reduction varies quite considerably at different transmural pressures and in different specimens. In general, there is a correspondence between the magnitude of the reduction of elastic modulus and the maximum value of active stress developed by the particular system.

The variation of theoretic values of characteristic impedance with transmural pressure is given in the right panel of Figure 3. Under passive conditions, characteristic impedance usually increases in a monotonic fashion with transmural pressure for most large arteries. Under activated conditions, there is a minimum value of characteristic impedance at approximately 120 mm Hg. At pressures above and below this value, characteristic impedance increases. Some vessels from some species show a different kind of behavior with passive smooth muscle [11]. Those vessels, such as the rat carotid artery, also exhibit under passive conditions a minimum value of characteristic impedance at some value of transmural pressure as occurs in the canine iliac arteries under activated conditions. This "U-shaped" variation of characteristic impedance with transmural pressure is a general characteristic of arteries with activated smooth muscle. It is interesting that all vessels studied appeared to possess a minimum value of characteristic impedance at a transmural pressure within the normal physiologic range.

In summary, two alternate approaches to evaluating and representing the response of the arterial wall to activation of its muscle have been described. In the first, the arterial wall is treated as a muscle and the effects of activation on active stress development and active shortening are quantitated. In the second approach, the effects of smooth muscle activation are quantitated in terms of its effect on the incremental elastic modulus of a blood vessel as well as on the theoretic value of its characteristic impedance. This latter approach is perhaps a more accurate representation of the physiologic function of large arteries in the circulation.

Series Elasticity

1. Methods and Results

Like other muscles, smooth muscle behaves mechanically as if passive tissue elements were coupled in series with its contractile elements [22]. It is possible to measure the properties of these series elastic elements (SE) experimentally by means of small length perturbations of various types applied to the active muscle [15, 20, 26]. One such method is shown schematically in Figure 4 [10]. During the time course of an isometric response to NE, small perturbations of internal pressure are introduced. These perturbations consist of small decreases and increases in pressure of about 5-15 mm Hg in amplitude, 150 ms in duration, and repeated 10-25 times/min. The diameter response to these pressure reductions consists of an instantaneous step response and a more slowly decreasing one. The initial elastic response represents the shortening of the SE while the slower decrease in diameter represents shortening of the contractile elements.

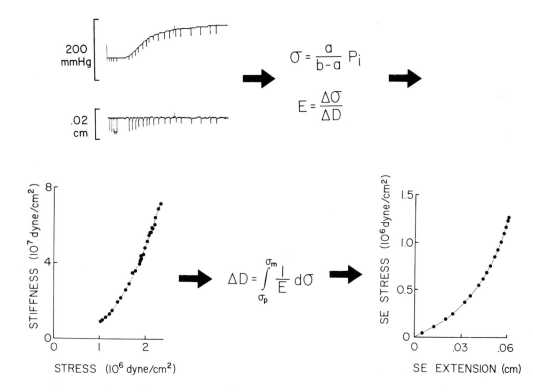

Fig. 4. Schematic summary of methods used for determining properties of series elastic elements in arterial smooth muscle. Pressure and diameter responses to periodic quick releases are converted to values of wall stress and incremental stiffness. This curve is then numerically integrated to yield series element stress-extension relations

The first panel in Figure 4 shows one such response; values of pressure are converted to values of wall stress as indicated. The incremental stiffness of the blood vessel is computed as the ratio of stress and diameter responses to each pressure step. The curve relating stiffness and stress is determined over the course of the entire isometric contraction. This incremental stiffness-stress curve is then numerically integrated by digital computer techniques to produce a curve of SE stress versus extension. It is necessary to assume a mechanical model to represent arterial smooth muscle in order to complete this latter integration. The models most usually employed are the three-element models of Hill that have been used in studies of striated muscle mechanics [4, 21, 22, 28]. It should be noted that it is only possible to compute an incremental stiffness not an incremental elastic modulus because the rest length of the SE is not determinable.

One of the characteristics of arterial smooth muscle SE is a variation with muscle length. The left panel of Figure 5 shows data on variation of incremental stiffness with wall stress in iliac artery smooth muscle at six different values of initial muscle length. If the "Voigt model" of Hill [22] was applicable to arterial smooth

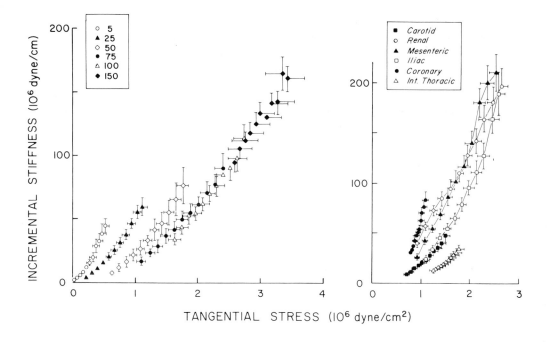

Fig. 5. Properties of series elasticity in arterial smooth muscle. Left: the variation of the relation between SE incremental stiffness and wall stress at different values of muscle length. Right: the variation of SE properties from different anatomic sites in the dog at a muscle length equivalent to L_{max}. Bars represent ±1 SEM

muscle, all of these curves for different muscle lengths would fall along a single unique curve. Since they do not, it is concluded that a Voigt type of model is not applicable to this arterial smooth muscle. If a "Maxwell model" were applicable, these curves would all be superimposable if translated to the origin of this graph, i.e., they would have the same slopes. Since they do not, it appears that a Maxwell type of model is not applicable either. This means that a different form of model must be developed to represent arterial smooth muscle or the properties based upon Hill's models must be made muscle length dependent.

In addition to this length dependence, the properties of the SE in arterial smooth muscle also demonstrate a marked anatomic variation. Results of experiments on six different arterial sites are summarized in the right panel of Figure 5. These measurements of SE were made at a muscle length corresponding to L_{max}, i.e., the optimum length for active stress development in these preparations. It is obvious that a wide variation in SE properties exist at these different arterial sites, with values for the carotid and internal thoracic being the most compliant and values from the coronary and mesenteric arteries being the stiffest. It is conceivable that a portion of these differences in SE mechanical properties is the result of differences in the rest length of SE in these preparations.

73

Experimental evidence exists to suggest that the major portion of SE in arterial smooth muscle resides outside of the contractile system [10, 16]. One potential candidate for a morphologic site for SE in arterial smooth muscle is the connective tissue matrix that couples individual smooth muscle cells in the media. Studies of blood vessel morphology indicate that both collagen and elastin exist in the media of large and medium-sized arteries [12, 17, 31]. It is possible, therefore, that the relative content of collagen and elastin may correlate with the mechanical properties of the SE. Table 2 summarizes the results of a study in which the connective tissue composition of arteries was compared with the properties of the SE. No clear correlation exists, however, between connective tissue composition of the blood vessel and the mechanical properties of the SE.

Table 2. Summary of mechanical properties data for arterial smooth muscle

Site	$\Delta L_{SE}/L_{max}$		$\Delta\sigma_{max}$	$-\Delta D/D_0$	Collagen
	Voigt %	Maxwell %	10^3 dyn/cm^2	%	Elastin
Carotid	8.41 ±.87	17.66 ±2.66	1085 ±135	36.9 ±4.0	2.10 ±.14
Coronary	1.80 ±.16	3.46 ±.62	387 ±57	20.6 ±2.9	3.00 ±.33
Iliac	3.76 ±.41	5.96 ±.99	1720 ±209	50.8 ±2.2	1.61 ±.18
Internal thoracic	7.92 ±.61	20.43 ±2.35	612 ±74	15.5 ±1.3	1.19 ±.11
Mesenteric	2.85 ±.31	3.71 ±.45	1722 ±143	57.0 ±2.3	1.43 ±.06
Renal	4.10 ±.58	5.26 ±.94	2142 ±270	63.1 ±3.3	1.97 ±.21

$\Delta L_{SE}/L_{max}$: SE strain for Voigt and Maxwell models; L_{max}: initial diameter for isometric response; $\Delta\sigma_{max}$: maximum active stress response; $-\Delta D/D_0$: maximum normalized diameter response; D_0: initial passive diameter.

Obviously, the true situation (i.e., the morphologic basis for SE in arterial smooth muscle) is more complicated than simply the relative amount of collagen and elastin. As indicated by the magnitude of the SE in these various arterial smooth muscles, the potential for a substantial distortion of the intrinsic properties of the contractile apparatus is present.

In comparing data from the coronary and internal thoracic arterial sites, given in Table 2, it appears that no significant difference exists between values of maximum diameter response for these two sites. The internal thoracic, however, generated a significantly larger maximum active stress response compared to the coronary. Values of SE strain at maximum isometric stress response were substantially larger in the case of the internal thoracic compared to the coronary arteries. That is, an arterial smooth muscle with relatively compliant SE had to generate a larger active stress response in order to produce an equivalent diameter response compared to an arterial smooth muscle with stiff SE. An analogous situation exists in the case of iliac and mesenteric arteries. No significant difference in the maximum active stress response was found for these two sites. However, mesenteric arteries did produce a larger maximal diameter response relative to the iliacs. The maximum extension of the SE in the mesenteric artery was significantly less than that of the iliac. That is, the mesenteric artery with a stiffer SE was able to generate a larger normalized diameter response for the same maximal active stress response than an arterial smooth muscle with a more compliant SE.

These results suggest that the mechanical properties of the SE in arterial smooth muscle may play an important role in determining the relationship between active stress response and active diameter response in a given blood vessel. Furthermore, these results suggest that changes in the relationship between active stress and diameter responses can be the result of changes in properties of the SE in addition to changes in the contractile elements per se.

Computer Simulation

The above discussion describes methods and results concerning the active responses of intact arterial wall to smooth muscle activation. These responses obviously represent the combined effects of the properties of the contractile elements of muscle and the passive tissue elements to which they are functionally connected. It is important to distinguish between changes in the contractile elements of muscle per se and those of changes in the properties of the passive elements [24]. In order to do this, it is necessary to develop a model representation of the blood vessel. An obvious starting point is the mechanical models that have been employed previously for the description of the mechanical properties of striated muscle, i.e., Hill's three-element models [22].

Hill has described two analogous models consisting of two nonlinear idealized elastic elements and one idealized contractile element. In the Voigt model, one elastic element (PE) is coupled in parallel with the idealized contractile elements (CE). The second elastic element is then coupled in series (SE) with this parallel combination. In the Maxwell form, one elastic element is coupled in series (SE) with the idealized contractile elements (CE). This series combination is then connected in parallel with the second elastic element (PE). While these two models are mathematically equivalent [18], the properties of the individual elements computed on the basis of a set of muscle responses is entirely different. As described above, it is not clear which, if either, of these two models is most appropriate for the representation of arterial smooth muscle mechanics. Consequently, results for the Maxwell form only will be presented since the properties of the individual elements for such a form are more easily computed from experimental data.

The equations describing the relationship between force and length in the individual elements of the Maxwell model have been programmed for digital computer computation. With values for the properties of series and parallel elastic elements and responses of the intact muscle, it is possible to compute values of properties for the contractile element. Figure 6 shows a summary of computed values of contractile element properties from this computer simulation. These data were

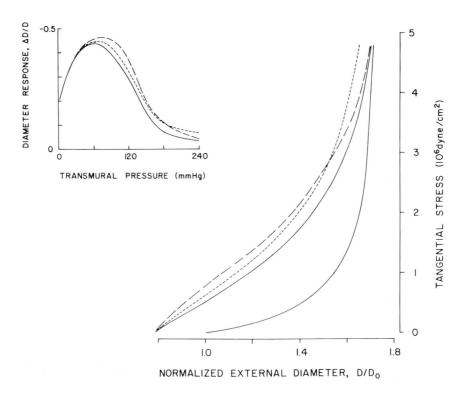

Fig. 6. Effects of series elasticity on computed values of contractile element properties. The upper left panel compares relative constriction responses of the whole muscle (solid curve) with that of the contractile elements computed using iliac SE data measured at various muscle lengths (long dashed curve) and iliac SE data for L_{max} only (short dashed curve). The lower right panel shows active stress-diameter relations computed using similar data

derived from experiments on canine iliac arteries. Results shown in this Figure illustrate the difference in active stress-strain relations for the total muscle and for the contractile elements only. As a result of the passive tissue elements, there is a reduction in the maximum value of force generated by the contractile apparatus as manifest by intact muscle responses. In addition, the intrinsic shorten-

76

ing capacity of the contractile system is also reduced by these passive tissue elements when represented as responses of the intact muscle.

Results of SE measurements from different arterial sites have been used to determine the influence of SE on computed contractile element properties. Table 3 represents a summary of the effects of using SE data from different sites on computed values of contractile element mechanical properties. It is obvious that the more compliant the SE, the larger the difference between maximum contractile element force development and maximum muscle force development. The same is true for the distortion of the maximum shortening capacity of contractile elements when represented as shortening of the intact muscle.

Table 3. Computed values of contractile element responses for different values of series elasticity stiffness

SE data source	$\dfrac{\Delta\sigma_{CE}}{\Delta\sigma_M}$	$\dfrac{\Delta D_{CE}}{\Delta D_M}$
Iliac artery data		
Iliac at L_{max}	1.56	1.09
Iliac at different muscle lengths	1.19	1.18
Renal artery data		
Coronary at L_{max}	1.08	1.03
Renal at L_{max}	1.22	1.09
Carotid at L_{max}	1.45	1.18

$\Delta\sigma_{CE}/\Delta\sigma_M$: maximum value of stress developed by contractile elements divided by maximum value of muscle stress development; $\Delta D_{CE}/\Delta D_M$: value of maximum shortening capacity of contractile elements at 100 mm Hg divided by maximum value of muscle shortening capacity.

Summary

Methods have been developed for the quantitation of vascular smooth muscle mechanics using intact segments of isolated arteries. These methods are based upon the differences in pressure-diameter relations determined using a slow inflation method for conditions of active and passive muscle. Active force-length and shortening-load relations obtained in this manner are qualitatively similar to those of other types of muscles. The length and load dependencies of these relations are what one would expect based on a sliding filament arrangement of contractile filaments. Pressure-diameter responses obtained with active muscle using slow inflation are not significantly different from active responses obtained using direct isometric (constant diameter) or isobaric (constant pressure) procedures.

Experimental methods have also been developed to study the properties of series elastic elements in these preparations. Load-extension relations of the SE are dependent on muscle length and anatomic source of the sample. With increasing muscle length, the SE appears to become stiffer. SE properties vary greatly in different preparations with a close correlation between SE stiffness and the maximum value of force development. Neither of Hill's models appear to be directly applicable in representing arterial SE.

Computer simulation methods have been developed for the computation of contractile element properties from active muscle responses and its elastic properties. The SE has a large effect on the relation between the properties of the muscle's contractile system and the responses of the whole artery.

References

1. Attinger, F.M.L.: Two-dimensional in-vitro studies of femoral arterial walls of the dog. Circ. Res. 22, 829-840 (1968)
2. Bargainer, J.D.: Pulse wave velocity in the main pulmonary artery of the dog. Circ. Res. 20, 630-637 (1967)
3. Bauer, R.D., Pasch, Th.: The quasistatic and dynamic circumferential elastic modulus of the rat tail artery studied at various wall stresses and tones of the vascular smooth muscle. Pflügers Arch. 330, 335-346 (1971)
4. Brady, A.J.: Length-tension relations in cardiac muscle. Am. Zoologist 7, 603-610 (1967)
5. Butler, T.M., Siegman, M.J., Davies, R.E.: Rigor and resistance to stretch in vertebrate smooth muscle. Am. J. Physiol. 231, 1509-1514 (1976)
6. Cliff, W.J.: The aortic tunica media in growing rats studied with the electron microscope. Lab. Invest. 17, 599-615 (1967)
7. Cox, R.H.: Three-dimensional mechanics of arterial segments in vitro: methods. J. App. Physio. 36, 381-384 (1974)
8. Cox, R.H.: Effects of norepinephrine on mechanics of arteries in vitro. Am. J. Physiol. 231, 420-425 (1976)
9. Cox, R.H.: Mechanics of canine iliac artery smooth muscle in vitro. Am. J. Physiol. 230, 462-470 (1976)
10. Cox, R.H.: Determination of series elasticity in arterial smooth muscle. Am. J. Physiol. 233, H248-H255 (1977)
11. Cox, R.H.: Comparison of carotid artery mechanics in the rat, rabbit and dog. Am. J. Physiol. 234; H280-H288 (1978)
12. Cox, R.H., Jones, A.W., Fischer, G.M.: Carotid artery mechanics, connective tissue, and electrolyte changes in puppies. Am. J. Physiol. 227, 563-568 (1974)
13. Dobrin, P.B.: Isometric and isobaric contraction of carotid arterial smooth muscle. Am. J. Physiol. 225, 659-663 (1973)

14. Dobrin, P.B.: Vascular muscle series elastic element stiffness during isometric contraction. Circ. Res. 34, 242-250 (1974)
15. Dobrin, P., Canfield, T.: Identification of smooth muscle series elastic component in intact carotid artery. Am. J. Physiol. 232, H122-H130 (1977)
16. Dobrin, P.B., Rovick, A.A.: Influence of vascular smooth muscle on contractile mechanics and elasticity of arteries. Am. J. Physiol. 217, 1644-1651 (1969)
17. Friedman, S.M., Scott, G.H., Nakashima, M.: Vascular morphology in hypertensive states in the rat. Anat. Rec. 171, 529-544 (1971)
18. Fung, Y.C.: Comparison of different models of the heart muscle. J. Biomech. 4, 289-295 (1971)
19. Furchgott, R.F.: Spiral-cut strip of rabbit aorta for in vitro studies of responses of arterial smooth muscle. In: Methods in Medical Research. Bruner, H.D. (ed.). Chicago: Year Bed. 1960, Vol. 8, p. 177
20. Halpern, W., Alpert, N.R.: A stochastic signal method for measuring dynamic mechanical properties of muscle. J. Appl. Physiol. 31, 913-925 (1971)
21. Hefner, L.L., Bowen, T.E. (Jr.): Elastic components of cat papillary muscle. Am. J. Physiol. 212, 1221-1227 (1967)
22. Hill, A.V.: Heat of shortening and the dynamic constants of muscle. Proc. R. Soc. Lond. (Biol.) 126, 136-195 (1938)
23. Hinke, J.A.M., Wilson, M.L.: A study of elastic properties of a 550-μ artery in vitro. Am. J. Physiol. 203, 1153-1160 (1962)
24. Johansson, B.: Determinants of vascular reactivity. Fed. Proc. 33, 121-126 (1974)
25. Jones, A.W., Swain, M.L.: Chemical and kinetic analyses of sodium distribution in canine lingual artery. Am. J. Physiol. 223, 1110-1118 (1972)
26. Loeffler, L., Sagawa, K.: A one-dimensional viscoelastic model of cat heart muscle studied by small length perturbations during isometric contraction. Circ. Res. 36, 498-512 (1975)
27. Murgo, J.P., Cox, R.H., Peterson, L.H.: Cantilever transducer for continuous measurement of arterial diameter in vivo. J. Appl. Physiol. 31, 948-953 (1971)
28. Pollack, G.H.: Maximum velocity as an index of contractility in cardiac muscle. Circ. Res. 26, 111-127 (1970)
29. Speden, R.N.: The maintenance of arterial constriction at different transmural pressures. J. Physiol. 229, 361-381 (1973)
30. Wiederhielm, C.A.: Distensibility characteristics of small blood vessels. Fed. Proc. 24, 1075-1084 (1965)
31. Wolinsky, H., Glagov, S.: Structural basis for the static mechanical properties of the aortic media. Circ. Res. 14, 400-413 (1964)

Models of the Arterial System

T. Kenner

Physiologisches Institut der Universität Graz, Graz/Österreich

Any attempt to effectively visualize a functional relation is a model. Models are abstractions of the reality which, in their structure, can have different degrees of agreement with the reality. It is often erroneously assumed that, with increasing complexity or with increasing computational effort, the quality of a model can be increased. In this study, some aspects of the yet unsolved problem of criteria for the choice of one or the other specific model will be discussed.

There are models in which the main emphasis is put on the structural and topographic agreement with the natural system. One historic example of such a model is the famous drawing of the arterial tree by Vesalius. In contrast, there are models in which there is no structural agreement with the reality whatsoever. The purpose of such a model is the visualization of a certain function. One most famous model of this kind is the description of the elastic storage function of the arterial system by comparison with an air chamber or with an elastic tube. The elastic tube model (fistula mollis et dilatabilis) shown in Figure 1 is taken from Borelli's book "de motu animalium" [4].

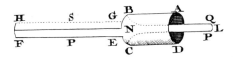

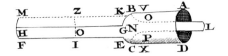

Fig. 1. Elastic tube model (fistula mollis et dilatabilis) by Borelli (1685)

The question which seems most important with respect to the choice and the use of a certain model is related to its information content. With increasing complexity of a system, the information content increases proportional to the logarithm of the complexity. Therefore, simplified models do have a relatively larger information content as compared with more complex models. The most

80

important example of such a simplified model is the air chamber model or windkessel model (Frank, 1899). Various modifications of this model have been used for the simulation of the most fundamental properties of the arterial system. Figure 2 shows the structure of one of the more elaborate windkessel models, first proposed by Broemser and Ranke [6] which has also been called the manometer model. In the recent past, this model has been revived by the work

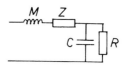

Fig. 2. Manometer model by Broemser and Ranke (1930)

of Westerhof et al. [22]. This model does not, of course, permit any simulation of pressure or flow distribution along the arterial tree. Only phenomena taking place at the aortic entrance can be simulated. The model is, therefore, especially useful for examining the relation between the heart and the arterial system and, furthermore, questions related to phenomena which take place at a frequency which is less than the heart rate.

The longitudinal resistance Z makes it possible to simulate the effect of the characteristic impedance of the arterial tube system. The inductance M improves the simulation of the frequency dependence of the central aortic input impedance which sometimes has been observed to have a minimum at a certain frequency and then increases with rising frequency. R and C correspond to the total peripheral resistance and the arterial compliance. The relation between Z and R can usually be assumed to be $Z/R = 0.1$.

Wetterer and Pieper [25] have measured the relation between the outflow from the arterial system and the arterial pressure using the so-called pressure slope method. By application of a piston pump to a large artery, pressure and flow in the arterial system could be varied sinusoidally by infusion and withdrawal of blood. A frequency between 0.2 and 0.3 Hz was chosen for the artificial variations. The results of the experiments demonstrated that the pressure flow relation in the whole arterial system is linear. However, the relation deviates very much from the proportionality which usually and tacitly is assumed in most model studies. The relation is schematically shown in Figure 3. As a consequence, the windkessel model has to be modified as shown on the right side of Figure 3.

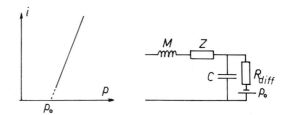

Fig. 3. Manometer model with nonlinear peripheral resistance

As has been shown by Ronniger [18] and by Kenner and Ronniger [14], the pressure flow relation can be described by the linear equation

$$i = (p - p_0) R_{diff}$$

where p_0 is the intercept pressure and

$$R_{diff} = dp/di$$

is the differential resistance value. In Figure 3, p_0 is simulated by a power source.

This property of the peripheral resistance has two consequences. First, the time constant of the model and, of course, of the arterial system depends on the differential value of the peripheral resistance

$$\tau = C R_{diff}$$

Second, the pressure decay during diastole tends toward the intercept pressure value p_0. Of course, this value is an extrapolated pressure, and in reality there will be a further decay of the pressure during a prolonged diastole according to some parabolic pressure flow curve. However, it is very surprising that, so far, this extremely important concept has not been evaluated and reexamined thoroughly with the exception of a thesis by Dujardin [7] from Pieper's lab. In this paper, the earlier findings by Wetterer and Pieper [25] were confirmed.

In recent papers related to the question of the determination of the time constant and of the diastolic pressure decay, the assumption is made that the time constant is related to the total peripheral resistance [5, 19, 20]. This implies that the pressure flow relation is assumed to be linear and proportional. Since this is certainly not the case, it can be concluded that such a simple question as the determination of the time constant of the windkessel model is still unsolved. It might be mentioned here that a nonlinear decay can be described by a sum of exponentials and that, according to Fung [10] "the separation of empirical data into a sum of exponentials is a highly unstable process."

The problem is complicated by the fact that during a prolonged diastolic decay, regulatory mechanisms of the circulation start to influence the process so that we cannot assume stationarity of the process. Thus, we need to introduce another addition to the windkessel model, as is shown in Figure 4. In order to describe the properties of the peripheral resistance under the influence of the baroreceptor control mechanism, the frequency response technique can be applied. Unfortunately, Wetterer and Pieper [25] had decided to chose just one frequency. Taylor [22] was the first to examine the low frequency input impedance of the arterial system by applying vagal stimulation in a random sequence. We later reexamined the problem using sinusoidal variations of the blood volume by a technique similar to the classic method of Wetterer and Pieper [25].

The results of this type of experiment are summarized schematically in Figure 4 (right side). Due to the reaction of the baroreceptors and of the autoregulatory

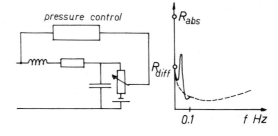

Fig. 4. Manometer model with nonlinear peripheral resistance and blood pressure control. On the right side the frequency dependent modulus of the input impedance is shown. The low frequency peak of the impedance is due to the pressure control. R_{abs} absolute value of the resistance, R_{diff} differential value of the resistance

mechanisms in the resistance vessels, the input impedance of the arterial system shows marked variations in the frequency region below the heart rate (Taylor, 1966; Kenner, 1971). In Figure 4, the dotted line corresponds to the frequency response of the passive, uncontrolled system. The solid line reflects the frequency-dependent influence of the control mechanisms.

For the interpretation of the results of the pressure slope method of Wetterer and Pieper [25] and of Dujardin [7] it is important that the frequency used in these experiments (0.2-0.3 Hz) is above the frequency region of the control mechanisms. Thus, it can be concluded that in these experiments no active influence by a control mechanism has taken place. This condition was assumed but not proven by Wetterer and Pieper [25].

It can be seen in Figure 4 that the low frequency input impedance of the arterial system, as measured in an anesthetized dog, has a maximum at about 0.05 Hz. This fact has the consequence that oscillations at this frequency might preferably be generated whenever some kind of excitation happens at this low frequency. As far as the model of Figure 4 is concerned, there is no reason to assume any low frequency component acting at the entrance. However, as soon as the model of the circulation is completed by the addition of a venous compliance, the generation of the oscillations at a frequency of about 0.05 Hz can be simulated. These so-called Mayer waves can be assumed, therefore, to be an expression of the instability of the closed circulatory system. The frequency of the oscillations is determined by the properties of the circulatory control systems [12] as indicated in Fig. 5.

One of the practical applications of models is their use for the estimation of parameters and variables. One example of such a determination is the calculation

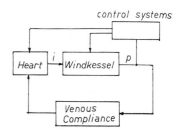

Fig. 5. Complete model of the circulatory system including venous return and feedback control loops

of arterial flow from pressure contours. It can be noted that the input impedance of the arterial system and of the windkessel model has the properties of a
low pass filter with respect to the transformation of flow to pressure. If during
a measurement the presence of a certain noise level has to be assumed, it can be
concluded that a certain amount of information is being lost in the higher frequency range as the flow pulse is being transformed into a pressure pulse by
virtue of the windkessel mechanism. Thus, it is quite simple to generate a pressure contour from a flow pulse by any model which is reasonably accurate in
the lower harmonic frequency range of the heart rate.

The reversal of the process, the calculation of a flow pulse from a pressure contour, is much more difficult and uncertain [23] and requires a more accurate
model of the system. Information, once lost, cannot be retrieved even by the
best model. The reversal of a low pass filtering would demand an amplification
of high-frequency components of a signal in the presence of noise. This fact ex-
plains why the measuring operation which is more interesting from a practical
viewpoint, the recording of flow, is more difficult to perform than the recording
of pressure. From these considerations, the conclusion can be drawn that, in
models used for the purpose of parameter estimation, unidirectional information
losses are to be expected. Parameter estimation, in principle, uses the continuous
and automated comparison between model and real system. The adjustment of
model parameters is performed by minimization of the difference between the
output of the real system and of the model, as shown schematicall in Figure 6.

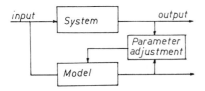

Fig. 6. Schematic diagram explaining the
use of a model for the purpose of parameter
estimation

Whether the comparison is performed by automatic process or by eye, there are
several important problems to be discussed. The first problem is related to the
fact that certain model computations may not be unique. For example, when
Wetterer and Kenner [24] simulated pressure pulses along the length of the
aorta by using a two part elastic tube model with only one outflow at the peripheral end of the system, it was easily possible to record quite natural pressure
contours. On the other hand, we can state that the flow pulses along this model
must have been quantitatively quite different from natural flow pulses along the
aorta. In the aorta, there is a continuous outflow along its length, whereas in the
model, this type of distributed losses was not taken into account. It can be concluded that a quantitatively and qualitatively excellent simulation of one variable
— pressure — does not ascertain that in the same model and at the same time
another variable — flow — is being simulated with equal accuracy.

Continuing along this line of thought, it can be concluded that certain circulatory models exist which allow, by adjustment of certain parameters, an excellent

simulation of a certain variable. And yet, such a model may possibly have no relation whatsoever to reality. A good example of this type is the model of Spencer et al. [21], which allows a surprisingly accurate simulation of central aortic and femoral pressures but otherwise has quite an odd structure.

In a generalized way, we can state that any input-output relation can be simulated in the time domaine by a polynome and equally in the frequency domaine by the corresponding Laplace transformed function. This simulation is independent of any relation to the real system. On the other hand, there are certain models in which the maximum agreement with the reality is attempted by taking into account any thinkable component irrespective of its role. Heinrich et al. [11] have recently discussed this problem in a general way.

An interesting example of such an extremely detailed model is the consideration of the so-called sleeve effect in an elastic transmission line. In spite of the highly increased difficulties and expenses for the simulation, there is nearly no measurable improvement of the result [15]. As Wetterer and Kenner [24] have discussed with respect to the simulation of the longitudinal impedance of a transmission line, the application of simplifications depends on the dimensions of the system. It seems logical to recommend the use of the most simple model for any purpose which still minimizes the deviation from reality.

One purpose of this discussion is to stress the fact that there is as yet no objective criterion available for the choice of a certain model for a certain purpose. This fact can be especially well demonstrated with respect to the question of whether nonlinear properties of the arterial system should be considered or not. In a study by Anliker and Rockwell [1] marked differences in the pulse contours were demonstrated using a nonlinear model as compared with a simplified linear solution. In general, the difference can be interpreted as demonstrating the importance of the nonlinear model. However, according to our subjective feeling, the linearized solution more closely resembles natural pulses.

In order to overcome the problem of applying subjective criteria, at least in certain problems, the application of minimization or maximization criteria seems possible [8]. One application, as mentioned above, is related to the parameter estimation technique as shown in Figure 6. Another application is the modeling of optimal functions in the organism, especially with respect to the circulatory system. Whenever a certain function is assumed to obey an optimization law, this law may be used to improve the simulation procedure. However, as discussed by Pfeiffer and Kenner [17], there might be a pitfall in the search for a solution in that the minimum might be rather faint and uncertain as shown in Figure 7 (left). Whereas such a minimum may lead to an ambiguous solution of a corresponding problem, a sharp minimum as shown in Figure 7 (right) will allow a unique solution.

Finally, I would like to discuss some problems related to the possibilities of alternate simulation procedures for the study of transmission line models. The first method of simulation consists in the use of hydrodynamic fluid-filled elastic tube models. The advantage of this type of model is the natural simulation of hydrodynamic events (Kenner and Wetterer [24]). The second possibility for simulating a transmission line is the application of the electric analogue elements. Such a line can be set up by a number of longitudinal inductance and

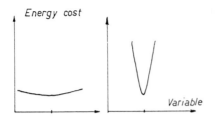

Fig. 7. The two diagrams are supposed to indicate that minimization of a cost functional may or may not bring a remarkable advantage

transverse capacitance elements and, possibly, further resistive components to simulate viscous losses. The result is a special purpose analogue computer [16]. The third possibility for simulating the same system is to translate the differential equations of wave propagation in a transmission line into difference equations and then to program these equations on a general purpose analogue computer [3]. The advantage of these analogue methods is the greater flexibility compared with a hydrodynamic model. The fourth possibility of simulation consists in the application of the linear solution of the wave equations, the so-called D'Alemberts solution. One way of applying D'Alemberts solution was first performed by Bauer et al. [2] using a digital computer. The method consists in the observation of the wave reflections which pass one certain location in the tube and the summation of these wave components to a resulting pressure or flow contour. With increasing complexity of the model, i.e., with increasing number of reflection sites in the line, the memory space used in the computation process increases. Another way of applying D'Alemberts solution [13] is similar to the method of characteristics and consists basically in following and summing the wave components at a certain time along the transmission line. With increasing complexity of the model in this type of simulation in a digital computer, the computation time per unit of wave propagation along the line increases. The latter method has the advantage that the events proceed in real time so that a hybrid computation by coupling the digital model to an analogue computer is possible. We have used such a hybrid system to simulate the interaction between heart and arterial system [13]. These two latter applications of the same equations demonstrate the complementarity of certain models. In any model, a certain economy and a certain cost-effectiveness relation can be defined. With respect to the linear transmission line models, the cost for a similar effect in one case is proportional to memory space, in the other case to the time unit of wave propagation.

Summary

In this discussion three topics have been selected. Using the most simple model of the arterial system, the so-called windkessel model, the most important hemodynamic principles are demonstrated step by step: the generation of the aortic input impedance, the effect of the nonproportionality of the total peripheral resistance, the frequency dependence of the control systems, and the possibility of generation of oscillations in the closed circulation by interaction of the venous return and the resonance of the baroreceptor control.

Secondly, an attempt is made to introduce the problem of subjective and objective criteria for the choice of a certain model. Since at least one purpose of models is their use in estimating parameters of the real system, minimization procedures play an important role. In certain problems, minimization processes themselves can be considered as models. In these cases, the effectiveness of the optimization can be described and used as criterion.

Finally, the possibilities of simulation of transmission line models is discussed. From the possibility of using real tubes or electric analogue systems to the calculation and solution of the corresponding equations, several modes of simulation exist. The two ways of realizing the simulation of D'Alemberts solution of the linear wave equations in Erlangen and in Graz make it possible to demonstrate the complementarity of time and computer memory space.

Acknowledgment: This work was supported by the Austrian Research Fund.

References

1. Anliker, M., Rockwell, R.L., Ogden, E.: Nonlinear analysis of flow pulses and shock waves in arteries: I. Derivation and properties of mathematical model. Z. Angew. Math. Phys. 22, 217-246 (1971)
2. Bauer, R.D., Pasch, Th., Wetterer, E.: Theoretical studies on the human arterial pressure and flow pulse by means of a non-uniform tube model. J. Biomech. 6, 289-298 (1973)
3. Beneken, J.E.W., Wit, B. De: A physical approach to hemodynamic aspects of the human cardiovascular system. In: Physical Bases of Circulatory Transport. Reeve, E.B., Guyton, A.C. (eds.). Philadelphia London: Saunders 1967 pp. 1-45
4. Borelli, J.A.: De motu animalium, pars secunda. Rom: Bernabo 1681
5. Bourgeois, M.J., Gilbert, B.K., Donald, D.E., Wood, E.H.: Characteristica of aortic diastolic pressure decay with application to the continuous monitoring of changes in peripheral vascular resistance. Circ. Res. 35, 56-66 (1974)
6. Broemser, P.H., Ranke, O.F.: Über die Messung des Schlagvolumens des Herzens auf unblutigem Wege. Z. Biol. 90, 467-507 (1930)
7. Dujardin, J.P.: Interaction between the Heart and the Vascular System. A circuit approach. Dissertation, Ohio State University 1976
8. Eykhoff, P.: System Identification, Parameter and State Estimation. London - New York: Wiley 1974
9. Frank, O.: Die Grundform des arteriellen Pulses. Z. Biol. 37, 483-526 (1899)
10. Fung, Y.C.B.: Stress-strain-history relations of soft tissues in simple elongation. In: Biomechanics. Fung, Y.C.B., Perrone, N., Anliker, M. (eds.). Prentice Hall: New Jersey 1972, pp. 181-208

11. Heinrich, R., Rapoport, S.M., Rapoport, R.A.: Metabolic regulation and mathematical models. Prog. Biophys. Mol. Biol. 32, 1-82 (1977)
12. Kenner, Th.: Dynamic Control of Flow and Pressure in the Circulation. Kybernetik 9, 215-225 (1971)
13. Kenner, Th.: The Central Arterial Pulses. Pflügers Arch. 353, 67-81 (1975)
14. Kenner, Th., Ronninger, R.: Untersuchungen über die Entstehung der normalen Pulsformen. Arch. Kreislaufforsch. 32, 141-173 (1960)
15. McDonald, D.A.: Blood Flow in Arteries. 2nd ed. Arnold: London 1974
16. Noordergraaf, A., Jager, G.N., Westerhof, N. (eds.): Circulatory Analog Computers. Amsterdam: North-Holland Publ. Company 1963
17. Pfeiffer, K.P., Kenner, Th., in this volume (1978)
18. Ronniger, R.: Zur Theorie der physikalischen Schlagvolumenbestimmung. Arch. Kreislaufforsch. 22, 332-373 (1955)
19. Rumberger, E., Schaefer, J., Reichel, H., Schwarzkopf, H.-J., Baumann, K., Schöttler, M.: Strömungswiderstand und diastolischer Abfall des arteriellen Druckes beim Hund unter dem Einfluß künstlich induzierter Herzfrequenz-änderungen. Verh. Dtsch. Ges. Kreislaufforsch. 40, 159-162 (1974)
20. Schöttler, M., Rumberger, E., Schaefer, J., Schwarzkopf, H.-J., Reichel, H., Baumann, K.: Mittlerer Druck und diastolischer Druckabfall im ateriellen System des Menschen unter dem Einfluß künstlich induzierter Frequenz-änderungen. Verh. Dtsch. Ges. Kreislaufforsch. 40, 163-166 (1974)
21. Spencer, M.P., Denison, A.B.: Pulsatile Flow in the Vascular System. In: Handbook of Physiology. Vol. II "Circulation". Hamilton, W.F., Dow, P. (eds.). Washington 1963, p. 839-864
22. Taylor, M.G.: Circ. Res. 18, 585-595 (1966)
23. Westerhof, N., Elzinga, G., Sipkema, P., Van den Bos, G.C.: Quantitative Analysis of the Arterial System and Heart by Means of Pressure-Flow Relations. In: Cardiovascular Fluid Dynamics and Measurement. Hwang, N.H.C., Norman, N.A. (eds.). Baltimore-London-Tokyo: U. Park Pr. 1977, pp. 403-438
24. Wetterer, E., Kenner, Th.: Grundlagen der Dynamik des Arterienpulses. Berlin-Heidelberg-New York: Springer 1968
25. Wetterer, E., Pieper, H.: Ein indirektes Verfahren zur Bestimmung des diastolischen Abstroms aus dem Arteriensystem und seine Anwendung zum Studium der Druck-Stromstärke-Beziehungen in vivo. Verh. Dtsch. Ges. Kreislaufforsch. 21, 430-439 (1955)

Separation of Time-Dependent and Time-Independent Terms in the Relation of Pressure and Diameter and of Pressure and Flow Velocity in Arteries

A. Schabert

Institut für Physiologie und Kardiologie der Universität Erlangen-Nürnberg, D-8520 Erlangen

In many cases of periodic events, for example in the arterial system, it is difficult to separate the quasistatic from the dynamic behavior of two variables. This is due to the fact that, because of viscosity or inertia, phase shifts occur between the variables so that when plotting one variable as a function of the other, a hysteresis loop appears which masks the quasistatic relationship. Two examples shall be used here to show how it may be possible in certain cases to obtain a friction-free or inertia-free relationship between two variables in the case of pulsatile flow.

The first example is concerned with the relationship between the flow velocity (u) and the pressure drop (Δp) at a stenosis in a rubber tube model. Apart from the rate of flow, the pressure drop along a stenosis is dependent on its geometric configuration [6, 11, 15]. An exact solution of the Navier-Stokes equations has not yet been obtained. Therefore, we have to work with empiric formulas whose usefulness has to be examined experimentally. Our model is shown in Figure 1.

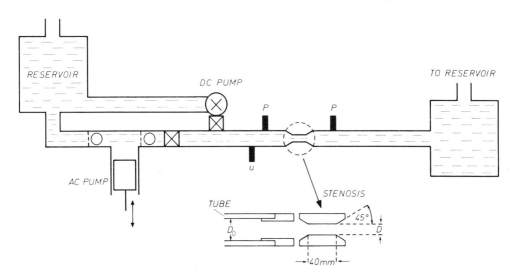

Fig. 1. Scheme of the apparatus. The pressures p are measured with Millar PC 350-A catheter tip manometers, the flow with a Statham SP 2202 electromagnetic flow meter. The system is filled with a 1% NaCl solution

The stenoses investigated were made of plexiglass tubes having a length of 40 mm and different internal diameters. The diameter of the entrance and exit of the stenoses is always 17.5 mm. The flow through the stenosis may be produced by an intermittently operating pump or a steady flow pump.

On the basis of steady and pulsatile flow tests, Young and Tsai [12, 13] have found that the pressure drop (Δp) at a stenosis as a function of the flow velocity can be described by the following equation

$$\Delta p = K_1 \cdot 8\,\pi\eta\,LuA_o/A^2 \qquad\qquad\qquad \text{I}$$

$$+ K_2 \cdot \rho\,((A_o/A) - 1)^a \cdot |u| \cdot u/2 \qquad \text{II}$$

$$+ K_3 \cdot \rho L\,du/dt \qquad\qquad\qquad\qquad \text{III} \qquad\qquad\qquad (1)$$

where K_1, K_2, and K_3 are dimensionless parameters, A_o and A are the cross-sectional areas of the tube and the stenosis, respectively, η is the viscosity of the fluid with the density ρ, and L the distance between the two pressure gauges. The first term (I) of Eq. 1 describes the pressure drop caused by the fluid viscosity; the second term (II) which contains the velocity in a quadratic form represents the pressure drop due to the convergence and the divergence of the flow in the stenosis associated with turbulence; the third term (III) is due to the inertia of the fluid. If the third term is neglected, the connection between the pressure drop and the flow velocity would be unequivocal. In the case of pulsatile flow, however, this term causes a phase shift between the two parameters and leads to a hysteresis loop in the Δp-u diagram. The form of the loop is mainly dependent on the respective pulse curves.

We carried out three series of experiments in order to obtain the dependence between the pressure drop and the flow velocity. In the first series, we used steady flows with different velocities. In this case, the last term equals zero. In the second series, we used pulsatile flows. By taking the means of the first two terms, the last term disappears once more. The results of these two series correspond well with each other. In the stenoses examined, we determined the factor K_2 to be 2 and the exponent a in the second term to be 1.87 [cf. 3, 4, 7, 14].

In the third series, we tried to find the contribution of the third term of Eq. 1 in the case of pulsatile flow. The method applied is independent of the shape of the flow pulse and might be described as a "loop closing method." An analogue computer (Fig. 2) substracts the time derivative of the flow velocity — employing a variable amplification factor (V) — from the pressure difference. The result thus obtained is shown on the screen of on oscilloscope in dependence on the instantaneous flow velocity. If V is zero, a loop is seen on the screen which is caused by the inertia term. By varying V, the opening of the loop can be diminished until a single line remains. In this case, the analogue computer will subtract the exact value of the inertia term from the pressure drop. The amplification factor (V) is then a measure for the factor K_3. In the left diagram of Figure 3, a Δp-u loop is shown, while in the right diagram, the closed curve obtained from this loop by the method described is shown. The considerable noise during this measure-

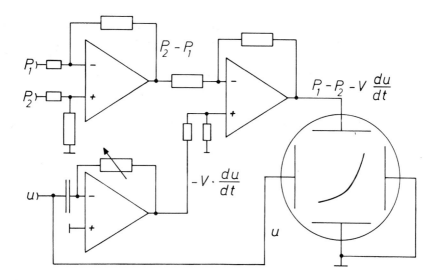

Fig. 2. Analogue computer for the determination of the inertia term

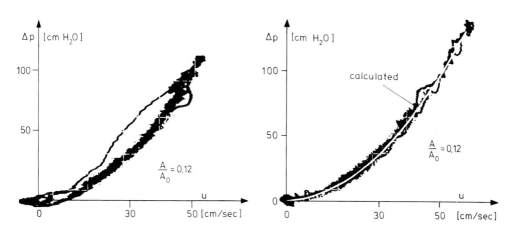

Fig. 3. Left: plot of the pressure drop against the flow velocity in the case of pulsa-tile flow. The loop rotates clockwise. Right: plot under the same conditions as in the left diagram but after subtracting the inertia term from the pressure difference

ment is caused by the electromagnetic flow meter. From several measurements based on this principle, an average value of 1.35 was obtained for the factor K_3 with a standard deviation of $\pm$ 4% [cf. 2, 4, 5]. The white curve plotted in the right diagram of Figure 3 has been calculated using the results of the first two series of experiments.

The essential aspect of this method is that it is possible to find the quasistatic relationship between the pressure drop along a stenosis and the flow velocity within the range of the flow pulse amplitudes.

In the second example, a method for finding the purely elastic pressure-diameter (p_{el}-D) relationship of arteries shall be discussed [1, 10]. The wall of the artery does not consist of purely elastic, but of viscoelastic material. Because of this, the counterforce of the wall of the artery against a change in diameter depends also on the strain rate. The consequence is that for the rhythmically changing natural pulses, the pressure-diameter relationship is not unequivocal. In a p-D diagram, a hysteresis loop results where the pressure precedes the diameter. The p_{el}-D relationship is obscured by the loop. In Figure 4, an example is shown which is obtained from in vivo measurements on a human common carotid

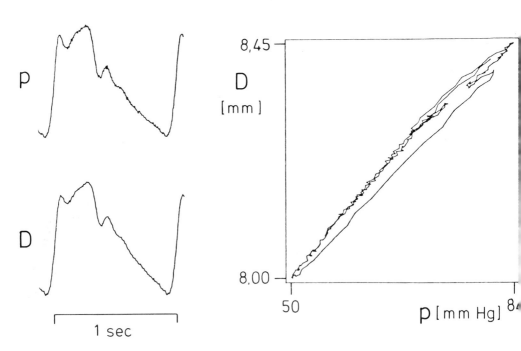

Fig. 4. Left: pressure (p) and external diameter (D) of a human carotid artery. The pressure was recorded with a catheter tip manometer (Millar PC 350 A), the diameter with a contact-free photoelectric device [9]. Right: pressure-diameter loop of the pulse of left side. The loop rotates counterclockwise

artery. In order to find the p_{el}-D relation, it is advantageous to start from a model for the arterial wall. The simplest mechanical model of an artery wall is the Voigt model [8] which consists of a spring representing the elastic properties and a parallel dashpot representing the viscous properties. In this model, a rhythmic change of the power of expansion leads to a hysteresis loop in the power-length diagram. When applying the model to an artery, the relation between the purely elastic pressure (p_{el}) and the diameter (D) can be formulated as follows

$$p_{el} = p - F \cdot dD/dt \qquad (2)$$

where p is the transmural pressure and F a coefficient in the second term which describes the pure viscous pressure. The Voigt model consists of linear elements. This means that the p_{el}-D relationship must show a linear behavior. A first variation of the Voigt model, which consists in the assumption of nonlinear elasticity of the spring, does not change the basic idea. Therefore, the pure elastic pressure can be determined by subtracting the rate of change in diameter multiplied by a suitable factor (F) from the transmural pressure. If the assumptions on which the calculation is based are correct, it should be possible to find a coefficient F such that the loop area in the p_{el}-D diagram is eliminated. The attempts to obtain a unequivocal curve in the p_{el}-D diagram and thus the purely elastic behavior of the arterial wall are not fully satisfactory. In every case, an area of the loop remains which is reduced to a minimum when the whole curve has the form of a flat eight.

A definite improvement is obtained by the assumption that, apart from the elasticity, the viscosity also shows nonlinear properties. The simplest form of nonlinear viscosity is to make it dependent on the rate of change of the diameter. Therefore, the factor F in the form

$$F = F_1 + F_2 \cdot |dD/dt| \tag{3}$$

was selected. The absolute value of dD/dt was taken into account, since the whole factor must remain independent of the sign of rate of change in diameter. The diagram in Figure 5 shows the p_{el}-D relationship which results from the p-D

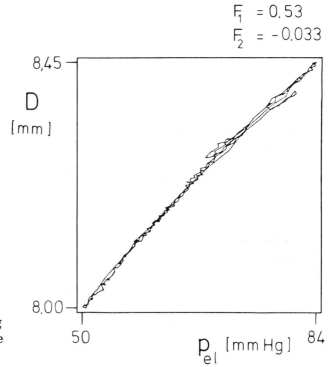

$$F_1 = 0.53$$
$$F_2 = -0.033$$

Fig. 5. p-D relationship of the same pulse as in Figure 4 after subtracting the viscous term from the measured pressure loop plotted in Figure 4 using Eq. 2 and 3. A slightly bent curve remains which represents the purely elastic behavior of the artery in the pressure range under consideration. It must be noted that in all experiments the factor F_2 becomes negative. This means that the vicosity decreases with increasing strain rate. Such behavior is called thixotropic.

References

1. Bauer, R.D.: Die quantitative Bestimmung der nichtlinearen Visko-Elastizität von Arterien in vivo: ein bisher ungelöstes Problem. Habilitationsschrift, Erlangen 1977
2. Fry, D.L.: The measurement of pulsatile blood flow by the computed pressure gradient technique. IRE Trans. Med. Electronics. ME 6, 259-264 (1959)
3. Klettner, W., Schabert, A., Summa, Y.: Pulsatile flow parameters of a stenosis inserted into an elastic tube. Proc. Int. Union Physiol. Sci. 13, 392 (1977)
4. Schabert, A., Bauer, R.D., Busse, R., Klettner, W., Summa, Y.: Die Bestimmung der charakteristischen Parameter von Stenosen an einem pulsierend durchströmten Schlauchmodell. Biomed. Tech. (Berlin) 22 [Suppl.], 295-296 (1977)
5. Schönfeld, J.C.: Resistance and inertia of the flow of liquids in a tube or open canal. Appl. sci. Res. A1, 169-197 (1948)
6. Seeley, B.D., Young, D.F.: Effect of geometry on pressure losses across models of arterial stenoses. J. Biomech. 9, 439-448 (1976)
7. Summa, Y., Schabert, A., Bauer, R.D., Busse, R.: Determination of pulsatile flow parameters of a stenosis inserted into an elastic tube. Pflügers Arch. 365, R8 (1976)
8. Wetterer, E., Kenner, Th.: Grundlagen der Dynamik des Arterienpulses. Berlin-Heidelberg-New York: Springer 1968
9. Wetterer, E., Busse, R., Bauer, R.D., Schabert, A., Summa, Y.: Photoelectric device for contact-free recording of the diameter of exposed arteries in situ. Pflügers Arch. 368, 149-152 (1977)
10. Wetterer, E., Bauer, R.D., Busse, R.: Arterial dynamics. in: Cardiovascular and Pulmonary Dynamics. M.Y.Jaffrin (ed.). Euromech. 92, (1977) (in press)
11. Young, D.F., Tsai, F.Y., Morgan, B.E.: Influence of geometry on flow in models of arterial stenoses. Proc. 24 th Ann. Conf. Eng. Med. Biol. 13, 325 (1971)
12. Young, D.F., Tsai, F.Y.: Flow characteristics in models of arterial stenoses — I. steady flow. J. Biomech. 6, 395-410 (1973)
13. Young, D.F., Tsai, F.Y.: Flow characteristics in models of arterial stenoses — II. unsteady flow. J. Biomech. 6, 547-559 (1973)
14. Young, D.F., Cholvin, N.R., Roth, A.C.: Pressure drop across artificially induced stenoses in the femoral arteries of dogs. Cir. Res.36, 735-743 (1975)
15. Young, D.F., Cholvin, N.R., Kirkeeide, R.L., Roth, A.C.: Hemodynamics of arterial stenoses at elevated flow rates. Circ. Res. 41, 99-107 (1977)

Determination of the Tangential Elastic Modulus of Human Arteries In Vivo

Y. Summa

Institut für Physiologie und Kardiologie der Universität Erlangen-Nürnberg, D-8520 Erlangen

Most of the determinations of the elasticity of the arterial wall are performed on excised arteries in vitro. This is done for the following reasons:

1. The parameters relevant to the calculation of the elastic modulus, e.g., wall thickness, wall radius, or transmural pressure, can be measured much easier in vitro than in vivo.

2. In vitro, all parameters can be adjusted easily and varied at will so that it is possible to study the elastic behavior of arteries over wide ranges of pressure and diameter.

3. To date, it has been possible to separate the elastic and the viscous behavior of arteries experimentally only in vitro.

The in vitro measurements have the disadvantage that the elastic behavior of excised arteries may differ from that of arteries in vivo. Therefore, in vivo measurements are preferable. For the determination of the elastic modulus of the arterial wall, stress-strain relations are needed [6]. The tangential stress σ_t is given by Eq. 1:

$$\sigma_t = \frac{P \cdot r_i}{h} = P \frac{(1 - \frac{4S}{\pi D^2})^{1/2}}{1 - (1 - \frac{4S}{\pi D^2})^{1/2}} = P \cdot f \tag{1}$$

where P is the transmural pressure, r_i the internal radius, h the wall thickness, $f = r_i/h$, D the external diameter, and S the cross-sectional area of the wall. The expression represented by f in Eq. 1 is obtained from the ratio r_i/h by a simple calculation. Assuming incompressibility of the arterial wall and longitudinal constraint of in vivo arteries, S is constant for a given artery. Thus, f depends only on the external diameter D.

Owing to viscoelasticity, the pressure-diameter recordings of pulsating arteries show hysteresis loops. In their contributions contained in this volume, Wetterer et al. [7] and Schabert [4] demonstrate that the pure elastic and pure viscous

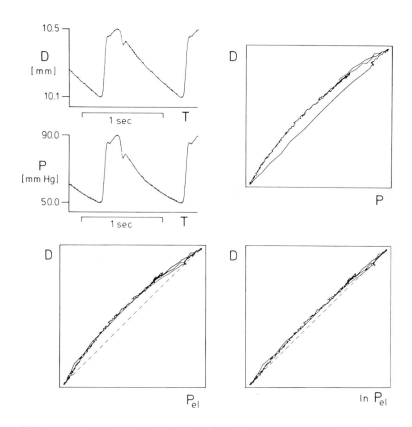

Fig. 1. Values obtained in the sclerotic common carotid artery of a 74-year-old patient during a surgical operation. Methods as described by Wetterer et al. [7] and Schabert [4]. Top: pulses of diameter (D) and pressure (P) (left), P-D loop of one pulse cycle (right). Bottom: P_{el}-D plot (left) and ln P_{el}-D plot (right) where P_{el} = elastic pressure

pressures can be separated from each other. An example is shown in Figure 1, which was obtained from the common carotid artery of a 74-year-old patient. The recordings were made during a surgical operation. The upper tracings on the left show the pressure and diameter pulses, while on the right the pressure-diameter loop of a single pulse cycle can be seen. The lower diagram on the left shows the result obtained from the upper diagram by the procedure described by Wetterer et al. [7] and Schabert [4]; p_{el} is the "purely elastic pressure." For the artery of Figure 1, the relative diameter change is about 4%, while the mean of the diameter changes obtained in the carotids of 13 patients (34-75 years) is 5.5%. This value is far smaller than those reported by Arndt [1] and Ungern-Sternberg [5].

In contrast to the canine carotids, the elastic pressure-diameter curves of human carotids (Figs. 1-3) show marked nonlinearity. To describe the nonlinearity of the p_{el}-D curve quantitatively, we approximate the elastic pressure-diameter curve of Figure 1 by the following second degree polynomial

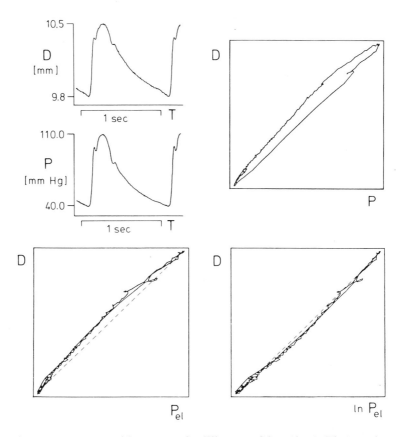

Fig. 2. Nonsclerotic common carotid artery of a 75-year-old patient. Plots as in Figure 1

$$p_{el} = 10494 - 2124\,D + 108\,D^2 \qquad (2)$$

(p_{el} in mm Hg, D in mm). In the case of Figure 1, the quadratic term is about 50% of the linear term. From numerous experiments performed in vitro on canine arteries, it is well-known that P-D relations show marked nonlinearity only if wide diameter ranges are covered. In the case of small diameter changes, however, the purely elastic behavior of canine arteries is almost linear [7]. Our findings show that this is not true for the human common carotid artery, so that the equations of the linear elasticity theory are not adequate even in the case of small diameter changes.

Under the assumption of strain-dependent moduli of elasticity, the linearized equations can also be applied to the determination of nonlinear elastic behavior. This procedure, however, is complicated if very large strains are to be considered. Under such circumstances, it might be preferable to apply the finite deformation theory [2, 3] which is generally valid. But it is not our purpose to apply this theory to the calculation of the tangential elastic modulus of arteries because, in the case we are dealing with, the calculation can be performed in a rather simpler manner with the aid of Eqs. 1 and 2, as will be seen below.

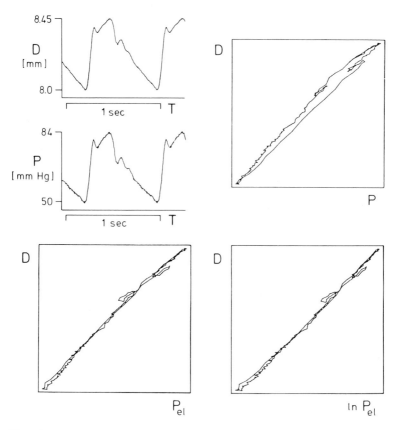

Fig. 3. Common carotid artery of a 37-year-old patient. Plots as in Figure 1

The shapes of the P_{el}-D curves might suggest that the diameter depends on pressure in a logarithmic way. To test this conjecture, the diameter is plotted against the logarithm of the elastic pressure. The result of this procedure applied to the P_{el}-D curve of Figure 1 is shown in the lower right of Figure 1. It can be seen that the ln P_{el}-D curve is not a straight line. The dashed straight line is drawn in order to illustrate the degree of deviation from linearity. We note that the logarithmic P_{el}-D curve shows a convex curvature toward the D axis. In the second example (Fig. 2), the logarithmic plot of P_{el} is also a curved line. In this case, the curvature is concave to the D axis. In contrast to these two examples, the ln P_{el}-D curve of the third example (Fig. 3) is a straight line, indicating a logarithmic relationship between elastic pressure and diameter. Indeed, all cases which we have examined so far show one of these three characteristics. S-shaped curves as sometimes described by other workers were not seen in our plots.

The deviation of the ln P_{el}-D curves from linearity cannot be attributed to a strain-independent active stress of the smooth muscle. This can be seen from the following consideration. The subtraction of a properly chosen constant pressure from the measured transmural pressure would abolish the convexity of a given

98

In P_{el}-D curve, but this procedure is obviously not possible in the case of curves which are concave to the D axis.

Finally, we should like to discuss the dependence of the tangential elastic modulus E_t on the strain for the example given in Figure 1. The elastic pressure-diameter curve, given by Eq. 2, can be written as

$$P = a - bD + cD^2 \tag{3}$$

D varies between 10.1 and 10.5 mm. Giving this equation another form, we obtain a relation in which only E_t and D are contained. This is done in the following way. Generally, we define

$$E_t = \frac{d\sigma_t}{(du/u)} \tag{4}$$

where σ_t = tangential stress, u = circumference of the mean wall layer = $2\pi\sqrt{r_i r_e}$ with r_i = internal radius and r_a = external radius. The relation between u and D is given by

$$u^2 = \pi^2 D (D^2 - \frac{4S}{\pi})^{1/2} \tag{5}$$

from which we obtain

$$\frac{du}{u} = \frac{(D^2 - \frac{2S}{\pi})}{(D^2 - \frac{4S}{\pi})} \frac{dD}{D} \tag{6}$$

Furthermore, we put

$$1 - \frac{4S}{\pi D^2} = e^2 \tag{7}$$

and obtain from Eq. 1

$$d\sigma_t = (\frac{dP}{dD} f + P \frac{df}{dD}) dD \tag{8}$$

Eqs. 6 and 8 give

$$E_t = \frac{d\sigma_t}{\frac{du}{u}} = \frac{D^3 e^2}{D^2 - \frac{2S}{\pi}} \left[(-b + 2cD) \frac{e}{1-e} + (a - bD + cD^2) \frac{4S}{\pi D^3 e (1-e)^2} \right] \tag{9}$$

99

$E_t(0)$ is obtained by making $D = D(0)$, where $D(0)$ is the smallest diameter contained in the recording.

Figure 4 shows, for the sclerotic carotid of the 74-year-old patient (curve 1), the relation between $E_t/E_t(0)$ and $D/D(0)$. It is seen that a relative diameter change of about 4% results in a relative change of E_t of more than 100%. In the two other cases (curves 2 and 3), the relative increases of E_t are far smaller.

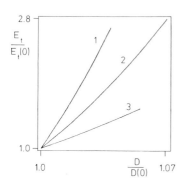

Fig. 4. Dependence of the relative tangential elastic modulus on the relative external diameter. The curves 1-3 refer to the patients of Figures 1-3. $D(0)$ = smallest external diameter contained in the recording. $E_t(0)$ = tangential elastic modulus calculated at $D = D(0)$

References

1. Arndt, J.O.: Über die Mechanik der intakten A. carotis communis des Menschen unter verschiedenen Kreislaufbedingungen. Arch. Kreislaufforsch. 59, 153-197 (1969)
2. Doyle, S.M., Dobrin, P.B.: Finite Deformation Analysis of the Relaxed and Contracted Dog Carotid Artery. Microvasc. Res. 3, 400-415 (1971)
3. Opatowski, I.: Elastic deformations of arteries. J. Appl. Physiol. 23, 772-778 (1967)
4. Schabert, A.: The separation of time-dependent and time-independent terms in the relation of pressure and diameter and of pressure and flow velocity in arteries. (In this volume).
5. Ungern-Sternberg, A.V., Traxel, W., Schuster, C.J.: Transkutane Messung altersbedingter Veränderungen der Gefäßelastizität der Arteria carotis communis des Menschen. Z. Kardiol. 64, 879-888 (1975)
6. Wetterer, E., Kenner, Th.: Grundlagen der Dynamik des Arterienpulses. Berlin-Heidelberg - New York: Springer 1968
7. Wetterer, E., Bauer, R.D., Busse, R.: New ways of determining the propagation coefficient and the visco-elastic behavior of arteries in situ. (In this volume).

Model of Nonlinear Viscoelastic Wall Rheology Applied to Arterial Dynamics

C. Oddou, P. Flaud, and D. Geiger

L. B. H. P.-Université Paris 7, 2 Place Jussieu - 75221 Paris Cedex 05

In modern cardiovascular research, one of the fundamental problems is the accurate determination of local flow patterns inside large arteries and their relation with pressure waves generated by the heart. Data for blood flow rates, wall shear stresses, and detailed velocity profiles (with localization of inflexion points, recirculation zone, and boundary layer separation) are necessary to study transport phenomena related to atherogenesis or instability and turbulence generation mechanism. Theoretic and experimental models for local hemodynamic studies, as they have most often been designed in the past, do not take into account the motion of the wall and, for analytic and experimental simplification purposes, consider only the rigid wall case. Nevertheless, in regard to the large strain generated inside the arterial tissues, radial motion of the boundary and associated convective effects in the blood dynamics have to be considered if a rigorous description of the hemodynamic events is required.

Among these events, generation by pressure wave propagation of unsteady flow patterns, under fully developed flow situation excluding stenotic, branched or curved type of flow, has been recently investigated [3]. Based upon the experimental observations of a locally developed flow profile generation as the pressure wave propagates along the artery, an approximate numeric method for calculating these flow profiles has been developed which takes into account nonlinear convective terms in the fluid dynamic equations and nonlinear wall rheologic behavior due to large deformations of the arterial wall. The velocity distribution and wall shear stresses at a given location along the arterial tree were determined from the measured values of pressure, pressure gradient, and pressure-radius relation at the same location. Such a simple indirect method for determination of velocity profiles is useful in cardiovascular research when direct anemometric measurements are rather difficult if not impossible. It was shown that, contrary to the theories based on the linearized long wave length approximation that failed to provide correct flow profiles and shear stresses, this nonlinear numeric approach gave results in good agreement with the corresponding experimental data. However, the comparison between results of linearized long wave length theory and such a nonlinear numeric approach does not answer some basic questions such as what type of flow profile should be assigned to the steady flow component in the linearized theory and what the effects are due to the tapered geometry of arteries. Moreover, in such a model, viscoelastic characteristics in the wall rheology have been omitted. These characteristics may play a determinant

101

role in the fluid wall interaction, although viscous loss moduli are generally rather small compared to the corresponding elastic storage moduli.

Due to its heterogeneous structure, made of a collection of cellules, elastin, and collagen fibrous elements embedded in a mucopolysaccharide medium, strain behavior of the vascular wall depends on the time course and history of stress application. It can be noted also that the properties of the arterial wall in its passive state can be modified by the contraction or relaxation of smooth muscle [2]. Moreover, from a histologic point of view, an arterial segment can be considered to have reasonably uniform local structure in the longitudinal and circumferential directions but not in the radial direction [9]. Nevertheless, from the point of view of pressure-volume relationship and pressure wave propagation, only the average properties of the blood vessel wall are relevant, and results based on overall homogeneity assumption are valid. When looking at the distinct rheologic contribution made by the different constituents such as elastin and collagen, it has been shown that the resistance to stretch at low pressure is almost entirely due to elastin and that at high pressure the behavior of the collagen fibers is the most important factor [7]. Therefore, the arterial wall material has to be characterized as an incompressible, orthotropic, viscoelastic nonlinear medium [6], the behavior of which has not yet been fully interpreted by the theory. Under physiologic conditions, such nonlinear viscoelastic rheologic properties of the arterial wall can be schematically illustrated by the pressure-radius relationship of a Kelvin-Voigt element (Table 1), where the wall inertia is neglected. It is assumed that the perivascular tethering prevents longitudinal motion and that the radial motion of the arterial wall is primarily didacted by the pressure wave.

In a first step of the study concerning the local hemodynamic properties, the nonlinear analytic model has been applied in the case of an idealized situation. In such a case, the local pressure is the result of a "quasilinear" pressure wave propagation in the downstream direction [8] neglecting wave reflection, dispersion effect due to blood viscosity, and distorsion effect due to tapering and change in nonlinear rheologic wall properties. Generally, such drastic conditions are not likely to occur everywhere in the arterial tree although it has been assumed to be the case in the ascending part of the aorta [4]. Nevertheless, they can be generated on a hydrodynamic model [1], where pressure wave shape can be easily controlled and reflection effects eliminated. With this hypothesis, entry data for the pressure wave and the pressure gradient wave are simply related. Then, for a given pressure gradient wave (Table 1), the effects of different mechanical behavior of the wall (rigid, $R = Ro$, purely elastic $\eta = 0$, viscoelastic) can be compared.

Details of the approximations underlying the simplification of the equation of fluid motion and elimination of all explicit dependance in the downstream coordinate are given in Table 2. By introducing radial coordinate transformation in order to simplify the equation concerning boundary conditions, one has to solve the following system of integral differential equation for the longitudinal v_z and radial v_r velocity component [3].

Table 1. Entry data of the arterial dynamics non linear model.

Wall rheologic law

$$\eta \frac{\partial R}{\partial t} + (R - R_0) = K (P - P_0)$$

Pressure gradient wave

$$-\frac{1}{\rho} \frac{\partial P}{\partial z} (\underline{z}, t) = A_0 + A_1 \cos (\omega t - k\underline{z})$$

Quasilinear pressure wave propagation

$$\frac{\partial \Delta P}{\partial z} = -\frac{1}{c} \frac{\partial \Delta P}{\partial t}$$

where $\qquad c^2 = \dfrac{R}{2\rho} \dfrac{dR}{dP} = \dfrac{\omega^2}{k^2}$

and $\qquad \Delta P = P(\underline{z}, t) - P_0(\underline{z})$

Dog aorta

$\eta = 4.10^{-2}s$;	$\rho = 1g/cm^3$;	$\nu = .036\ cm^2/s$;	$T = .8\ s$;
$\overline{v_z} = 20\ cm/s$;	$R_0 = .68\ cm$;	$P_0 = 100\ mm\ Hg$;	$K^{-1} = 400\ mm\ Hg/cm$;
$\dfrac{\overline{v_z}}{c_0} = .05$;	$a = 10$;	$\lambda = 3$;	$\overline{Re} = \simeq 750$.

$$v_r = \left[\frac{\partial P}{\partial z} \frac{\partial R}{\partial P} \right] \left[xv_z - \frac{2}{x} \left(\int_0^x x'v_z dx' - \frac{\int_0^1 x'v_z dx'}{\int_0^1 x|v_z| dx'} \int_0^x x'|v_z| dx' \right) \right.$$

$$\left. + \frac{1}{x} \frac{\partial R}{\partial t} \frac{\int_0^x x'|v_z| dx'}{\int_0^1 x'|v_z| dx'} \right. \tag{1}$$

$$\frac{\partial v_z}{\partial t} = -\frac{1}{\rho} \frac{\partial P}{\partial z} + \left(\frac{x}{R} \frac{\partial R}{\partial t} - \frac{v_r}{R} \right) \frac{\partial v_z}{\partial x} + \frac{v_z}{R} \left(\frac{\partial v_r}{\partial x} + \frac{v_r}{x} \right) + \frac{\nu}{R^2} \left(\frac{\partial^2 v_z}{\partial x^2} + \frac{1}{x} \frac{\partial v_z}{\partial x} \right) \tag{2}$$

Table 2. Basic hypothesis for the local and nonlinear hemodynamical analysis.

small   radial   velocity   approximation

$$\frac{\partial R}{\partial t} \ll V_z \longrightarrow V_r \ll V_z \longrightarrow p\,(z,t)$$

large   wavelength   hypothesis

$$\lambda \gg R \longrightarrow \frac{\partial^2}{\partial z^2} \ll \frac{\partial^2}{\partial r^2}$$

radial   coordinate   transformation

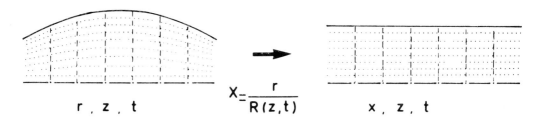

r , z , t $X = \dfrac{r}{R\,(z,t)}$ x , z , t

longitudinal   velocity   gradient   approximation

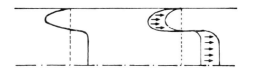

$$\frac{\partial V_z}{\partial z} \simeq \mathrm{sgn}\left(\frac{\partial V_z}{\partial z}\right) \left| (k-1)V_z\,(x,z,t) \right|$$

$$V_z\,|_{x=1} = 0 \tag{3}$$

$$\left.\frac{\partial V_z}{\partial x}\right|_{x=0} = 0 \tag{4}$$

Solution of such a system is obtained by numeric integration using the finite difference method with a rectangular mesh in the normalized radius-time space (x, $\tau = t/T$). If dx $\cdot$ dτ is the elementary mesh size, necessary conditions for numeric stability and convergence require that the equivalent radial velocity of the calculation should be greater than the radial velocity for vorticity diffusion

$$\frac{Rdx}{Td_\tau} > 2 \, (^\nu/Td_\tau)^{1/2} \tag{5}$$

Considerations of accuracy are more difficult to handle and should be tested using different mesh size: taking into account the necessity of a fine mesh size in the radial direction (dx = .02) in order to have an accurate determination of the wall shear stress and the effect of cumulative truncature errors, an optimal value of $d_\tau = 4.10^{-4}$ has been experimentally found, a value lower by an order of magnitude than the one calculated from Eq. 5, the numeric results of which are significantly different.

Some of the instantaneous velocity profiles and associated flow rate and wall shear stresses computed by such a method are shown in Figure 1, which gives

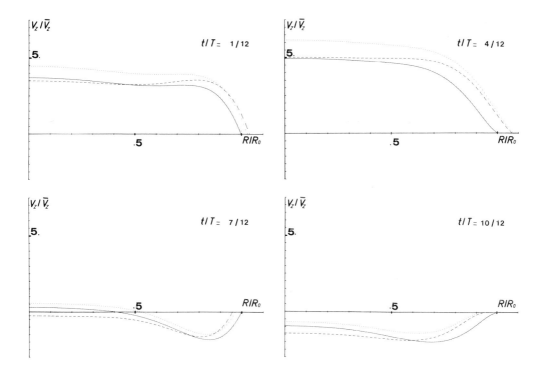

Fig. 1. Computed instantaneous velocity profile: rigid (———), elastic (– – – –) and viscoelastic (. . . . . . .) tube.

a detailed comparison between results obtained assuming different behavior of the wall rheology. It is to be noted that velocity profiles, in the rigid case, agree perfectly with those obtained from linear calculation [5], the analytic expression of which is given by·

$$v_z = 2\bar{v}_z (1 - x^2) + \tilde{v}_z \left\{ \frac{1 - \dfrac{J_0 (axi^{3/2})}{J_0 (ai^{3/2})}}{1 - \dfrac{2J_1 (ai^{3/2})}{ai^{3/2}J_0(ai^{3/2})}} \right\} e^{i\omega t} \tag{6}$$

where J_0 and J_1 are the Bessel function and $\bar{v}_z$ and $\tilde{v}_z$ the steady and harmonic components of the velocity. These profiles are determined by the following data (cf. Table 1):

Mean Reynold's number $\qquad \overline{Re} = \dfrac{2 R_0 \bar{v}_z}{\nu}$ $\hfill (7)$

Amplitude parameter $\qquad \lambda = \dfrac{\tilde{v}_z}{\bar{v}_z}$ $\hfill (8)$

Unsteadiness parameter $\qquad a = R_0 \sqrt{\dfrac{\omega}{\nu}}$ $\hfill (9)$

In the rigid tube case, computed instantaneous normalized mean velocity (or flow rate) and wall shear stress values have also been found to be the same as those analytically derived [10] by integration of (6)

$$\frac{< v_z >}{\bar{v}_z} = 1 + \frac{A_1}{A_0} \sigma_v \cos (\omega t - \delta_v) \tag{10}$$

$$\frac{\tau}{\frac{1}{2}\rho \, \bar{v}_z^{2}} = \frac{16}{\overline{Re}} \left[1 + \frac{A_1}{A_0} \sigma_\tau \cos (\omega t - \delta_\tau) \right] \tag{11}$$

where σ_v, δ_v, σ_τ, and δ_τ are normalization coefficients, the function of a, which were tabulated by Womersley.

Under such a simple situation (no static tapering of the wall, harmonic variation of the pressure gradient, simple model for the rheologic behavior of the wall), the comparison between linear and nonlinear theory is renderered easier. In particular, it is shown that nonlinear effects (both in the elastic and viscoelastic case) increase the fluid velocity during systole and to a lower extent during diastole. On the contrary wall, shear stress data are not significantly different from these obtained in the linear case.

The physical process at the origin of such an important effect in the fluid dynamics is thought to be related to the radial motion and tapering of the wall

106

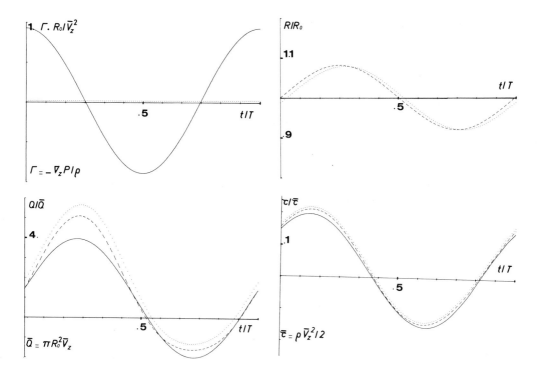

Fig. 2. Numerical results for rigid (————), elastic (- - - - - - -) and visco-elastic (. . . . . . .) tube.
upper left: applied pressure gradient wave
upper right: resultant wall radial strain
lower left: resultant flow rate
lower right: resultant shear stress.

induced by the pressure wave. It is interesting to note that, during the early accelerative phase of the applied pressure gradient, an acceleration of the fluid inside the distensible tube is greater than in the case of the rigid wall tube. During this phase, the radial velocity, even though of small magnitude, tends to fall toward the positive direction and is directly responsible for the convective acceleration. Thus, through this induced convective acceleration, phase relations between time variations of pressure gradient, induced tapering, and radial motion of the wall are hemodynamically important factors in the fluid-wall interaction and pressure flow relationships. This effect is particularly important in the case of viscoelastic wall rheology. An experimental study on a hydrodynamic model including a viscoelastic silicon rubber section is under way to test the validity of such a physical interpretation.

Summary

Nonlinear rheologic wall properties and radial convection in fluid dynamics have a large effect upon the details of the local flow pattern. Assuming particular characteristics of wave propagation, local relations between pulsatile pressure gradient and flow can be analyzed by means of an approximative theoretic arterial dynamics model. For a given pressure gradient, resulting flow patterns, shear stresses, and flow rates are compared when assuming different mechanical behavior of the wall: rigid, purely elastic, and viscoelastic wall in a uniform artery model. By numeric analysis of approximate fluid mechanics equations, based on the finite difference method, it is found that nonlinearity due to radial convective term and radial motion of the wall significantly enhance the flow rate, and to a minor degree, the wall shear stress. These effects are more sensible in the viscoelastic case.

References

1. Flaud, P., Geiger, D., Oddou, C., Quemada, D.: Dispositif expérimental pour la modélisation de l'écoulement sanguin dans les artères. Rev. Phys. Appl. 10, 61-67 (1975)
2. Gow, B.S.: The influence of vascular smooth muscle on the viscoelastic properties of blood vessels. In: Cardiovascular Fluid Dynamics. Bergel, D.H. (ed.). New York: Acad. Pr. 65-110, 1972, Vol. II
3. Ling, S.C., Atabek, H.B.: A nonlinear analysis of pulsatile flow in arteries. J. Fluid Mech., 55, 493 (1972)
4. McDonald, D.A.: Blood Flow in Arteries. London-Edinburgh: Edward Arnold, 1974
5. Oddou, C., Flaud, P., Geiger, D.: Rheologie des parois et hydrodynamique artérielle. J. Physiol. (Paris) 72, 663-681 (1976)
6. Patel, D., Vaishnav, R.N.: The rheology of large blood vessels. In: Cardiovascular Fluid Dynamics. Bergel, D.H. (ed.). New York: Acad. Pr. 1972, Vol. II 1-64
7. Roach, M.R., Burton, A.C.: The reason for the shape of the distensibility curves of arteries. Can. J. Biochem. Physiol. 35, 681-690 (1957)
8. Wetterer, E., Kenner, T.: Die Dynamik des Arterienpulses; Heidelberg-Berlin-New York: Springer 1968
9. Wolinsky, H., Glagov, S.: Structural basis for the basic mechanical properties of the aortic media. Circ. Res., 14, 400-413 (1964)
10. Womersley, J.R.: An elastic tube theory of pulse transmission and oscillatory flow in mammalian artery. Wright Air Dev. Ctr. Tech. Rep WADC TR 56-614 (1957)

Validity of the Moens-Korteweg Equation

D. L. Newman, and S. E. Greenwald

Guy's Hospital Medical School, London, SE1 9RT. The London Hospital, London E1.

The pulse wave velocity (c) in an infinitely thin-walled elastic vessel may be predicted from its viscoelastic properties using the so-called Moens-Korteweg equation

$$c^2 = Eh/2Rp \qquad (1)$$

where E is the Young's modulus of the wall, h the wall thickness, R the internal vessel radius, and p the density of the wall material. In thicker walled vessels, a commonly quoted variation (1) of Eq. 1 is

$$c^2 = Ep\,(1 - \gamma)/2p \qquad (2)$$

where γ is the ratio of wall thickness to external vessel radius and Ep is the pressure elastic modulus [7] defined as

$$Ep = \Delta P \cdot R/\Delta R \qquad (3)$$

where ΔR is the change in external radius of the vessel associated with a pressure change ΔP and R is the mean vessel radius. The validity of Eq. 1 or 2 have not been fully explored in vivo, but they would be expected to apply only in vessels in which there are no wave reflections [3]. This paper presents some results of simultaneous measurements of arterial elasticity and pulse propagation velocity in the abdominal aorta of anesthetized dogs under both vasodilated and vasoconstricted conditions.

Materials and Methods

Experiments were carried out on the exposed abdominal aorta of six anesthetized greyhounds. Pulse propagation velocities were determined by simultaneous measurement of flow (three dogs) and pressure (three dogs) at each end of a segment of the abdominal aorta bounded by the left renal artery and the aortic termination. The flow wave forms were measured with closely fitting electromagnetic cuff probes placed around the vessel and connected to flow meters. The pressure wave forms were measured through cannulae inserted via the left renal artery and the femoral artery. Near the midpoint of the segment, a mercury in silastic strain gauge was placed around the vessel to measure changes in diameter. Pulsatile pressure was measured by inserting a 21 G hypodermic needle into the vessel approximately 5 mm upstream of the strain gauge. The needle was connected via a saline-filled cannula to a pressure transducer. The needle was passed through a loose fitting PVC cuff in order to hold it steady and at right angles to the flow.

The measurements were carried out during continuous infusion of noradrenalin to produce vasoconstriction and subsequently under vasodilated conditions by perfusion of isoprenaline. The mean diameter of the aorta at the mean pressures corresponding to the vasoconstricted and vasodilated condition was determined from radiographs obtained after injection of 15 ml of radio-opaque material (60% Hypaque) through a cannula in the renal artery. The strain gauge was calibrated postmortem against measured radiographs obtained by injection of barium sulfate suspension (Micropaque) into the aorta with stepwise pressure increments.

Following this static calibration of the strain gauge, the vessel segment was removed, blotted dry, stripped of loosely adhering adventitial material, and weighed. Knowing the weight, density, and internal diameter of the vessel at various pressures, the thickness of the wall was calculated assuming a circular cross-section and isovolumetric expansion. Following Bergel [1], the thickness of the vessel wall was expressed as its ratio to the external radius (γ).

Selected trains of three cardiac cycles were subjected to Fourier analysis on a digital computer programmed to print out modulus and phase values for each of the measured variables up to the tenth harmonic. The measured phase velocity (C_m) was calculated from the phase lag between corresponding harmonics of the pressure or flow waves recorded at each end of the segment. The calculated phase velocity (C_c) was determined for each harmonic using Eq. 2, using the experimentally determined values of Ep and γ. A third estimate of the propagation velocity (C_{ff}) was obtained by direct measurement of the time delay between the feet of corresponding pulses from the two sites.

In one of the dogs, the modulus and phase of the local impedance was obtained for the first ten harmonics from pressure and flow recordings obtained at the midpoint of the segment

Results

Table 1 shows the mean values ($\pm$ SD) of blood pressure, heart rate, the modulus and phase of Ep, external radius R_o and relative wall thickness (γ) calculated for the six dogs. The modulus and phase of Ep for each dog was calculated as the mean of the first ten harmonics.

The mean values of the measured and calculated phase velocities of flow and pressure obtained from the six dogs (three for pressure and three for flow) during vasoconstriction and vasodilation are shown in Figure 1.

During both vasoconstriction and vasodilation, the calculated phase velocities (broken line) show very little frequency dependence. At high frequencies

110

Table 1. Mean values (± SD) for all the dogs of mean blood pressure (BP), heart rate, pressure strain elastic modulus (Ep), and phase (ϕ), external aortic radius (R_O), and relative wall thickness (γ)

	Vasoconstriction	Vasodilation
BP (mm Hg)	118 ± 23.6	61.5 ± 5.5
Heart rate (Hz)	2.6 ± 0.3	3.4 ± 0.5
Ep ($Nm^{-2} \times 10^4$)	15.90 ± 4.0	9.49 ± 1.8
ϕ (degrees)	+ 2.0 ± 2.0	-1.0 ± 5.0
R_O (mm)	5.5 ± 0.9	4.4 ± 0.6
γ	0.12 ± 0.03	0.17 ± 0.02

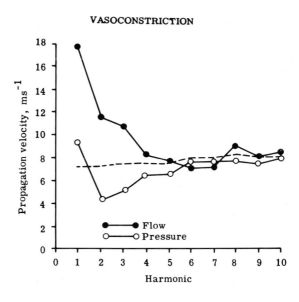

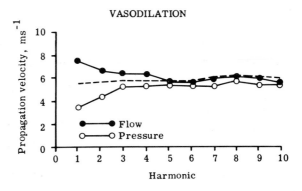

Fig. 1. Variation of flow and pressure wave propagation velocities and calculated propagation velocities (broken line) with harmonic number during vasoconstriction and vasodilation. Results shown are mean values for all the dogs

(harmonics $\geqslant$ 5th), the measured phase velocities of the pressure and flow waves tended toward the calculated values for both vasoconstriction and vasodilation. At lower frequencies, the measured phase velocities of pressure and flow did not agree with the calculated values, and this was more marked during vasoconstriction, suggesting that the lack agreement is due, at least in part, to the presence of peripheral reflections. During vasoconstriction, the impedance modulus (measured in one of the dogs, Fig. 2) falls from a value of 19×10^7 Nm^{-5} s at zero frequency to a minimum of 4.5×10^7 Nm^{-5} s at $\sim$ 7 Hz, and increases to a value of 9×10^7 Nm^{-5} s at higher frequencies. During vasodilation, the impedance modulus at zero frequency was 12.0×10^7 Nm^{-5}s, there was a less obvious minimum at $\sim$ 4 Hz, and less overall variation with frequency when compared to the vasoconstricted state.

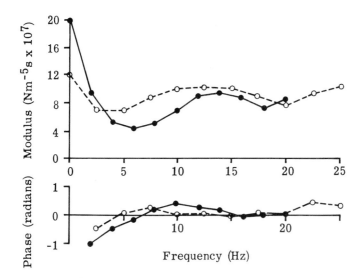

Fig. 2. Variation of modulus and phase of local fluid impedance with frequency during vasodilation (broken line) and vasoconstriction (solid line)

Assuming a lumped peripheral termination, the distance of the measurement site from the termination may be calculated since the quarter wave length position occurs when the phase passes through zero [3]. For vasoconstriction, the calculated distance is 333 mm while for vasodilation it is 345 mm.

Table 2 shows the values for the measured and calculated propagation velocities for each dog. The calculated values were averaged over all ten harmonics, and the mean values for the measured velocities were obtained by averaging from harmonics five through ten. The third column shows foot-to-foot velocities calculated from ten successive heartbeats.

The Student's t test was used to compare corresponding means of the measured and calculated velocities for each dog. No significant differences were observed at the 5% level. Similarly, comparison between mean foot-to-foot and calculated wave velocities also failed to show any significant differences.

Table 2. Comparison of pulse wave velocities for each dog during vasoconstriction (VC) and vasodilation (VD). Mean values ± SD m s^{-1}

Dog	Vasoactive state	Measured (C_m)	Calculated (C_c)	Foot-to-foot (C_{ff})
1	VC	8.16 ± 0.55	7.72 ± 1.15	8.67 ± 0.72
	VD	6.03 ± 0.41	6.04 ± 0.68	6.07 ± 0.42
2	VC	9.41 ± 1.23	9.00 ± 1.22	8.81 ± 0.12
	VD	7.33 ± 1.00	7.02 ± 1.01	6.91 ± 0.12
3	VC	7.16 ± 1.40	8.59 ± 1.52	7.80 ± 0.47
	VD	5.75 ± 0.96	6.03 ± 1.05	5.75 ± 0.24
4	VC	6.10 ± 0.25	6.23 ± 0.24	6.39 ± 0.18
	VD	3.89 ± 0.16	4.08 ± 0.24	4.03 ± 0.31
5	VC	9.32 ± 0.63	8.97 ± 0.45	7.61 ± 0.15
	VD	5.47 ± 0.15	6.04 ± 0.54	5.36 ± 0.15
6	VC	8.11 ± 0.27	8.08 ± 0.54	8.12 ± 0.96
	VD	6.82 ± 0.23	6.80 ± 0.34	6.63 ± 0.23

Discussion

Few detailed in vivo studies concerning the validity of the Moens-Korteweg equation in arteries have been reported. The effect of peripheral reflections on the frequency dependence of the apparent pulse wave velocity has been discussed by McDonald and Taylor [4] who concluded that foot-to-foot velocity correlated well with values predicted by elasticity measurements. More recently, Nichols and McDonald [5] have shown that phase velocity values averaged over the first ten harmonics were in close agreement with the velocity of the wave front. However, in their study, measurements were made in the ascending aorta where peripheral reflections will most probably have been greatly attenuated. In a study on the anisotropic elastic properties of the aorta in living dogs, Patel et al. [6] compared measured foot-to-foot propagation velocities with values predicted from static elasticity measurements in the descending thoracic aorta. The agreement between the theoretic and measured values was surprisingly close, although no assessment was made of the degree of reflection from the periphery and vessel junctions.

The frequency spectrum of the impedance modulus measured at a certain distance from the reflection site closely resembles the frequency variation of the apparent phase velocity, since in large vessels the impedance modulus (Z_i) is related to the apparent propagation velocity (C_a) by Eq. 4.

$$|Z_i| = \frac{\rho C_a}{\pi R^2} \qquad (4)$$

In the impedance spectrum obtained in one of the dogs (No. 5), it may be seen that at higher frequencies for both vasoconstriction and vasodilation the impedance modulus is relatively constant and the phase angle is close to zero. This indicates that the contribution from peripheral reflections is small at high frequencies and in such circumstances the input impedance (Z_i) is close to the characteristic impedance (Z_c). Thus, the measured propagation velocity will be close to the true value.

At lower frequencies, particularly during vasoconstriction, the presence of reflections causes the appearance of maxima and minima in the frequency spectrum of the impedance modulus and a variation in the phase such that it passes through zero at successive maxima and minima. The frequency at which this occurs corresponds to quarter wave length distances from a lumped peripheral termination. From Eq. 4, it may be seen that the frequency variation in the apparent phase velocity will be similar to that of the impedance modulus. However, the difference between the true and apparent propagation velocities of the pressure and flow waves will be of the opposite sign because the phase angles of these waves reflected from the termination are in antiphase.

The results of the impedance measurements indicate that $Z_i = Z_c$ for all harmonics above the first during vasodilation. For the higher harmonics, it may be seen that the measured propagation velocity changes little with frequency and is close to the value calculated from the Moens-Korteweg equation. From Eq. 4, one may calculate a value for the true propagation velocity for dog 5 from the average impedance modulus of these higher harmonics. During vasoconstriction, the value calculated is 8.52 ± 0.94 ms^{-1} and during vasodilation 5.88 ± 0.97 ms^{-1}. These values compare well with those obtained by direct measurement and those calculated from the Moens-Korteweg equation (Table 2).

The results presented in this study show that in the abdominal aorta during vasodilation the measured and calculated phase velocites (C_m and C_c) agree to within a few percent for all harmonics above the first; while during vasoconstriction, agreement is only found at the higher harmonics. In the absence of reflections, the so-called true propagation velocity for both pressure and flow waves will be determined solely by the elastic properties of the vessel. If reflections are present, these interact with the incident waves in such a way that the measured or apparent propagation velocity fluctuates around the true value when plotted against frequency or distance from the reflection site [8].

References

1. Bergel, D.H., Schultz, D.L.: Arterial elasticity and fluid dynamics. Prog. Biophys. Mol. Biol. 22, 3-36 (1972)
2. Gow, B.S., Taylor, M.G.: Measurement of viscoelastic properties of arteries in the living dog. Circ. Res. 23, 111-122 (1968)

3. McDonald, D.A.: Blood Flow in Arteries. London: Edward Arnold, 1974
4. McDonald, D.A., Taylor, M.G.: The hydrodynamics of the arterial circulation. Prog. Biophys. 9, 107-173 (1959)
5. Nichols, W.W., McDonald, D.A.: Wave velocity in the proximal aorta. Med. Biol. Eng. 10, 327-335 (1972)
6. Patel, D.J., Janicki, J.S., Carew, T.E.: Static anisotropic elastic properties of the aorta in living dogs. Circ. Res. 25, 765-779 (1969)
7. Peterson, L.H., Jenson, R.E., Parnell, J.: Mechanical properties of arteries in vivo. Circ. 8, 622-639 (1960)
8. Taylor, M.G.: An approach to an analysis of the arterial pulse wave. I. Oscillations in an attenuating line. II. Fluid oscillations in an elastic pipe. Phys. Med. Biol. 1, 258-329 (1957)

Time Domain Reflectometry in a Model of the Arterial System

P. Sipkema and N. Westerhof

Laboratorium voor Fysiologie, Vrije Universiteit Amsterdam/Holland

Introduction

The arterial tree can be characterized by means of its frequency response function (the input impedance) and by means of its time response function (the impulse response function). These descriptions are Fourier transforms of each other. If the impulse excitation is supplied by a special generator that has an impedance matched to that of the characteristic impedance of the ascending aorta, then the analysis is called time domain reflectometry.

The input impedance of a uniform tube can be determined by sinusoidal excitation; its modulus and phase angle oscillate as a function of frequency. The first minimum of the modulus of the impedance is found at a frequency equal to $f = c/(4l)$, where c is the wave velocity and l is the length of the tube.

The impulse response function for this uniform tube is the pressure measured due to a flow that is a δ-function and consists of a series of equidistant peaks. The time interval between peaks being $2l/c$.

In case of a matched source, the reflected wave is absorbed in the source. The impulse response function at the entrance of a uniform tube consists of only two peaks $2l/c$ s separated from each other. The first peak is due to the δ-function sent into the system and the second peak is the reflected wave. This reflected wave is then absorbed in the source.

The determination of the location of the reflection points will be illustrated on a model described by Wetterer and Kenner [3] consisting of two uniform tubes with different properties in series loaded at the end with a resistor such that positive pressure reflection occurs.

Methods

The impulse response function is the pressure response of a system resulting from a flow that is a unit impulse function (infinitely short in duration and infinitely high with unit area). In the case of the arterial system, application of this excitation is not desirable and the impulse response function should preferably be obtained from the measured pressure drop [p(t)] over and the flow [f(t)] into the arterial system. Fourier transformation of p(t) and f(t) gives $P(n\omega_0)$

and $F(n\omega_0)$, where $\omega_0 = 2\pi/T$ with T the heart period and n is the harmonic number. Input impedance $[Z(n\omega_0)]$ of a linear system is defined by

$$P(n\omega_0) = Z(n\omega_0) \cdot F(n\omega_0) \qquad (1)$$

Laplace transformation of Eq. 1 gives

$$p(t) = \int_0^t z(t-\tau)\, f(\tau)\, d\tau \qquad (2)$$

where $z(t)$ is the impulse response function of the linear system under study. The impulse response function may also be derived from $Z(n\omega_0)$ as follows

$$z(t) = \sum_0^\infty |Z(n\omega_0)| e^{j[n\omega_0 t + \Phi(n\omega_0)]} \cdot \Delta\omega \qquad (3)$$

where $\Phi(n\omega_0)$ is the phase angle of the impedance.
Thus, the impulse response function is periodic and can be calculated both via Eq. 2 and Eq. 3. Because the deconvolution procedure gives rise to a set of unstable equations, we have chosen Eq. 3. To perform the calculation according to Eq. 3, we must know an infinite number of impedance values while in practice only a limited number is known. This means that the summation in Eq. 3 is truncated, which gives rise to superimposed oscillations at the cutoff frequency. The details of the filtering procedure are described elsewhere [1]. The necessary steps to perform the procedure are:
1. Discrete Fourier transformation (N harmonics) of one pair of pressure and flow waves
2. Division of moduli and subtraction of phases of $P(n\omega_0)$ and $F(n\omega_0)$
3. Multiplication of $Z(n\omega_0)$ by Dolph-Chebychev filter of the order 2N
4. Inverse Fourier transformation
The effectiveness of the filter is shown [1] on the impedance of a four-element windkessel model. The theoretic impulse response function of a four-element windkessel is composed of a δ-function plus a doublet (positive and negative δ-function), and an exponentially decaying function with a time constant equal to Rp $\cdot$ C (Rp is the peripheral resistance and C is the total arterial compliance of the four-element windkessel model). Transformation of the truncated input impedance of the model gives rise to oscillations. The filter removes all the oscillations due to the truncation but broadens the initial peak indicating that high frequency information is lost.

Results

Two tubes (a and b) with different properties (Table 1) were connected in series. The distal tube (b) was loaded with a resistor (5000 g cm^{-4} s^{-1}). The specifications in Table 1 are from rubber tubing used in our laboratory and are different from those given by Wetterer and Kenner [3]. The pulse wave velocity in both tubes was approximately the same. With the weighted average value (1004 cm/s)

Table 1. Specifications of the model system

Tube	a	b	
Internal radius	0.95	0.55	cm
Compliance	2.83	1.02	$10^{-6}\,g^{-1}\,cm^4\,s^2$
Length	80	30	cm
Characteristic impedance	407	1189	$g\,cm^{-4}\,s^{-1}$
Wave velocity	1017	970	$cm\,s^{-1}$

of the velocities (1017 and 970) and the frequency of the first minimum, (2.75 Hz) of the modulus of the input impedance (Fig. 1), a length of 91 cm is found, which is an approximation of the total length (110 cm) [2]. The reason that the actual length is not found is that we assumed a uniform tube with an averaged velocity, while in reality a reflection point is present at the connection point. In fact, the reflected wave arriving at the pump is the sum of a wave that returns from the point where the two tubes are joined together (local reflection coefficient: 0.49) and of a wave that returns from the load end of the tube (local reflection coefficient: 0.61). The amplitude and phase of the backward wave, measured at the entrance of the proximal tube, depends on the amplitudes of both the reflected waves and their phase difference and the frequency of the sinusoidal pump. As frequency is varied, this backward wave determines where a minimum in impedance modulus is found. The estimate of total length as described above is the only information about the geometry that we can derive easily from the imput impedance plot. More information is present but is difficult to obtain.

The impedance as shown in Figure 1 was subjected to the filter mentioned above, and the transformation to the time domain was performed with the assumption that the frequency of the first harmonic was 1 Hz (i.e., the impedance is only known at multiples of 1 Hz). The result is shown in Figure 1 (left side). The first main peak is due to reflection at the connection point. The time elapsed since the δ-pulse was sent into the system is 0.16 s, and this is the time a wave traveling with 1017 cm/s needs to run forth and back in a tube of 80 cm length. The second main peak is found at t = 0.22 s. The difference in time between this peak and the previous peak is equal to the time the wave needs to run from the connection point to the load end and back. Thus, the location of the connection point and the load end are easily found with this method. The subsequent positive and negative peaks are due to multiple reflections at the connection point, the load end, and the source and do not contribute to the knowledge about the geometry of the system. They give information, together with the two peaks already discussed, about the reflection coefficients and the damping characteristics of the system.

The question arises: how do we know from the impulse response function that the first two peaks are due to reflection sites in the system and that the subsequent peaks are due to the same two sites and thus the result of multiple reflections.

118

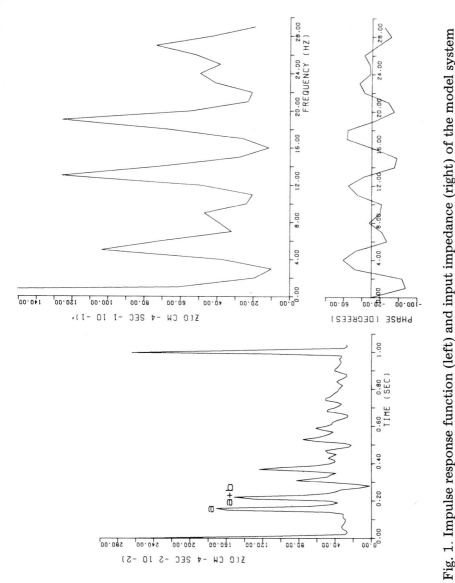

Fig. 1. Impulse response function (left) and input impedance (right) of the model system (source not matched) consisting of two tubes (Table 1) connected in series. The peripheral resistance is 5000 g cm^{-4} s^{-1}. The first two peaks in the impulse response function are due to reflection at the connection point of the two tubes and the load end, respectively. Other peaks are due to mulple reflections

In a system with two reflection sites in series, a peak in the impulse response function is found at:

$$T_p = kT_a + mT_b \qquad k = 1, 2, 3, \ldots ; \qquad m = 0, 1, 2, 3, \ldots$$

with positive or negative polarity, where T_a and T_b are the times required for a wave to travel forth and back in the tubes with lengths a and b, respectively. The first step is to read the time T_a of the first peak and to check if the times when subsequent peaks are found are all multiples of this value (i.e., k assumes all values while m = 0). If this is not the case, a second reflection point is present, and again one checks all the multiples but now also all possible combinations of k an m have to be taken into consideration. If necessary, a third reflection point must be added and the formula above extended accordingly.

The situation would be less complex if we were able to eliminate multiple reflections, then all peaks would be the result of reflections at different sites. This is partly possible. We are able to match the source. i.e., all waves returning to the source are absorbed at the source. However, multiple reflections between other reflection sites connot be prevented. Results for the two-tube system are shown in Figure 2. The input impedance of the matched system is shown on the right, while the impulse response function with matched source is shown on the

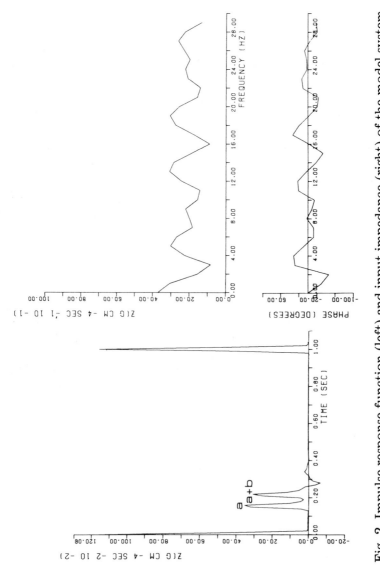

Fig. 2. Impulse response function (left) and input impedance (right) of the model system (source matched) consisting of two tubes (Tables 1) connected in series. Notice that the number of peaks in the impulse response function is considerably reduced, while the input impedance function is still complicated

left. The number of peaks is considerably reduced. A system consisting of one tube with a load at the end gives only one reflected peak in its time domain impedance. More peaks are visible in Figure 2; thus, we have to assume at least one reflection point more. The impulse response function can again be explained with two reflection points.

Conclusions

The impulse response function of a system is the time domain equivalent of the input impedance in the frequency domain and is the pressure measured at the entrance of the system as a result of a flow that is a unit impulse function. Both have a complicated pattern, but from the time domain response function, one can determine where the major reflection points are located, while in the frequency domain, with the assumption of a uniform tube, only an approximation is found for the location of the load end of the system. The pattern in the time domain becomes less complicated if we match the source. Both the locations are now easily found.

The accuracy of the distance for the location of the connection point from the impulse response function is good because it is the local reflection coefficient [2] and not the global reflection coefficient that determines the shape and timing of the reflected peak. Peaks of the time domain impedance function may be the result of summation of different peaks. This will be the case in the arterial system where several parallel ways are present. In that case, one finds an effective length, and the relation with the geometry is not as simple as it is in the case of the two-tube system.

References

1. Laxminarayan, S., Sipkema, P., Westerhof, N.: Characterization of the arterial system in the time domain. IEEE, Trans. Biomed. Eng. BME 25, 177-183 (1978)
2. Sipkema, P., Westerhof, N.: Effective length of the arterial system. Ann. Biomed. Eng. 3, 296-307 (1975)
3. Wetterer, E., Kenner, Th.: Grundlagen der Dynamik des Arterienpulses. Berlin-Heidelberg-New York: Springer, 1968

New Approaches to Electromagnetic Measurement of Blood Flow and Vasomotion Without Recourse to Surgery*

A. Kolin

University of California, Los Angeles, CA 90024 USA

Introduction: Beginnings of Electromagnetic Rheometry

In view of the occasion which honors our friend and colleague, Professor Eric Wetterer, I will go back to the beginnings of the electromagnetic flow meter, i.e., to the middle 1930s when he and I were racing full steam ahead on a collision course toward the same goal, unaware of each other's existence.

Figure 1 shows Wetterer's magnet [29]. It was applied from above to a rabbit's aorta. My first magnet [7], by contrast, was ugly, heavy, and clumsy (a rebuilt, old-fashioned electric motor). We had to put a dog face-down over it and pull the carotid artery out of the neck to fit it between the pole pieces. The second magnet which was completed late in 1936 or at the beginning of 1937 is shown in Figure 2. It weighed about 140 pounds. It could be applied from above with-

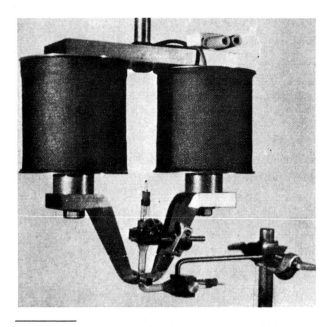

Fig. 1. Wetterer's magnet and electrode assembly. [29]

* This work was supported in part by USPHS Grant HL 17591, by the Alexander von Humboldt Foundation and Medical Testing Systems, Inc.

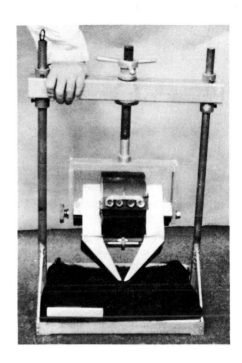

Fig. 2. Kolin's second magnet with adjustable pole pieces (1936-37)

out the need for excessive displacement of the artery from its normal position. It yielded a magnetic field in excess of 10 kG for a gap large enough to accommodate a canine carotid artery. We should keep this image in mind to appreciate the subsequent developments in miniaturization.

Wetterer performed his classic experiments on a rabbit's aorta [29, 30], whereas I used dogs' carotid arteries in my early work [6, 7, 18]. Both of us proceeded in the same way. The exposed artery was sandwiched between the poles of the DC electromagnet, which gave a field in the order of several thousand gauss. A pair of nonpolarizable electrodes, applied externally to the intact artery wall along a diameter perpendicular to the magnetic field, picked up the electric signal induced by the magnetic field in the bloodstream. Figure 3 shows the record of blood flow in a rabbit's aorta obtained by Wetterer in 1937 [29] which is of a quality

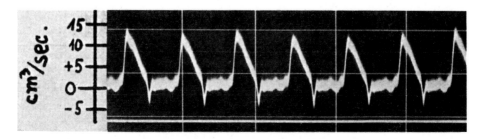

Fig. 3. Tracing of blood flow in rabbit's ascending aorta [29]

that surpasses anything that I have or anybody else has ever achieved subsequently with more elaborate electronic equipment.

Exciting as the early results were, the hopes and enthusiasm of the early workers
were soon damped by the formidable experimental difficulties. The exposure and
exteriorization of the artery were physiologically undesirable conditions and the
"nonpolarizable" electrodes were not performing their function ideally. The
zero-flow base line was not stable due to variable electrochemical potentials, and
it soon became clear that some drastic innovations were necessary to secure the
survival of the method.

Circumstances and/or new interests turned Professor Wetterer's attention toward
fundamental hemodynamic work for which he is being honored today, as well as
for his earlier pioneering work on the electromagnetic flow meter. After Wetterer's
diversion to other fields, a great deal of methodologic development remained to
be done on the electromagnetic flow meter. It was almost literally a voyage along
a river of blood, sweat, and tears, rowing against the current. My present report
will describe a harbor which I recently found on this voyage; but I am not sure
that it is the end of the road. We will see, however, how the greatest obstacle to
the development of the electromagnetic flow meter was turned into a beneficial
asset which opened new avenues to hemodynamic research.

Solution of the Polarization Problem and Emergence of the Transformer EMF Problem

The survival of the method required elimination of electrode polarization and of
the perception of drifts in DC potentials. This was achieved by substitution of
an alternating magnetic field [8, 16] for the constant field of the original approach
[7, 29]. This was a costly victory; while it suppressed polarization and DC drifts,
it introduced a new formidable disturbance, the transformer EMF, which occupied researchers for decades in attempts to eliminate it. While this struggle still
continues, this paper will show how the transformer EMF was turned into a
bonus as the foundation of a new hemodynamic method: induction angiometry.

Two Aspects of Electromagnetic Induction

The term electromagnetic induction is often used quite loosely. It is, however,
essential for us to distinguish two distinct phenomena labelled by this term
which are described by different equations

Lorentz equation: $\qquad \vec{E} = [\vec{v} \times \vec{B}]$ $\qquad\qquad\qquad\qquad$ (1)

Maxwell equation: $\qquad \text{Curl } \vec{E} = \dfrac{d\vec{B}}{dt}$ $\qquad\qquad\qquad$ (2)

Only the first of these equations contains a velocity term $(\vec{v})$. It states that a
moving electric charge "sees" an electric field $\vec{E}$ which is given by the vector
product of the velocity vector $\vec{v}$ and the magnetic field vector $\vec{B}$. Thus, the

Lorentz field $\vec{E}$ is perpendicular to the plane which contains the vectors $\vec{v}$ and $\vec{B}$. It is this equation which describes the law on which the electromagnetic flow meter is based. From it follows the flow meter equation for the configuration of a circular tube in a perpendicular magnetic field (Fig. 4)

$$V_O = 10^{-8} \ B_O d \ \bar{v} \tag{3}$$

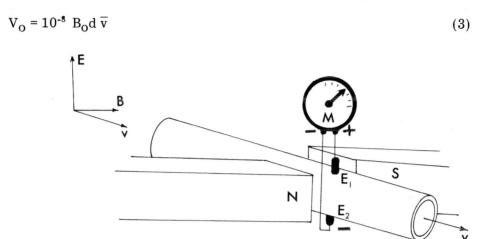

Fig. 4. Scheme of electromagnetic flow meter. E: electric field; B: magnetic field; v: fluid velocity; N, S: magnet poles; E_1, E_2: electrodes; M: sensitive volt meter

(where V_O is the flow signal in volts, B_O the magnetic field in gauss, and d the tube diameter perpendicular to $\vec{B}_O$). Eq. 2, on the other hand, does not contain a velocity term and, hence, cannot give information about fluid flow. It states that in a closed circuit an EMF/unit area (Curl $\vec{E}$) is induced whose magnitude is equal to the rate of change of the magnetic field. Thus, this velocity-independent term does not play a part in flow measurements in a constant magnetic field. However, the introduction of an alternating magnetic field to suppress polarization introduces this disturbing Maxwell term which adds to the flow signal a velocity-independent voltage that can only be determined by stopping the flow, which is not always possible in physiologic observations and is, as a rule, undesirable whenever it is possible.

The closed circuit, in which the "transformer EMF" based on the Maxwell term of Eq. 2 is induced, comprises the blood vessel and the loop formed by the electrode leads conveying the flow signal to the detector input. Due to unavoidable imperfections in flow-sensor construction, there is always a noticeable magnetic field component perpendicular to this loop, which gives rise to a transformer EMF that is given by

$$V_L = -A \frac{dB}{dt} \ 10^{-8} \tag{4}$$

(where V_L is measured in volts, A, the projection of the loop area on a plane perpendicular to the magnetic field, in cm^2, t in seconds, and the magnetic field

125

B in gauss). It is this flow-independent error-voltage against which the electro-magnetic flowmetricians have been waging a 40 years' war since 1938 in order to secure a reliable zero-flow base line.

The first approach to the solution was the use of phase-sensitive detection [17]. This idea is based on the fact that when the magnetic field is sinusoidal

$$B = B_0 \sin \omega t \tag{5}$$

The transformer EMF (quadrature voltage) of Eq. 4 will be given by a cosine function

$$V_L = -10^{-8} A \frac{dB}{dt} = (-10^{-8} A \omega) B_0 \cos \omega t \tag{6}$$

The flow signal of Eq. 3 will, however, be given by a function

$$V_F = (10^{-8} d \bar{v}) B_0 \sin \omega t \tag{7}$$

The waves describing the flow signal and transformer EMF will be 90° out of phase so that the flow signal will be maximal when the transformer EMF is zero. Thus, if we sample electronically the flow signal at its peak, the transformer EMF will be zero at this point, and we will have avoided a falsification of the zero-flow base line level. Unfortunately, the alternating magnetic field does not eliminate electrode polarization completely at the frequencies normally used. This results in a small phase-shift between the flow signal and transformer EMF which are, as a result, not exactly in phase quadrature. To allow the polarization EMF to decay more effectively, a new type of current wave form was introduced which amounts to cutting the sine wave at its apices, moving the segments (a, b, c, d) apart and joining them by horizontal segments (A, B, C) as shown in Figure 5. The detection of the flow signal is then performed near the end of the horizontal sections (A, B, C) while dB/dt = 0. This "interrupted resonance" magnetic field wave form has given us the nearest approach to perfect elimination of the

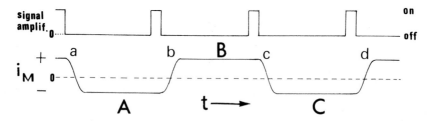

Fig. 5. Magnetic field and magnet current wave form (lower tracing i_M and timing (upper tracing) of signal-sensing in the interrupted resonance scheme. a, b, c, d: intervals of sinusoidal current change; A, B, C: plateaus of constant current and magnetic field. The upper tracing shows when the flow-sensing amplifier is activated ("on"). [22]

transformer EMF [19, 22]. We shall show below how we not only used the segments A, B, C of this new wave form but the alternating field segments, a, b, c, d as well.

Metamorphosis of the Electromagnetic Flow Meter into a Catheter Sensor of Blood Flow and Vasomotion

The initial evolution of the electromagnetic flow meter proceeded from the monstrous dimensions seen in Figure 2 toward miniaturization for adaptation to clinical use and implantation in chronic animal experiments [9, 10, 11]. Figure 6 shows examples of such miniaturization.
This trend of development was abruptly changed by the advent of catheterization techniques in connection with angiography [12]. Mills [13, 25] was the first to take advantage of the new materials and procedures to introduce intravascular devices. He designed a catheter, the tip of which terminated in an inside-out electromagnetic flow sensor [25] shown in Figure 7. He was thus able to introduce such a catheter by a cutdown through a peripheral blood vessel and to obtain flow records in major human blood vessels [26] as shown in Figure 8. It was a breakthrough but not without drawbacks. The device was not an inappreciable obstruction to flow, especially in smaller blood vessels, having a diameter of about 2.7 mm. The ideal orientation at the center of a blood vessel parallel to the flow could not be assured, and whipping motions of the sensor in the pulsating blood stream could occur, thus affecting the flow velocity record. This device was not a flow meter, strictly speaking, but rather a velometer. Its aim was to measure the blood velocity at the center of a vessel. The volume rate of flow had to be inferred from it. This could be done by multiplying the average velocity by the artery cross-section. Unfortunately, one could not take it for granted that the

Fig. 6. Stages in the evolution of the electromagnetic perivascular flow meter.
A: Single-coil coreless flow probe [23]. E_1, E_2: electrodes; Eg: ground electrode; G: ground lead; T: tubing; W_1, W_2, M_1, M_2: electrode- and magnet-coil lead wires; C: magnet coil; S: removable shutter admitting artery through slit.
B: Implantable iron-core flow probe usd in chronic dog preparations. [10] C_2: cylindrincal channel harboring blood vessel; S_2: shutter closing the slot in channel C_2; L_E, L_M: electrode and magnet-leads.
C: Implantable coreless flow probe used in chronic cat preparations. (Reference as in B above). C_1: cylindrical channel (1.5 mm i.d.) harboring the blood vessel; S_1: shutter sealing the slot; T: lead wires.
D: Tracing of phasic blood flow in cat's carotid artery obtained with transducer shown above in C. (From reference cited above in B).
E: Miniature iron core blood flow transducer (1 mm i.d.) compared to underlying aspirin tablet. [2]
F: Tracing of phasic blood flow in rat's carotid artery obtained with the flow sensor in E above. (reference as above in E)

127

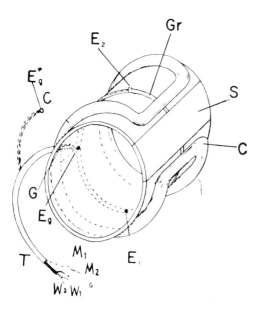

Fig. 6 A, B, C

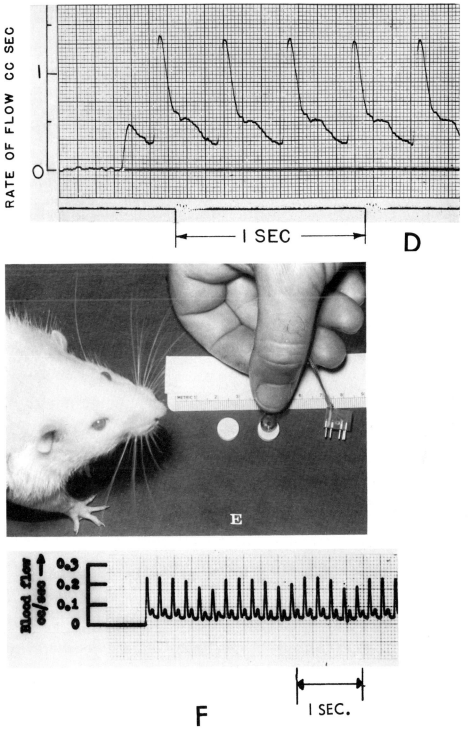

Fig. 6 D, E, F

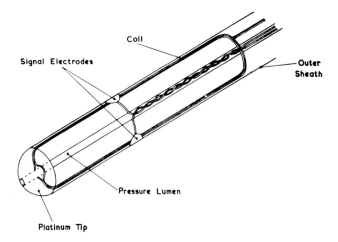

Signal Electrodes

Coil

Outer Sheath

Pressure Lumen

Platinum Tip

Fig. 7. Mills' intravascular catheter velometer. [25]

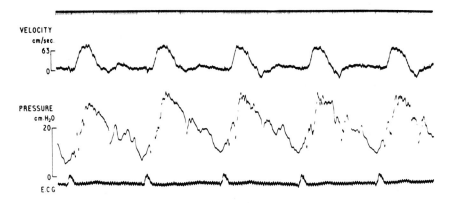

VELOCITY
cm/sec.
63
0

PRESSURE
cm·H₂0
20
0
E.C.G

Fig. 8. Blood velocity in human pulmonary artery (upper tracing) obtained with Mills' catheter probe. [26]

instrument reading yielded the average velocity in the actually prevailing velocity profile. Such an approximation was more valid near the root of the aorta than in the terminal aorta and would have been totally erroneous in a vein.

Loop Sensor With an Extracorporeal Magnetic Field

The above problems as well as the necessity of a cutdown, which represented an undesirable surgical intervention, stimulated me to tackle the problem of measurement of the volume rate of blood flow in deep-seated human blood vessels without surgical intervention. The Seldinger technique permits the introduction of a #7 French angiographic catheter (2.7 mm o.d.) into a peripheral artery through a needle puncture in the skin. This catheter can then be targeted toward various branches of the aorta so that an intravascular sensing device could be introduced through it into a branch artery supplying an organ of interest, e.g., into the renal artery, or the catheter can be used as an access to the aorta to measure flow in it.

The design of a sensor that could be introduced through such a relatively small opening to measure flow in an artery of the size of the aorta faces a paradoxic requirement: it must be small enough to pass through a lumen of about 2 mm and large enough to contact two diametrically opposed points of the artery lumen, which may be as much as 25 mm apart, in order to measure the average flow in the manner of the standard electromagnetic flow meter across a blood vessel diameter.
This problem was solved by a combination of two ideas.
1. The magnet, being the bulkiest part of a flow sensor, was separated from it. The magnetic field was provided by a large magnet coil external to the body [13].
2. The sensor electrodes were mounted on a resilient loop which could be collapsed as it passed through a narrow catheter lumen and expanded spontaneously emerging from the tip of the catheter into the target artery [13].
Figure 9 shows the scheme with an extracorporal magnet and Figure 10 shows photographs of such loop probes as they pass through catheter tubes down to 1 mm in internal diameter. Figure 10 E shows how such a probe can be used to measure flow to a chosen organ. Figure 11 shows examples of blood flow obtained in different arteries in this fashion [19, 21, 28].

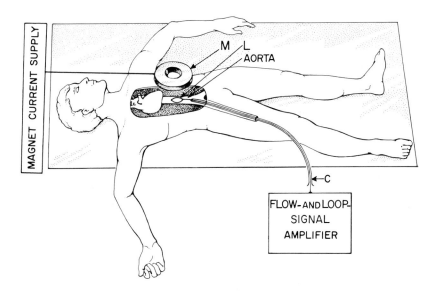

Fig. 9. Scheme for intravascular blood flow and vascular diameter measurement with loop sensor L and magnetic field generated by extracorporeal magnet coil M. [21]

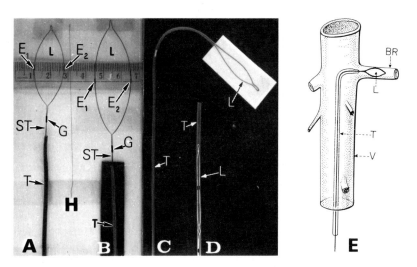

Fig. 10. Flow- and vascular diameter- sensing loop probes L compared in wire thickness to human hair H as viewed against a metric scale. T: angiographic catheters ranging from about 2 mm i.d. in A to 1 mm i.d. in B and C. The loop probe is inside the catheter in D and has partly emerged from a curved catheter in C. E illustrates introduction of a loop probe L into a branch BR of the aorta V through a curved catheter T. [21]

Calibration for Arbitrary Configuration

A self-evident immediate concern when viewing Figure 9 is the question as to how we can calibrate the instrument in view of the variability of distance and relative orientation between the magnet coil and loop sensor. The problem of calibration found a simple solution through the loop-shape of the frame that holds the electrodes. The EMF induced by an alternating magnetic field in the loop depends on the amplitude and orientation of the magnetic field vector in the same fashion as the EMF induced in the fluid flowing between the electrodes. In both cases, it is the component of the magnetic field which is perpendicular to the plane of the loop which is effective in inducing the flow, or the loop-signal. For convenience, we rewrite Eq. 3 by writing $b = (B_0 d)$. We need not know for absolute flow measurement the field amplitude B_0 or the artery diameter d individually. We need only their product b. We obtain thus for the flow signal amplitude

$$(V_F)_0 = 10^{-8} \, g \, b \, \overline{v} \tag{3a}$$

The factor g which we introduced (calling it "Gessner factor") has the following meaning. Eq. 3 is valid for a flow of a conductive fluid through a nonconductive conduit where $g = 1$. When the conduit, like a blood vessel, is electrically conductive and, especially when it is imbedded in a conductive medium, then the flow signal in the blood-stream is reduced due to shunting by ambient tissues by

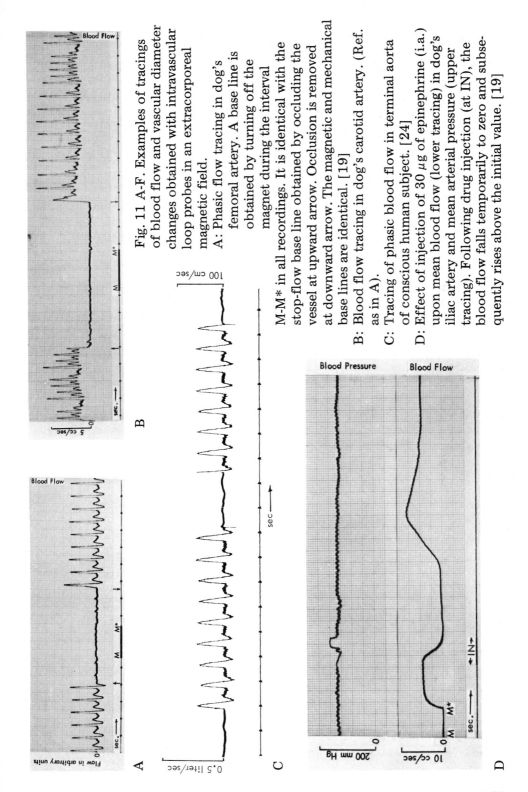

Fig. 11 A-F. Examples of tracings of blood flow and vascular diameter changes obtained with intravascular loop probes in an extracorporeal magnetic field.

A: Phasic flow tracing in dog's femoral artery. A base line is obtained by turning off the magnet during the interval M-M* in all recordings. It is identical with the stop-flow base line obtained by occluding the vessel at upward arrow. Occlusion is removed at downward arrow. The magnetic and mechanical base lines are identical. [19]

B: Blood flow tracing in dog's carotid artery. (Ref. as in A).

C: Tracing of phasic blood flow in terminal aorta of conscious human subject. [24]

D: Effect of injection of 30 μg of epinephrine (i.a.) upon mean blood flow (lower tracing) in dog's iliac artery and mean arterial pressure (upper tracing). Following drug injection (at IN), the blood flow falls temporarily to zero and subsequently rises above the initial value. [19]

133

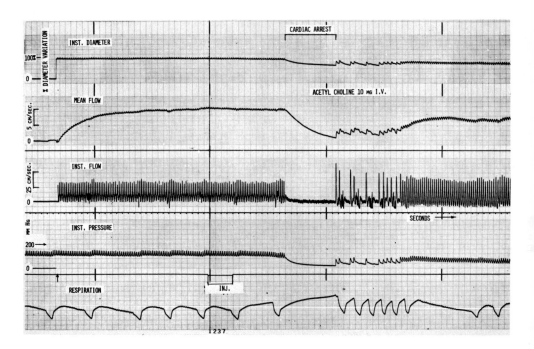

E: Multichannel recording in canine terminal aorta during cardiac arrest of (from top to bottom): instantaneous internal vascular diameter, mean blood flow, inst. arterial blood pressure, and respiration; 10 mg of acetylcholine (i.v.) temporarily stops the heart. The vascular diameter drops with the arterial pressure as does the blood flow. The base line of the instantaneous flow record during cardiac arrest is identical with the base line at the beginning of the record when the magnetic field is zero at full flow. [21]

134

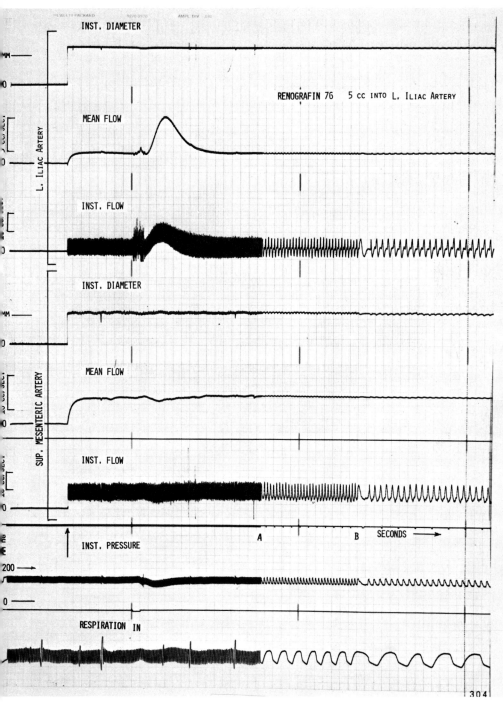

F: Simultaneous recording (with two magnet coils) in two widely separated arteries of blood flow and vascular diameter changes in response to an injection of contrast medium (Renografin 76) into the iliac artery. [21]

135

the factor g which can be inferred from Gessner's calculations [3, 21]. It has the value of 0.8 for the commonly assumed conductivity ratio of $\sigma_2/\sigma_1 = 1/4$ where σ_1 is the conductivity of blood and σ_2 that of the surrounding tissues.

$$g = \frac{\sigma_1}{\sigma_1 + \sigma_2} \quad . \tag{8}$$

In Eq. 6, we do not have the factor $(B_o d)$, but we do have the factor $(B\ A)$ in $V_L = -10^{-8}\ d(BA)/dt$. Thus, the signal derived from the loop is

$$V_L = -10^{-8}\ \omega\ (B_o\ A)\ \cos\ \omega\ t \tag{6a}$$

Since the shape of the loop is such that its area A is very nearly (within about 3%) proportional to the width d of the loop (for compressions not exceeding 1/3), we can write $(B_o A) \cong K\ d$ and obtain

$$V_L \cong -10^{-8}\ \omega\ (B_o\ d\ k)\ \cos\ \omega t = K'b\ \cos\ \omega t, \tag{6b}$$

(where we set $B_o\ d = b$ and $10^{-8}\ K\ \omega = K'$).
The amplitude of the loop signal is then

$$(V_L)_o = K'\ b \tag{9}$$

and the amplitude of the flow signal is from Eq. 3a

$$(V_F)_o = (10^{-8}\ g)\ b\bar{v} = K''\ g\ b\ \bar{v}. \tag{10}$$

From Eq. 10 follows the flow velocity sensitivity S

$$S = (V_F)_o/\bar{v} = K''g\ b\ . \tag{10a}$$

We see from this equation that the quantity b (which is measured by the loop output given in Eq. 9) is a measure of the flow velocity sensitivity of the instrument. Thus, the measurement of b takes into account at once the variability in the artery diameter in the animal as well as of the relative distance and orientation between the sensor loop and the magnet coil, which affect the intensity of the signal-determining magnetic field component.
We can now proceed as follows to calibrate a given flow sensor in an artificial flow system when a known flow traverses a plastic tube in a perpendicular magnetic field generated by a magnet coil fixed at a standard distance from the tube. We shall assign starred symbols to quantities measured in this calibrating setup: S* stands for flow- velocity sensitivity and b* for the loop- output reading. The corresponding quantities measured in the animal in the course of an experiment are S and b. We have then, according to Eq. 10a from measurements in the artificial system and in the animal (remembering that g = 1 in the plastic tube) the following proportion

$$\frac{S}{S*} = \frac{K''g\,b}{K''b*} \tag{11}$$

so that the flow velocity sensitivity in the animal is

$$S = g\left(\frac{b}{b*}\right) S* \tag{11a}$$

Thus, in addition to measuring the flow-induced voltage in the animal, we must simultaneously record the loop output. If we desire to obtain the volume rate of blood flow, we must multiply the mean velocity measured by the instrument by $(\pi/4)d^2$, where d is the radiologically determined diameter of the artery.

Induction Angiometry

In addition to providing a means of calibrating the intravascular flow-sensor, the formerly useless, and in fact disturbing, transformer EMF became the foundation of a new method of studying vasomotion with the same loop sensor that measures blood flow.

We can consider the combination of an AC magnet coil and sensor loop as a transformer in which the magnet coil plays the role of the primary and the loop of the secondary if the spatial relation (i.e., distance and orientation) between the magnet coil and the sensor loop is fixed. Variations in the voltage induced in the loop will indicate variations in the loop area and thus in the diameter of the blood vessel in which the loop dwells, in accordance with Eq. 6b which we can simplify to Eq. 6c for the signal amplitude

$$(V_L)_0 \cong \omega\, c\, d \tag{6c},$$

where c is constant under the assumed conditions and $\omega = 2\pi f$ is proportional to the AC frequency f which does not change. We thus have an angiometer whose output amplitude $(V_L)_0$ is proportional to the blood vessel diameter d. If we assign the value of 100% to the initial diameter, we have the relative measure of all subsequent diameters without the need for a calibration or for knowledge of the absolute diameter value. Of course, if the latter is known, the absolute values of the subsequent diameter dimensions are determined.

The proportionality of the loop signal to the AC frequency shows that one can diminish the strength of the alternating magnetic field, as one makes a compensatory increase in its frequency, without diminishing the angiometer sensitivity. Even at a moderate frequency of 1000 Hz, using a standard sine wave phase-sensitive electromagnetic flow meter channel to detect the loop signal, one can record diameter variations in the order of a micron in a blood vessel of the size of a canine femoral artery. The induction angiometer thus permits one to perform microscopy of vascular diameter changes in situ with a magnification rivaling a good high-power optical microscope [13, 14, 20]

137

The following illustrations demonstrate the capabilities and the sensitivity of the induction angiometer. Figure 12 shows a simultaneous recording of phasic arterial pressure and the concomitant diameter pulsations in a canine terminal aorta [24].

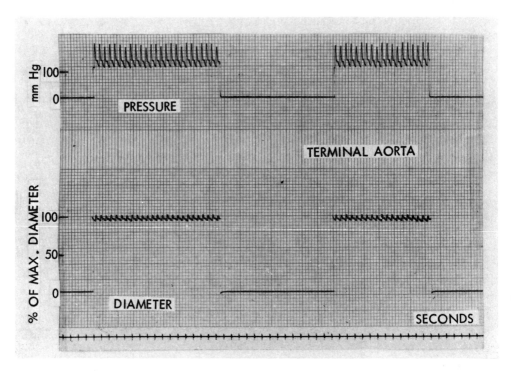

Fig. 12. Pulsatile diameter variations (lower tracing) and instantaneous blood pressure in canine terminal aorta. The blood pressure signal is short-circuited during the intervals when the magnet is turned off to obtain a base line. [20]

When the magnet is turned on, we obtain a deflection which consists of a constant component representing the minimum diastolic diameter with a superimposed pulsating component representing the phasic diameter changes throughout the cardiac cycle. By suppressing the constant component, we can record a greatly amplified diameter pulse [20] which parallels the pressure pulsations as shown in Figure 13. By strong filtration on both sides of the pulsatile tracing, we obtain a recording corresponding to the mean diameter value. By removing the filtration, we visualize the deviations of the pulsatile diameter value from the mean.

Recording of mean diameter values can be accomplished by use of filter circuits with a high signal-to-noise ratio. Figure 14 illustrates the effect of an intra-arterial injection of adrenaline upon the mean diameter of a canine descending aorta. It has also proved possible to simultaneously record the blood flow and diameter changes in an artery and a vein as illustrated in Figure 15.

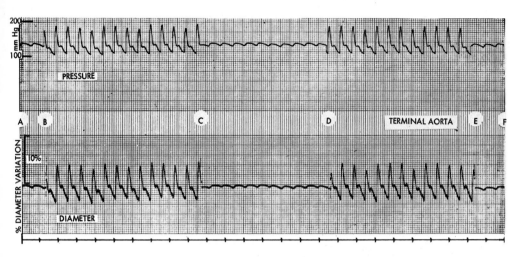

Fig. 13. Magnified pulsatile diameter changes recorded with the induction angio-meter in canine terminal aorta (lower tracing) below tracing of pulsatile arterial pressure changes. The sections A-B, C-D, and E-F are recorded at a high time-constant to establish a reference base line. [21]

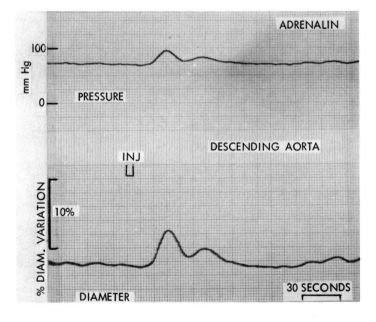

Fig. 14. Effect of adrenaline (40 μg i.v.) upon the mean blood pressure and mean diameter of the canine descending aorta. Diameter changes as low as 0.1% can be perceived in this record. [20]

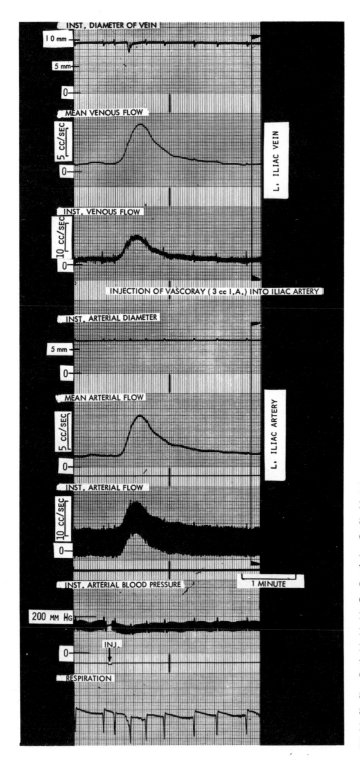

Fig. 15. Simultaneous recording of blood flows and vascular diameter changes in an artery (iliac A.) and the homologous vein (iliac V.) using one extracorporeal magnet coil. Effect of intra-arterial injection of a contrast medium (Vascoray 3 cc into the iliac artery at the arrow marked INJ). The venous as well as the arterial blood flows show an approximately five-fold transient increase. [21]

The following figures illustrate physiologic and pharmacologic observations in animals and man of vasomotion in veins obtained recently in collaboration with Professor E. Bassenge and Dr. J. Holtz in Munich (to be published in detail elsewhere [1, 4, 5]).

Figure 16 shows diameter variations in the inferior vena cava of an anesthetized dog (bottom tracing). The venous and arterial pressure tracings are shown above. While pulsatile changes in venous pressure are barely discernible, concomitant changes in venous diameter in synchrony with pulsatile changes in arterial blood pressure are clearly visible in the first portion of the tracing superimposed upon

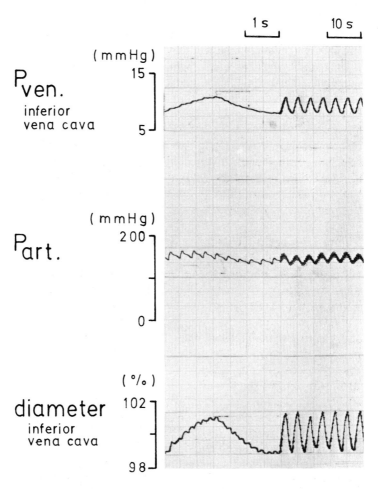

Fig. 16. Induction angiometer tracing (bottom) of the diameter of the canine inferior vena cava below tracings of arterial (P_{art}) and venous pressure ($P_{ven.}$) Pulsatile diameter changes in the rhythm of the heart beat are clearly discerned in the initial fast portion of the record, whereas respiratory diameter changes only are seen in the second, slower portion of the tracing. Diameter variations in the order of 1 μm can be detected. [4]

141

a slow (respiratory) pressure-related vasomotion. The second half of the record, taken at slow paper speed, depicts the respiratory changes in venous diameter and arterial as well as venous blood pressure. This recording demonstrates the sensitivity of the angiometric method (which was by no means maximal in this experiment). One small-scale division represents a diameter change of 0.1% for a 3-mm diameter artery. This corresponds to a diameter variation of 3 μm. Since a deflection of 1/3 mm is still perceptible, we can detect microscopic diameter changes in the order of 1 μm.

Figure 17 shows, at lower recording speed, a tracing of venous diameter variations in a femoral vein of an anesthetized dog (chloralose anesthesia [27]). One clearly sees slow periodic vasomotion. The faster variations are of respiratory origin. They correlate with the respiratory venous pressure variations most clearly seen in the pressure tracing in the thoracic vena cava and are clearly recognizable in the arterial pressure tracing. Respiratory changes in the distal femoral vein pressure (top tracing) are small. The slowest rhythm of venous diameter changes is correlated with the Traube-Hering waves clearly seen in the tracings of arterial pressure. It is worth noting that the venous diameter and arterial pressure Traube-Hering waves are in phase opposition, i.e., the venous diameter is lowest when the arterial pressure is at its peak.

Figure 18 shows dose-response tracings for intravenously administered nitroglycerin in a canine femoral vein (chloralose anesthesia). The active nature of the elicited vasomotion is clearly visible from the fact that the venous diameter rises as the venous pressure falls. The biologic sensitivity of the method is apparent from the magnitude of the venous diameter change recorded for a dose of 0.1 μ g/kg.

Figure 19 is again a Nitroglycerin dose-response tracing, but this time in a canine vena cava. In this case, there is no evidence of active vasomotion; rather, the changes in venous pressure and venous diameter parallel each other. The latter ones are thus passive responses to the changes in venous pressure.

The following two recordings illustrate venous vasomotion in a conscious human subject. In this case, the diameter of a superficial vein does not remain as constant as in an anesthetized dog. There are spontaneous changes, which may, in part, be due to thermal stimuli of air currents or changes in concentration and relaxation of the subject.

In Figure 20, we see the effect upon the diameter in the human cubital vein (a few centimeters above the elbow) of a minute dose (0.4 μ g/kg) of nitroglycerin (administered intravenously). Although the venous pressure is falling slightly, the original downward drift of the venous diameter is reversed abruptly by a steep rise in response to the drug injection. As the nitroglycerin response declines, a Valsalva maneuver is performed which again causes a reversal of the downward trend of the venous diameter, but only initially and briefly, as a passive response to the venous pressure rise. Immediately following, a strong active venoconstriction (at a venous pressure restored to the original value) causes a sharp diameter reduction which drives the recording pen off the scale. The recording shows two venous diameter tracings because an orthogonal loop sensor (as shown in Figure 22) has been used. The two tracings are derived from the two mutually perpendicular loops of this sensor.

142

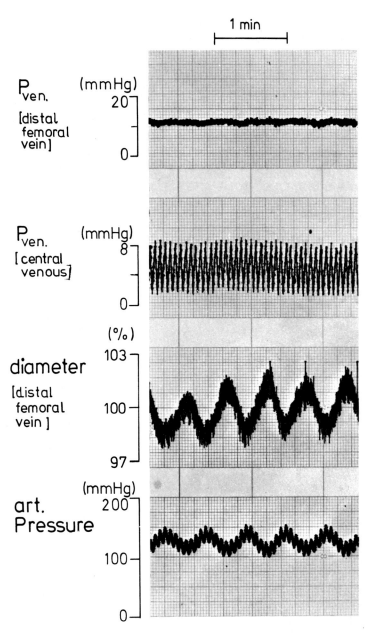

Fig. 17. Variations in the diameter (as recorded with the induction angiometer) of the canine distal femoral vein (second tracing from bottom) correlated with variations in arterial, central venous, and distal femoral vein pressures. The tracing reveals in addition to passive vasomotion in the respiratory rhythm, active venous vasomotion in the rhythm of the Traube-Hering waves clearly seen in the arterial pressure tracing. The latter waves are in phase opposition with respect to the venous diameter undulation pattern. [1]

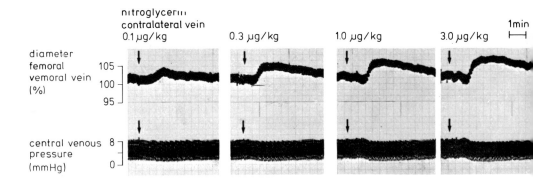

Fig. 18. Correlation between dose and vasomotive response to nitroglycerin as recorded with the induction angiometer in the canine femoral vein. The consistent increase in vascular diameter with concomitant fall in central venous pressure demonstrates active vasomotion in the peripheral vein. [1]

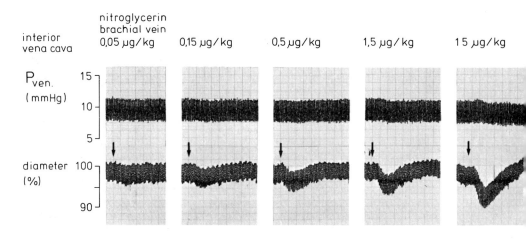

Fig. 19. Correlation between dose and vasomotive response to nitroglycerin as recorded with the induction angiometer in the canine inferior vena cava. Unlike the responses in the femoral vein, the vasomotion in the vena cava is passive exhibiting diminution in vascular diamter with falling venous pressure. [1]

Figure 21 shows the response in the right human cubital vein to a thermal stimulus. The left tracing (A) shows active venous vasoconstriction at a rising venous pressure in response to application of an ice bag to the back of the subject between the shoulder blades. The right tracing (B) again shows active vasoconstriction of nearly constant (only slightly elevated) venous pressure upon submersion of the left (contralateral) hand of the subject into ice water.

144

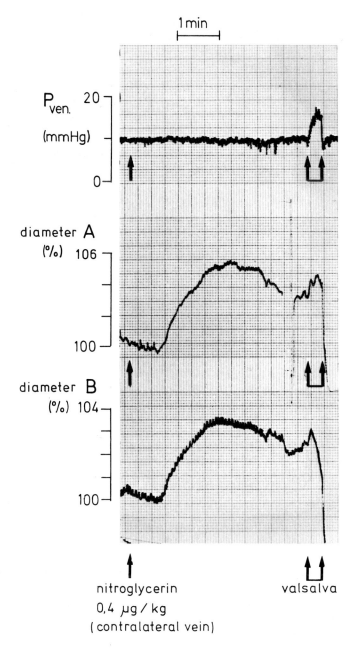

Fig. 20. Vasomotion in the cubital vein of a conscious human subject (Dr. J. Holtz). Response to 0.4 μg/kg of nitroglycerin (i.v.) is recorded for two mutually perpendicular diameters of the vein with an orthogonal induction angiometer sensor (tracings A and B). Active venous vasomotion is clearly seen as the venous diameter increases at nearly constant (slightly declining) venous pressure. A subsequent Valsalva maneuver causes a transient increase of venous pressure and diameter followed by an active venoconstriction at a restored original venous pressure. [5]

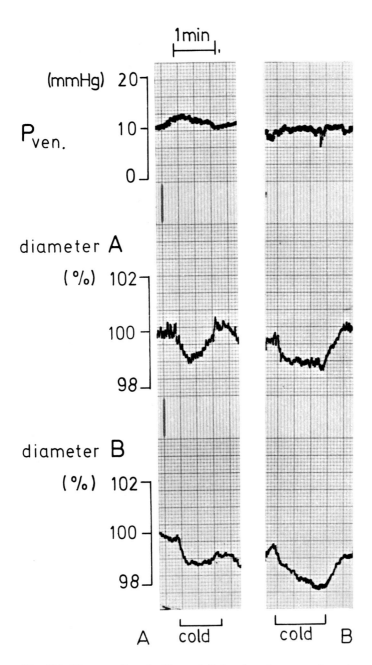

Fig. 21. Vasomotion in the cubital vein of a conscious human subject (Dr. J. Holtz) in response to thermal stimuli.

A: Active venous vasoconstriction at rising venous pressure in response to application of ice bag to subject's back.

B: Active venous venoconstriction at constant venous pressure in response to immersion of contralateral hand into ice water

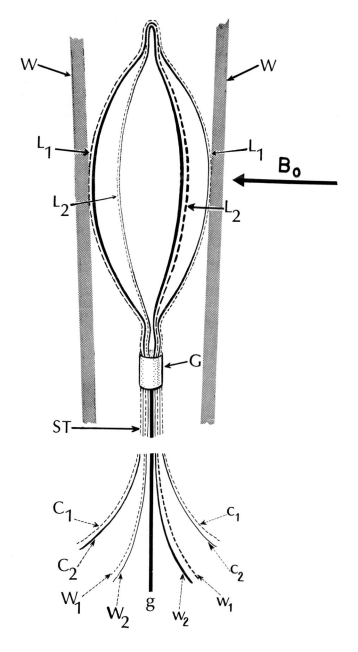

Fig. 22. Orthogonal loop sensor. L_1, L_2: two mutually perpendicular loops; G: ground electrode; St: probe stem; W: vascular wall; B_0: magnetic field vector; C_1, C_2, W_1, W_2; g: lead wires from loops and ground electrode

"Eggbeater" Sensor

We have to explain now how it has been possible to simultaneously record vascular dimensions in two mutually perpendicular directions. This capability is a by-product of an attempt to solve the following experimental difficulty. While one can obtain a flow- as well as diameter-sensing signal from a loop probe in any orientation relative to the magnetic field in which there is a magnetic field component normal to the loop, it is desirable to optimize the orientation. This is advisable not only for the purpose of maximizing the signal, but also for minimizing sensitivity to rotational artifacts.

Unfortunately, it is almost never possible to alter the orientation of the loop continuously by twisting the probe stem or by rotating the catheter. The loop orientation either remains unchanged or jumps into a new unpredictable plane. To circumvent this problem, the following new type of loop sensor has been devised, as shown in Figure 22.

It consists of two mutually perpendicular loop sensors which have been united into one unit. This can be done for flow sensors which are equipped with electrodes as well as for angiometer loops which have none [15]. If the magnetic field is oriented so as to bisect the two loop planes, for instance, we obtain equal angiometer signals from both loops. It is by means of such a sensor that vasomotion has been recorded in Figures 19-21 in two mutually perpendicular planes. It has also been shown that the flow and diameter signals obtained from the two loop components of the eggbeater sensor can be combined vectorially so as to obtain an orientation-independent flow or diameter signal in a round vessel [15].

Outlook on Future Developments

The flow- and diameter sensors have been usually made of "Elgiloy" wires 0.1 mm in diameter. The smallest probes were made of Elgiloy wires as small as 0.075 mm in diameter. The probes are very smooth and flexible, and no injuries to blood vessels have been detected. The method is thus "mildly invasive" and may be suitable for research and diagnostic use in human subjects [5, 24]. This opens new possibilities for studies in human vascular physiology in conscious subjects during routine cardiovascular diagnosis. It also creates the possibility of examining the effect of a drug or other types of treatment on the individual patient instead of relying on statistical inferences based on experimental results derived from observations on nonhuman species and from scanty data on effects in heterogeneous human group samples.

References

1. Bassenge, E., Holtz, J., Kolin, A.: Induction angiometer studies of venous vasomotion in response to Vasoactive Agents (In preparation).
2. Cox, P., Arora, H., Kolin, A.: Electromagnetic determination of carotid blood flow in the anesthezioted rat. IEEE Trans. Biomed. Electronics 10, 171-173 (1963)

3. Gessner, U.: Effects of the vessel wall on electromagnetic flow measurement. Biophys. J. 1, 627-637 (1961)

4. Holtz, J., Restorff, W. v., Bassenge, E., Kolin, A.: Phasic registration of venous diameter changes in-situ with the induction angiometer. Pflügers Arch. (submitted)

5. Holtz, J., Bassenge, F., Kolin, A.: Venous Vasomotion in Man in Response to Pharmacological and Sensory Stimuli. (In preparation).

6. Katz, L.N., Kolin, A.: The flow of blood in the carotid artery of the dog under various circumstances as determined with the elctromagnetic flow meter. Am. J. Physiol. 122, 788-797 (1938)

7. Kolin, A.: An electromagnetic flow meter. Principle of the method and its application to blood flow measurements. Proc. Soc. Exp. Biol. Med. 35, 53-56 (1936)

8. Kolin, A.: Electromagnetic rheometry and its application to blood flow measurements. Am. J. Physiol. 122, 797-804 (1938)

9. Kolin, A.: Electromagnetic Blood Flow Meters. Science, 130, 1088-1097 (1959)

10. Kolin, A.: Blood flow determination by electromagnetic method. In: Medical Physics. Glasser, O. (ed.). Chicago: Year Bk. Med. 1960, Vol. III, p. 275

11. Kolin, A.: Evolution of electromagnetic blood flow meters. In: Pathophysiology of Congenital Heart Disease. UCLA Forum Med. Sci. 10, 383-405 (1970)

12. Kolin: A.: Approaches to Blood Flow Measurement by Means of Electromagnetic Catheter Flow Meters. IEEE Trans. Mag. MAG-6 , 308-314 (1970)

13. Kolin, A.: A New Approach to Electromagnetic Blood Flow Determination by Means of Catheter in an External Magnetic Field. Proc. Natl. Acad, Sci. USA 65, 521-527 (1970)

14. Kolin, A.: Recent trends in approaches to electromagnetic determination of blood flow and outlooks for the future. In: Modern Techniques in the Physiological Sciences. Gross, E., Kaufmann, R., Wetterer, E. (eds.). New York: Acad. Press 1973, p. 81

15. Kolin, A.: A System for intravascular, radially orientation-independent electromagnetic flow- and diameter- sensing. Pflügers Arch. 372, 109-111 (1977)

16. Kolin, A.: An, A.C.: Induction flow meter for measurement of blood flow in intact blood vessels. Proc. Soc. Exp. Biol. Med. 46, 235-239 (1941)

17. Kolin, A., Kado, R.T.: Miniaturization of the elctromagnetic blood flow meter and its use for the recording of circulatory responses of conscious animals to sensory stimuli. Proc. Natl. Acad. Sci. USA 45, 1312-1321 (1959)

18. Kolin, A., Katz, L.N.: Observation de la vitesse instantanée du sang a l'aide du rhéomètre electromagnétique. Ann. Physiol. Physicochimie Biol. 13, 1022-1025 (1937)

19. Kolin, A., MacAlpin, R.N., Snow, H.D., Coster, I.R., Stein, J.J.: Dependability of the non-occlusive baseline of the interrupted resonance electromagnetic blood flow meter system. Life Sci. 16, 501-516 (1975)

20. Kolin, A., MacAlpin, R.N.: Induction angiometer: electromagnetic magnification of microscopic vascular diameter variations in-vivo. Blood Vessels 14, 141-156 (1977)

21. Kolin, A., MacAlpin, R.N., Steckel, R.J.: Electromagnetic rheo-angiometry: An extension of selective angiography. Am. J. Roentgenol. 130, 13-23 (1978)

22. Kolin, A., Steele, J.R., Imai, J.S., MacAlpin, R.N.: A constant field interrupted resonance system for percutaneous electromagnetic measurement of blood flow. Proc. Natl. Acad. Sci. USA 71, 1294-1298 (1974)

23. Kolin, A., Wisshaupt, R.: Single-Coil Coreless Electromagnetic Blood Flow Meters. IEEE Trans. Biomed. Electronics 10, 60-67 (1963)

24. MacAlpin, R.N., Kolin, A., Stein, J.J.: The external field intravascular electromagnetic flow meter system as applied to standard arteriographic catheters and conscious humans. Cathet. Cardiovasc. Diagn. 2, 23-37 (1976)

25. Mills, C.J.: A catheter tip electromagnetic velocity probe. Phys. Med. Biol. 11, 323-324 (1966)

26. Mills, C.J., Shillingford, J.P.: A Catheter Tip Electromagnetic Velocity Probe and its Evaluation. Cardiovasc. Res. 1, 263-273 (1967)

27. Restorff, W.v., Bassenge, E.: Evaluation of a neurogenic rapid coronary dilatation during an excitatory response in conscious dogs. Pflügers Arch. 367, 157-164 (1976)

28. Steckel, R.J., Kolin, A., MacAlpin, R.N., Snow, H.D., Juillard, G.J.F., Tesler, A.S., Metzger, J.: Continuing studies with an intravascular blood flow and vascular diameter sensor: physiologic correlations with radiation protection. Am. J. Roentgenol. (in press)

29. Wetterer, E.: Eine neue Methode zur Registrierung der Blutgeschwindigkeit am uneröffneten Gefäß. Z. Biol. 98, 26-36 (1937)

30. Wetterer, E., Deppe, B.: Vergleichende tierexperimentelle Untersuchungen zur physikalischen Schlagvolumenbestimmung. Z. Biol. 100, 437-474 (1941)

Control Theory and Regulation

Regulation of Blood Volume

Otto H. Gauer

Physiologisches Institut der Freien Universität Berlin 1 Berlin 33 (Dahlem)

In 1850, Ernst H. Weber [18] analyzed the propagation of pulse waves in elastic tubes using a model made of jejunum. This pioneer work on arterial hemodynamics is to my knowledge also the first paper which discusses fundamental problems of volume control without, however, mentioning this section of the treatise in the title. He clearly stated that the transport of fluid through a circulatory system depends not only on the pumping capacity of the heart but also on the adequate filling of the vascular system. As it turned out much later, he made a remarkable contribution toward the quantitative analysis of problems related to volume control when he introduced (on the advice of his brother Edward — as he wrote in a footnote) the term "mittlerer Druck." This entity first reappeared about 100 years later as "mean circulatory filling pressure" [6] or "static pressure" [16]. This pressure can best be measured when the heart is not beating. It is independent of cardiac output and, at a given distensibility of the total vascular bed, a function of blood volume alone. He was also the first — and for many years to come — the only hemodynamicist, who realized the clos interdependence of circulatory function and fluid balance of the organism. His model afforded a very simple demonstration of the fact that, as in the animal circulation, the intravascular volume results from the equilibrium between fluid uptake and fluid excretion; the jejunum was leaky, so he had to continuously replenish the fluid which was lost. This was done with the help of a little funnel, inserted into the system. He was so fascinated by this side issue of his main topic that he tried water infusions into the vascular bed of corpses while measuring presurres. The results were disappointing because the water dissipated quickly into the tissues. At that time, the role of blood colloids had not yet been discovered.

Encouraged by Weber's paper and taking it as a model for this Symposium, I accepted the challenge to briefly present the comparatively unsophisticated problems of blood volume control as an addendum to the brilliant analytic studies of arterial hemodynamics which we have heard.

Definition of Volume Control

When speaking of volume control, we do not mean the homeostatic control of blood volume but the adjustment of the volume to the ever changing size of the

153

vascular bed to assure an adequate filling pressure of the heart which forms the basis of cardiac performance and arterial dynamics.

Principle Mechanisms of Volume Control

The regulation of blood volume comprises the regulation of plasma fluid volume with the electrolytes, plasma protein mass, and the volume of the erythrocytes. There is little known about the regulation of plasma proteins and erythrocyte volume in response to volume stimuli. However, the regulation of plasma volume is accessible to quantitative analysis. As an integral part of the extracellular fluid volume, it results from fluid uptake through the intestines and fluid elimination through kidney, skin, and lungs. Therefore, at a rigidly controlled fluid uptake, the kidney represents an ideal indicator organ for any volume regulatory effort of the organism; blood loss is followed by oliguria, and an isosmotic expansion of blood volume by a blood transfusion results in a diuresis.

Figure 1 depicts the possible pathways for the control of blood volume [3]. The rectangular frame of the diagram is taken from an analogue model of the overall regulation of the circulation [5]. This model, proposed by Guyton and Coleman, is based on the assumption that urine flow is a function of arterial blood pressure. Starting in the upper right corner, the events following a forced increase in blood volume can be described as follows. The increase in blood volume will involve an increase of plasma fluid volume and extracellular fluid volume (ECFV). At a given distensibility of the circulation, the filling pressure of the heart, and hence cardiac output, will rise. As long as total peripheral resistance (TPR) remains constant, arterial blood pressure will increase and induce an increase in urine excretion. Provided fluid intake remains constant, the ECFV will decrease. Thus, blood volume will finally become normal again although with a raised hematocrit.

This scheme will certainly function when there are great changes of blood volume. However, there is now good evidence that under normal conditions the filling pressure of the heart is monitored through mechanoreceptors which control renal function (II) and influence the thirst mechanism (I) via the autonomic nervous system. These two factors together regulate ECFV. Finally, by affecting capillary filtration pressure, this reflex shifts the dividing line between the interstitial fluid volume and the plasma volume to the left or to the right (III). Working through routes I, II, and III, the mechanoreceptors responding to subtle changes in the cardiac filling pressure will induce corrections in plasma volume before the less sensitive mechanism that influences arterial pressure and urine flow via a change in cardiac output has taken effect. Only when the volume gain is large enough to significantly affect cardiac output (mean arterial pressure and/or pulse pressure) will the arterial baroreceptors contribute to the above reflex control mechanism. This is indicated by the thin dotted line connecting the arterial pressure with receptors and the CNS. The following conditions must be fulfilled in order for these low-pressure monitoring mechanisms to function.

154

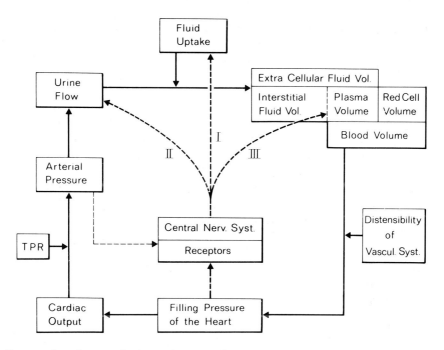

Fig. 1. Pathways for the regulation of extracellular fluid volume and plasma volume by a mechanical feedback mechanism (solid arrows) and by reflex mechanisms involving the autonomic nervous system (broken arrows). Both mechanisms can only function if the filling pressure of the heart is a well-defined function of blood volume. Arrows I and II signify the major efferent pathways by which extracellular fluid volume is controlled; arrow III indicates that, with a constant extracellular fluid volume, plasma volume can still be changed by shifting the dividing line between plasma volume and interstitial fluid volume to the left or to the right (for details see text) [3]

Properties and Location of Receptor Sites for a Reflex Control of Volume

1. Compliance of the Low-Pressure System

Regardless of whether we subscribe to the classic theory of a mechanical feedback mechanism or to the hypothesis of a reflex control involving receptors, the filling pressure of the low pressure system near the heart should be a clear-cut function of blood volume. This is indeed the case. It turned out that the effective compliance Δblood volume/Δ central venous pressure [1] as determined by several groups has the character of a biologic constant. Depending on posture, the effective compliance of man varies between 2.3 and 3.3 ml/(mm Hg · kg BW).

2. Intrathoracic Location of Receptor Sites

Stretch receptors must exist which are very sensitive to changes in intravascular volume. There are two possibilities. The first is that the receptors are uniformly distributed throughout the vascular bed and their input is integrated somewhere in the central nervous system. The second possibility is that — as in the arterial system — an appropriate area monitors the whole system.

While little is known about stretch receptors in the peripheral circulation, all four chambers of the heart are densely populated with a variety of mechanoreceptors, which for many years have been held responsible for reflex changes in heart rate and peripheral resistance [10]. Owing to their great distensibility, the atria with their receptors appear to be ideally suited to record the filling of the low pressure system at this strategically most important section. Especially Paintal's B receptors [13] in the atria have been shown to respond very sensibly to minute changes in passive wall tension induced by small changes of total blood volume [8]. Furthermore, unmyelinated fine endnets [15] are distributed throughout the whole heart, especially the ventricles. Among other functions they seem to record ventricular filling [12]. The major afferent pathways from these receptors lie in the vagal nerves [8, 17]. Nervous activity from mechanoreceptors is, however, also found in cardiac sympathetic fibers [11].

If the hypothesis is correct that the crucial receptor site for a volume control reflex lies in the heart, it should be possible to produce the diuresis of isotonic blood volume expansion not only by a blood transfusion but by any measure leading to increased filling of the intrathoracic vascular compartment alone at the expense of the peripheral capacitance vessels. The most innocuous method of increasing intrathoracic blood volume is by application of mild negative pressure breathing (NPB). This procedure induces an increase in urine flow in anesthetized dogs as well as in men [4, 14] (Fig. 2). In most cases, this was a water diuresis. The early suggestion that this effect was mainly due to a reduction in ADH activity was later confirmed by numerous authors [3]. To determine the volume-sensitive area more precisely, a cherry-sized inflatable balloon was placed into the left atrial appendix of dogs and the chest closed. Inflation of the balloon for 30-45 min produced clear-cut diuresis [7]. The diuresis of left atrial distension could be eliminated by vagus cooling [8] (Fig. 3).

Neurohormonal Effector Mechanisms

In the past 20 years, the balloon technique has been used by numerous groups in many modifications and in both atria. It furnished suggestive evidence that the regulation of ADH activity originates mainly in the left atrium while distension of the right atrium affects more the suprarenal cortical hormones [3].

The NPB technique has been replaced by the technique of whole body immersion. It allows distension of the intrathoracic circulation for hours and even days without significantly disturbing the subjects. Figure 4 demonstrates the change in heart volume [9] and Table 1 the primary and secondary effects on hemodynamics [3]. Immersion to the neck proved to be a very powerful tool to induce strong

156

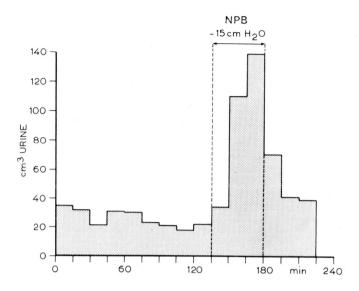

Fig. 2. Induction of diuresis in man by negative pressure breathing (NPB) of
-15 cm H_2O. The slow onset of the effect and its persistence after cessation of
the stimulus suggested that a hormonal factor, probably ADH, is involved [14]

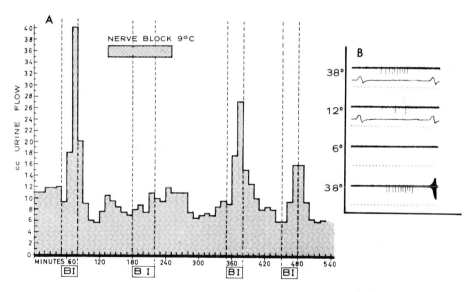

Fig. 3. A: Induction of diuresis in the dog by inflation of a small balloon in the
left atrium (BI). The effect was blocked when the vagi were cooled to below 9°C.
B: Neural activity of an atrial B-receptor recorded from a single fiber in the vagus
at normal temperature and during cooling to 12° and 6°C, respectively. The simultaneously recorded ECG in the upper two traces indicates that the B-receptors
discharge during the passive distention of the atria during diastole [8]

157

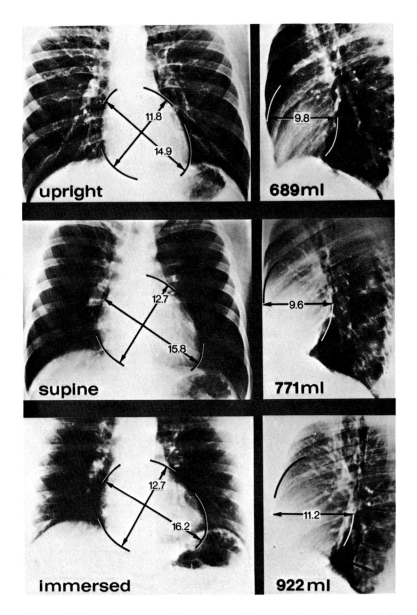

Fig. 4. Effect of postural changes and immersion of the upright standing subject on heart volume. The volumes calculated from the diameters (cm) are given in the right panels [9]

volume regulatory responses of water and mineral metabolism in which all related neurohormonal systems seem to be involved (Fig. 5).

Immersion of 6-8 h leads to a considerable loss of water and sodium and to a reduction of plasma volume by 8%-15%. For a comprehensive documentation of pertinent data, the reader is referred to recent reviews by Epstein [2] and Gauer and Henry [3]. Since the described mechanisms reside at the root of cardiac dynamics and fluid volume regulation, they are ideally suited to decisively contribute to the control of the numerous conditions which are characterized by the interference of hemodynamics and fluid balance [2, 3].

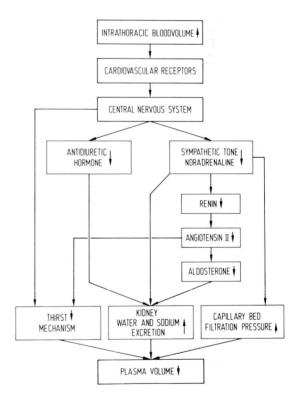

Fig. 5. Major pathways for the reflex control of plasma volume following an expansion of the intrathoracic blood volume. An increase in intrathoracic blood volume will stimulate cardiovascular receptors, thus conveying information to the central nervous system (CNS). The water and sodium regulatory mechanisms are activated via decreased ADH on one hand and sympathetic and renin-angiotensin control of kidney function on the other. Fluid uptake is diminished both due to action in the CNS and via decreased angiotensin effect on thirst. Restraint from fluid uptake and increased fluid excretion together decrease ECFV and hence plasma volume; furthermore, it is possible to affect plasma volume by changing the capillary filtration pressure via the sympathetic outflow. For the sake of clarity, several important points have been omitted, e.g., a possible diuretic and saliuretic hormonal factor, the interaction between the ADH and sympathetic renin-aldosterone system, as well as the possible effects of the various hormones on vascular tone [3]

Table 1. Effects of whole body immersion on circulatory parameters [3]

CIRCULATORY CHANGES INDUCED BY WHOLE BODY IMMERSION*

Primary Effects

Δ Central Blood Volume (L)**	+ 700 ml
Δ Heart Volume (G)**	+ 180 ml
Δ Central Venous Pressure (G, L)	+ 12 to + 18 mm Hg
Δ Intrathoracic Pressure (G, L)	+ 4 to + 5 mm Hg
Δ Transmural Pressure (G, L)	+ 8 to + 13 mm Hg

Secondary Effects

Δ Stroke Volume (L)	+ 35 % ***
Δ Cardiac Output (L)	+ 32 % ***
Δ Total Peripheral Resistance (L)	− 30 %
Δ Peripheral Venous Tone (G)	− 30 %
Δ Arterial Pressure (L)	+ 10 mm Hg****

*Subject standing or sitting erect in air versus standing or sitting in water

**(G) Gauer and Co-workers; (L) Lundgren and Co-workers.

***Heart rate was unchanged

****The arterio-venous pressure gradient was not changed since CVP was increased by the same amount.

Acknowledgment: The editorial help of Miss L. Schepeler is gratefully recognized.

References

1. Echt, M., Düweling, J., Gauer, O.H., Lange, L.: Effective compliance of the total vascular bed and the intrathoracic compartment derived from changes in central venous pressure induced by volume changes in man. Circ. Res. 34, 61 (1974)
2. Epstein, M.: Cardiovascular and renal effects of head-out water immersion in man. Application of the model in the assessment of volume homeostasis. Circ. Res. 39, 619 (1976)
3. Gauer, O.H., Henry, J.P.: Neurohormonal control of plasma volume. In: Cardiovascular Physiology II. Guyton, A.C., Cowley A.W. (eds.) Baltimore-London-Tokyo, U. Park Pr., 1976, p. 145
4. Gauer, O.H., Henry, J.P., Sieker, H.O., Wendt, W.E.: The effect of negative pressure breathing on urine flow. J. Clin. Invest. 33, 287 (1954)

5. Guyton, A.C., Coleman, T.G.: Longterm regulation of the circulation: Inter-relationships with body fluid volumes. In: Physical Bases of Circulatory Transport. Regulation and Exchange. Reeve, E.B., Guyton, A.C. (eds.). Philadelphia-London: Saunders 1967 p. 179

6. Guyton, A.C., Polizo, D., Armstrong, G.G.: Mean circulatory filling pressure measured immediately after cessation of heart pumping. Am. J. Physiol 179, 261 (1954)

7. Henry, J.P., Gauer, O.H., Reeves, J.L.: Evidence of the atrial location of receptors influencing urine flow. Circ. Res. 4, 85 (1956)

8. Henry, J.P., Pearce, J.W.: The possible role of cardiac atrial stretch receptors in the induction of changes in urine flow. J. Physiol. 131, 572 (1956)

9. Lange, L., Lange, S., Echt, M., Gauer, O.H.: Heart volume in relation to body posture and immersion in a thermo-neutral bath. A röntgenometric study. Pflügers Arch. 352, 219 (1974)

10. Linden, R.J.: Function of cardiac receptors. Circulation 48, 463 (1973)

11. Malliani, A., Recordati, G., Schwartz, P.J.: Nervous activity of afferent cardiac sympathetic fibres with atrial and ventricular endings. J. Physiol. 229, 457 (1973)

12. Öberg, B., Thorén, P.: Studies on left ventricular receptors, signalling in non-medullated vagal afferents. Acta.Physiol. Scand. 85, 145 (1972)

13. Paintal, A.S.: Vagal sensory receptors and their reflex effects. Physiol. Rev. 53, 159 (1973)

14. Sieker, H.O., Gauer, O.H., Henry, J.P.: The effect of continuous negative pressure breathing on water and electrolyte excretion by the human kidney. J. Clin. Invest. 33, 572 (1954)

15. Sleight, P., Widdicombe, J.G.: Action potentials in fibres from receptors in the epicardium and myocardium of the dog's left ventricle. J. Physiol. 181, 235 (1965)

16. Starr, I.: Role of the "static blood pressure" in abnormal increments of venous pressure, especially in heart failure. (II. Clinical and experimental studies.) Am. J. Med. Sci. 199, 40 (1940)

17. Szczepanska-Sadowska, E.: The activity of the hypothalamo-hypophysial antidiuretic system in conscious dogs. II. Role of the left vagosympathetic trunk. Pflügers Arch. 335, 147 (1972)

18. Weber, E.H.: Über die Anwendung der Wellenlehre auf die Lehre vom Kreislaufe des Blutes und insbesondere auf die Pulslehre. Verh. Königl. Sächs. Ges. Wiss. Leipzig, 3, 164 (1850)

Changes in Blood Flow-Distribution During the Application of Multiple Stresses

E. O. Attinger and F. M. L. Attinger

Division of Biomedical Engineering, University of Virginia, Charlottesville, VA 22901, USA

Until recently, the quantitative analysis of the cardiovascular system was focused primarily on the mechanical properties of the heart and the cardiovascular tree, as well as on the physicochemical properties of the blood. A variety of models were developed dealing either with overall input-output relationships (mostly lumped parameter models) or with the pulsatile nature of blood flow and pressure (mostly distributed parameter models). The investigation of cardiovascular control systems by means of such models was limited largely to isolated control functions such as cardiac and blood volume control, chemo- and baroreceptor reflex loops, and autoregulation [4, 10, 14, 16, 18].

As this work progressed, it became increasingly clear that the proposed, relatively simple control schemes based on such models could not account for many changes in cardiovascular performance, particularly under conditions of multiple mental or physical stresses [12, 21]. One of the major reasons for the discrepancy between model predictions and experimentally observed changes relates to the large variety of complex and variable interactions between and within components and subsystems of any biologic system functioning within its natural environment.

Guyton [11] has attempted to integrate many different control functions into a comprehensive model of the cardiovascular system. While the predictions of this model are fairly accurate for the simulation of the development of arterial hypertension, it is not clear how the model would respond to multiple disturbance applied simultaneously.

Since the transportation of fuel and waste represents not only an essential task of the cardiovascular system but also involves other biologic subsystems, we chose the oxygen transport system (O_2-TS) as the basis for our analysis. We hypothesized that the design of the O_2-TS was based on performance optimization and that maximal delivery at the site of need at minimal cost and without interference with other body functions represented the optimization criterion [3, 15]. While it is intuitively obvious that cost (O_2 requirements of the cardiac and respiratory pumps) can become performance limiting, particularly during severe stress, and that changes in flow distribution and O_2 extraction rates represent a much more efficient mechanism for an increase in local O_2 delivery, little attention has been paid by previous investigators to the need for protecting other "consumers," if

Supported in part by PHS grants HL 11747 and GM 01919

such a scheme were really adopted. The presence of multiple consumers in different states of activity competing for the same limited resources also implies a hierarchy of control systems in which decisions are made at different levels depending upon changing local and overall (global) priorities. In order to test our hypothesis, we designed a series of experiments in which we studied the redistribution of blood flow between muscle, leg, and other organ systems when the muscles were electrically stimulated.

Methods

The basis of our approach is diagrammatically illustrated in Figure 1. We chose a muscle group in the hind leg as the bed under investigation and monitored its blood flow and blood composition as it was electrically stimulated (5-10 V, 5 Hz for 2 min). Since our hypothesis postulated that the increase in blood flow would, at least initially, be achieved by a redistribution of flow between "nutrient" and "shunt" flow channels, we also monitored the total blood flow to the leg. In the first series, we used the gracilis muscle and studied the blood flow distribution in one leg only. In the second series, we chose the biceps muscle, which has two inflow channels, and monitored in addition the blood flow to the contralateral leg. In the third series, we stimulated the sciatic nerve and hence most of the muscles in one leg and simultaneously measured cardiac output, blood flow to the forepart of the animal, the gut, the kidneys, and to the contralateral leg. As more global variables were added to the experimental protocol (blood flows to other beds), some of the local variables were discarded, since their response pattern had been established in the earlier experiments (local oxygen consumptions and venous blood composition).

The experimental technique has been described in detail elsewhere [5] and is only summarized here. All experiments were carried out in dogs anesthetized with chloralose-urethane. Blood flow was measured by means of electromagnetic flow meters and arterial pressure through Statham pressure transducers. Venous oxygen content was monitored continuously either by means of a densitometer (O_2 saturation) or a radiometer analyzer using a flowthrough cuvette (pO_2). Arterial blood was analyzed for pO_2, pCO_2, and pH by means of a second radiometer system. In all cases, ventilation (tidal volume and respiratory rate) and total oxygen uptake were monitored by a servocontrolled spirometer system. Heart rate was obtained on-line from the electrocardiogram.

Data Analysis

All the data were sampled at 250 Hz and averaged over one or more cardiac cycles. Control values were obtained over a 60-s interval. Four parameters were used to characterize the response: time delay, initial slope of the response, maximum (or minimum) of the response, and the average value during the 2-min stimulation [1, 5]. Since most of the variables were nonnormally distributed, we used primarily nonparametric statistics (cluster and principal component analysis) for

163

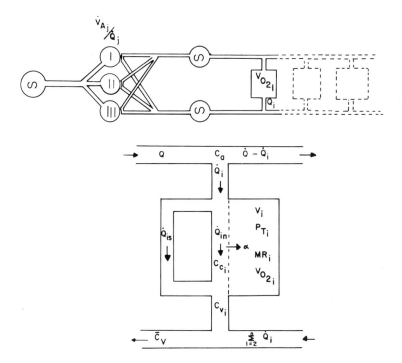

Fig. 1. A distributed parameter model of the oxygen transport system (top) and details of one model block representing the ith peripheral vascular bed (bottom). $\dot{V}_{Aj}|\dot{Q}_j$: local ventilation-perfusion ratio; $\dot{Q}$: blood flow (l/min); $\dot{Q}_i$: blood flow into the ith vascular bed; $\dot{Q}_{is}$: "shunt flow" through the ith bed; $\dot{Q}_{in}$: "nutritive flow" through the ith bed; C_a: arterial oxygen content; C_{ci}: oxygen content in nutritive capillaries of ith bed; C_{vi}: oxygen content of venous blood leaving the ith bed; C_v: oxygen content of mixed venous blood; V_i: volume of tissue supplied by ith bed; P_{Ti}: tissue oxygen tension of ith bed; MR_i: metabolic rate of tissue supplied by ith bed; $\dot{V}_{O_{2t}}$: oxygen uptake from ith bed; a: local extraction rate for O_2. The three circles ⊙ represent the respiratory pump, the left and right heart, respectively; the other three circles represent lung regions with different ventilation-perfusion ratios.

the analysis [1, 6], having verified their validity by means of a simulated, hierarchically structured model [8].

The analytic approach was aimed at reducing the dimensionality of the system in order to obtain a parsimonious, hierarchical representation of its behavior in terms of intrinsic or latent dimensions which are smaller in number than the observed or manifest variables. In practice this involves the combination of various measurements in the different dimensions making up the system's profile at a given moment and under different conditions of stress by means of some multivariate statistical technique.

Cluster analysis is, of course, not a statistical method in the strict sense. Each individual of a multivariate sample may be represented by a point in a multidimensional Euclidean space. Cluster analysis attempts to group these points into disjoint sets which, hopefully, correspond to characteristic features of the sample. Different methods of cluster analysis of the same sample may assume different geometric distributions of the points or may employ different clustering criteria or may differ in both respects. But the criteria underlying most clustering methods can be interpreted in terms of the distances between the centroids of the clusters. Classic linear factor analysis assumes independent, unique factors responsible for changes in a set of variables, i.e., the factors are an unknown combination of latent variables. In contrast, in principal component analysis, the factorization is unique, for the component coefficients have been chosen to partition the total variance orthogonally into successively smaller portions, and if the positions are distinct, only one set of coefficient vectors will accomplish this purpose. By inverting the principal component analysis, one can arrive at the factors obtained by the traditional factor analysis. Since both of these methods are based on linear equations, differences between the results may cautiously be interpreted as nonlinear interactions.

Results

Table 1 summarizes the most important data. Since our monitoring system was not capable of following the dynamics of changes in oxygen uptake, these data represent average values (Means and standard deviation) for control and response. The response values are normalized with respect to the control data, but the statistical significance of the difference between control and response values was obtained from pairwise comparision of the absolute values. The first column represents the experiments carried out in mongrel dogs on the gracilis muscle. The second and third columns contain the data from experiments involving the stimulation of the biceps or the entire leg carried out in racing greyhounds, and the last column represents the data obtained in large mongrel dogs where blood flow to the major organ systems was monitored. (The size and type of dogs used probably accounts for the difference in leg blood flow [9] between the different series). During the early part of the preparation, heart rates were usually in the order of 120 beats/min but rose to around 190 during the 5th and 6th hr of preparation. These high heart rates, indicating an increase in sympathetic tone, may account for the smaller than expected changes in this variable. In all series, there was a significant increase in ventilation and oxygen consumption during stimulation. The gracilis data indicate a marked increase in muscle flow and muscle oxygen consumption with a decrease in the O_2 content of the muscular venous outflow. There was no corresponding increase in the blood flow to the leg. As larger muscle masses were stimulated (columns 2 and 3), blood flow to the stimulated leg increased, while that to the contralateral leg decreased. The O_2 content of the venous outflow of the leg fell significantly while there was no consistent change in the composition of the venous outflow of the stimulated muscle. The sum of these changes implies a significant increase in the O_2 consumptions of the stimulated muscle as well as of the leg. The last column indicates that these changes were achieved without a significant increase in cardiac output, thus validating

Table 1. Effect of electric stimulation of different leg muscle groups on the O_2 transport system

	Stimulation of muscle				Stimulation of leg			
	Gracilis		Biceps		Biceps		Flow distribution	
	control	response	control	response	control	response	control	response
	(No. = 11)		(No. = 13)		(No. = 12)		(No. = 19)	
HR	193.8 ± 15.6	1.04	193.2 ± 5.4	.92	201.3 ± 8.1	1.1[b]	155 ± 7.65	1.04
C.O.	—	—	—	—	—	—	3.56 ± .34	1.04
RR	21.8 ± 3.4	1.65	16.7 ± 1.03	1.28	17.5 ± 8.45	1.13	29.6 ± 2.48	1.14[b]
MV	6.9 ± .96	1.59[b]	8.07 ± 1.0	1.37[c]	8.45 ± 1.06	1.89[c]	9.68 ± 1.21	1.30[b]
Pa	209.1 ± 5.0	.97[b]	231 ± 8.75	.97[b]	226 ± 4.8	.99	162 ± 8.5	.94
PaO_2	157.7 ± 10.9	1.06	115 ± 5.1	1.02	112 ± 6.8	1.03	95 ± 8.7	1.01
PvO_{2L}	53.5 ± 4.0	.95	63.7 ± 2.7[a]	.9[c]	69.7 ± 5.7[a]	.85[b]	—	—
PvO_{2M}	43.6 ± 3.2	.86[b]	31.9 ± 3.4	1.13	34.7 ± 1.9	1.11	—	—
$\dot{Q}_L$	51.7 ± 8.3	1.076	246 ± 28.8	1.17[c]	193.5 ± 2.1	1.77[c]	159 ± 21.3	1.83[b]
$\dot{Q}_M$	8.1 ± 2.0	1.965[b]	66.1 ± 12.86	2.95[c]	53.6 ± 8.4	3.14[c]	—	—
$\dot{V}O_{2T}$	223.1 ± 10.5	1.062[b]	343.8 ± 19.8	1.15[c]	336 ± 20.4	1.25[c]	192 ± 8.1	1.11[c]
$\dot{V}O_{2L}$	3.0 ± .5	1.269	—	—	—	—	—	—
$\dot{V}O_{2M}$	.6 ± .1	2.58	—	—	—	—	—	—
$Q_{Lcontra}$	—	—	197 ± 34.2	.82	157.8 ± 9.8	.97	69 ± 10.5	.93[b]

[a] Venous O_2 saturation. [b] $a < .05$. [c] $a < .01$.

166

the hypothesis that redistribution of blood flow represents a preferential mode for increased O_2 delivery under the conditions of our experiments. It also should be noted that arterial pressure decreased only during stimulation of the muscle but not during stimulation of the entire leg.

In order to assess the relationships between the changes in the individual variables, we used Pearson's product moment correlation. Table 2 represents the results in terms of statistical significance for the gracilis data. The variables are divided into five groups:

1. Central variables: (heart rate, respiratory rate, minute ventilation, and arterial pressure)
2. Supply variables: arterial pO_2, blood flow to the leg, and to the muscle
3. Demand variables: total O_2 consumption, O_2 consumption of the leg, and of the muscle
4. Criterium variables: AV O_2 differences for the leg and for the muscle, and venous pO_2 for both the leg and muscle
5. Control variables: the ratios of muscle to leg flow and of muscle to leg O_2 consumption

The lower half of the matrix is based on both control and response data, while the upper half represents only response data. It is apparent that the criterion variables are strongly correlated with the first three central variables. So are the supply and demand variables. The control variables correlate strongly with demand variables, the AV O_2 difference across the leg (a criterium variable), and arterial pressure.

Both cluster and principal component analysis yielded similar results as indicated in Figures 2 and 3. The data are plotted in the factor space (indicating the intrinsic dimensions of the system). The contours around the different variables represent the results of the cluster analysis, the dash-dot lines between the cluster configurations indicate that the separation between clusters is statistically significant ($a < .05$, Mountford B statistic [8]). For the control data, three factors account for 87.5% of the variance. The first factor (40.5% of the variance) is loaded positively by the AV O_2 differences and heart rate, and negatively by the venous pO_2 tensions and the local control variables. The second factor (31.5% of the variance) represents all the supply and demand variables. The third factor (15.5%) is characterized by the respiratory variables in the positive and by arterial pressure in the negative region. During stimulation, the picture changes considerably. Four factors are now needed to account for 89% of the variance. The first factor (35% of the variance) contains the local supply and demand variables as well as arterial pressure. The general demand variable O_2 consumption loads on factor 4 (7.2% of variance). Factor 2 (32% of variance) contains the venous pO_2s in its negative region and the central variables heart rate and respiration in its positive region. The local control variables load on factor 3 (14% of variance). We interpret these results as follows: in the control state, the system can be characterized by three dimensions as far as average values are concerned. The most important one represents a local control dimension, with which heart rate is also associated. The second is characterized by supply and demand variables. The third, and least impor-

Table 2. Electrical stimulation of gracilis. Pearson moment correlation: levels of significance of correlation coefficients [upper half: stimulation; lower half: both control and response data]

	1	2	3	4	7	10	11	12	13	14	5	6	8	9	15	16
1 HR								.001	.002							(.08)
2 RR			.001			(.1)	(.06)	(.1)			(.08)		(.08)		(.07)	
3 V	.05	.001				(.08)	(.07)				(.08)		(.06)	.05		
4 Pa						.04		.03	.001		.03		(.06)		(.07)	.004
7 P_{aO_2}						(.1)				.03						
10 $\dot{Q}_L$		.04	.03	.01	.05		.03		.001	.001		.004				
11 $\dot{Q}_G$		.04	(.07)		.02	.001			.02	.001		.003				
12 $\dot{V}_{O_2 T}$		(.09)		.002	.01	(.08)	.01				.003	(.1)				
13 $\dot{V}_{O_2 L}$	.05			.007		.001	.002			.02	(.1)	(.1)	.05			
14 $\dot{V}_{O_2 g}$		(.08)			.03	.001	.001	.02	.001			.02			.02	.04
5 Av_L	.02	.04	.03	.1		.023	.026	(.06)	.006				.004	(.07)	.02	.02
6 Av_g		(.07)	.04		(.07)			(.08)			.007					.02
8 $P_{vO_2 L}$	.001	.05	.03						.001		.001	.05		.001		
9 $P_{vO_2 G}$	.001	(.07)	.03						.03		.009	.001	.001			
15 $\dot{Q}_G/\dot{Q}_L$		(.09)		.007				.006	.001	.001	.03					.002
16 $\dot{V}_{O_2 G}/\dot{V}_{O_2 L}$	.07			.001				.04	.04	(.09)	.02		.04		.001	

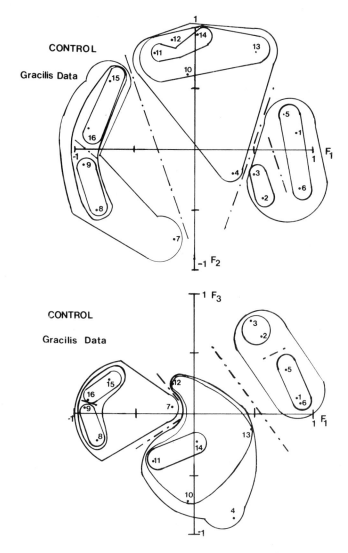

Fig. 2. Results of principal component analysis (on gracilis data control state). The data can be reduced to three intrinsic dimensions, labeled here F_1, F_2, and F_3. The contours around the different variables (represented by numbered dots) show the results of the cluster analysis on the source data. Dash-dot lines between the cluster configurations indicate that the separation between clusters is statistically significant ($a < .05$). The key for the variables is as follows:

central variables: heart rate 1, respiratory rate 2, ventilation 3, arterial pressure 4;

supply variables: arterial pO_2 7, leg flow 10, muscle flow 11;

demand variables: total O_2 consumption 12, leg O_2 consumption 13, muscle O_2 consumption 13;

criterium variables: AV difference leg 5, AV difference muscle 6, Pv_{O_2} leg 8, Pv_{O_2} muscle 9;

control variables: muscle flow/leg flow 15, V_{O_2} muscle/V_{O_2} leg 16

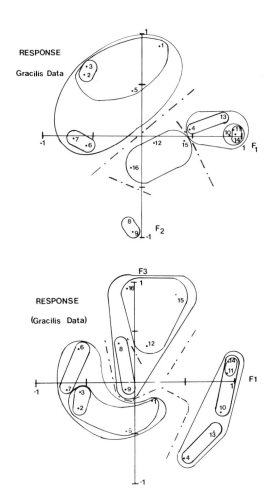

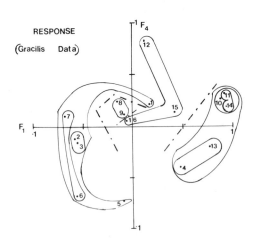

Fig. 3. Results of principal component analysis and cluster analysis for gracilis data (response state). A fourth dimension, characterized by total V_{O_2} (12) has emerged. (symbols as in Fig. 2)

tant, represents a central control dimension. During stimulation, local supply and demand dimensions assume a major importance. The importance of central control has increased and is also coupled to local performance criteria (factor 2). The importance of local control has decreased (factor 3) and a new dimension, general demand, is emerging.

Figure 4a shows the results of the cluster analysis of the biceps data during muscle stimulation (column 2 in Table 1). Both control and response data were clustered together. The first cluster group (top) represents the demand-supply dimension. Note that local and general supply variables are separated, oxygen consumption being associated with the former and the pO_2 of the outflow from the muscle with the latter. The next group of variables represents a central dimension. The first five variables indicate central outputs subject to the influence of the O_2 saturation of the venous outflow from the leg (dimension 3 in Fig. 3). The central control of the resistance of the contralateral leg is clearly separated from the other central outputs. The last cluster group at the bottom represents local control at two levels: control of muscle flow and control of the supply to the corresponding leg.

During stimulation of the leg (Fig. 4b), a considerably larger stress, the supply-demand dimension contains all blood flows (with the exception of the flow to the contralateral leg) without the separation seen in Figure 4a. The central outputs, arterial pressure and flow to the contralateral leg, are separated from those which are under the influence of local inputs (HP, RP, and O_2 saturation in the leg vein). Central control (R_o) is again differentiated from the two local control levels.

The picture becomes somewhat more complex if one considers the cluster analysis of the 23 variables monitored during the flow distribution experiments (Fig. 5) [8]. The two main clusters for both control and response values represent a supply-demand dimension and a control dimension respectively. The first subcluster of the former links total O_2 uptake with the ventilation-perfusion ratio and the ratio of flow to the stimulated leg to cardiac output. A partial regression analysis showed that the change in VO_2 was most highly correlated with the change in the ventilation-perfusion ratio, both during normoxia and hypoxia. Renal flow (Q_{23}) is also associated with this cluster although it never changed significantly between control and stimulation. The second cluster contains cardiac output (Q_0) and blood flow to the forepart of the animal (Q_{01}) on the one hand, flow to the stimulated leg (Q_4), the gastrointestinal tract (Q_{12}), and the contralateral leg (Q_5) on the other hand. Note that Q_{12} and Q_5 represented the primary suppliers for the increased blood flow in the stimulated leg. As in the previous series, blood flow to the contralateral leg is closely linked with arterial pressure.

The control dimension consists of three cluster groups. The one on top represents local control (R_4 and R_4/R_0) and, as in the previous series, is associated with a central variable (heart rate in the control state, respiratory rate during stimulation). Next follows a cluster of intermediate control, characterized primarily by the resistance to the contralateral leg. The central control cluster contains, of course, R_0, the total peripheral resistance as well as the resistance to the forepart of the animal.

171

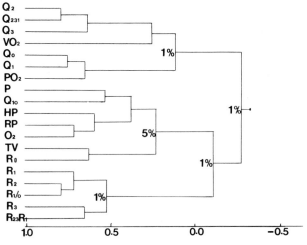

BICEPS(Muscle) control and response data

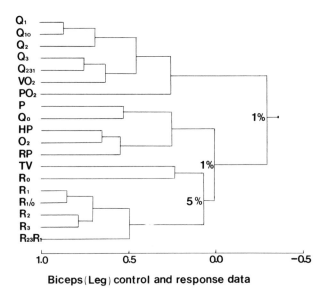

Biceps(Leg) control and response data

Fig. 4. Cluster analysis of biceps data.
a) Control and response data during muscle stimulation.
b) Control and response data during leg stimulation.
Q_0: flow to contralateral leg; Q_1: Flow to stimulated leg; Q_2 and Q_3: upper and lower inflow to the biceps muscle; $Q_{1/0}$: ratio of both leg flows; $Q_{23/1}$: ratio of muscle to leg flow; V_{O_2}: total O_2 consumption; P: arterial pressure; HP: heart period; RP: respiratory period; TV: tidal volume; P_{O_2}: O_2 tension of muscle outflow; O_2: O_2 saturation of leg outflow. The subscripts of the resistances (R) correspond to those of the flows (the numbers separating the different cluster configurations indicate the significance levels of the dissimilarities)

172

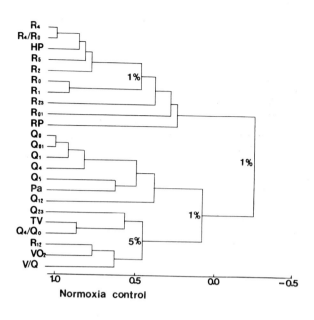

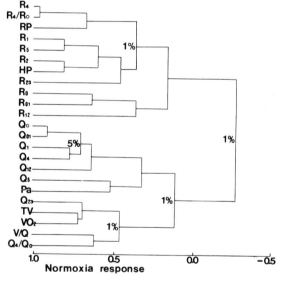

Fig. 5. Cluster analysis of the blood flow distribution data during control and stimulation of the leg (normoxia). Q_0: cardiac output; Q_1: aortic flow above diaphragm; Q_2 and Q_3: aortic flow above and below renal arteries; Q_4: flow to stimulated leg; Q_5: flow to contralateral leg. The Qs with two subscripts represent the differences between two actually measured flows, i.e., Q_{01}: flow to forepart of the animal; Q_{12}: flow to the GI tract; Q_{23}: flow to the kidneys; Q_4/Q_0: ratio of flow to stimulated leg to cardiac output. The subscripts of the resistances (R) correspond to those of the flows. V_{O_2}: total O_2 consumption; V/Q: ventilation perfusion ratio; Pa: arterial pressure; HP: heart period; RP: respiration period; TV: tidal volume (the numbers separating the different cluster configurations indicate the significance levels of the dissimilarities)

Thus far, we have only discussed how the different variables are connected in the factor space as far as their steady-state responses are concerned. While such results are important for the interpretation of the goals of control hierarchies, they shed little light on the actual mechanisms by which these goals are achieved. Inference about mechanisms must rely primarily on the dynamics of a response. As already stated, our measurement system precluded a dynamic analysis of the O_2 uptake, which is thus excluded from the results reported in the next section.

We characterized the dynamics of the response for all the other variables by three parameters: time delay, initial slope, and maximum (or minimum). We screened the relative importance of these parameters by means of a functional proposed by Andrews [1, 6] and carried out cluster and principal component analysis using vectors composed of those components suggested by the results provided by the functional. Using primarily time delays and slopes on the data of the biceps experiments, we were able to identify four dynamic dimensions: central versus local control, rate versus magnitude control, cardiovascular versus respiratory control, and finally a measure of tightness of control (or coordination) [6, 8].

The flow distribution experiments were carried out under four different conditions: normoxia, hypoxia (produced by the administration of a 15% O_2, 85% N_2 mixture), hypertension (produced by a continuous infusion of norepinephrine), and a combination of hypoxia and hypertension. A cluster analysis of all the variables, based on time delays and slopes only, produced four clusters. The first comprised respiratory rate and blood flow to the stimulated leg, which was to be expected on the basis of the steady-state data of all three series. The second cluster consisted of cardiovascular variables, the third of tidal volume, and the fourth of mixed venous blood O_2 saturation. The first cluster remained identical under all four experimental conditions, while the variables in the cardiovascular cluster shifted depending upon the experimental condition with one single exception (renal flow), which was unaffected by either hypoxia or hypertension.

Figure 6 shows the results of the principal component analysis for all the variables (the vectors consisting of control values and standard deviation, average response value and standard deviation, time delay, and initial slope) under the four experimental conditions. During normoxia, most of the variables load on factor 1 (accounting for 75% of the total variance). R_0, TV, V/Q, and R_{12} load on factor 2 (22% of the variance). During hypoxia, the loading on factor 1 increases to 82% since both V/Q and TV become dissociated from factor 2. During the infusion of norepinephrine, factor 3 assumes increasing importance, since Q_{23} and R_{23} now load on it. In the combination norepi-hypoxia, factor 3 still retains its importance (V/Q, TV, and R_{23}), while only R_0 remains as a load factor for the second dimension.

Assuming that the degree of lack of significant changes in a variable between either the four experimental conditions or between rest and simulated exercise indicates the level of independence of that variable, we ranked the variables on an "independence" scale and used this ranking to identify the underlying systems dimensions resulting from either cluster or principal component analysis. We thus obtained three control levels: a central coordinating level (occupied by the vari-

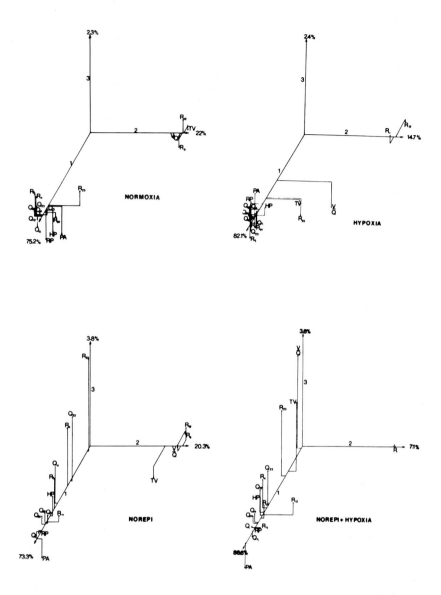

Fig. 6. Principal component analysis of the blood flow distribution data during normoxia, hypoxia, hypertension (norepi), and hypertension plus hypoxia. For each variable, a vector (consisting of control value plus standard deviation, average response value plus standard deviation, time delay and initial slope for each individual experiment) was constructed as input to the computer program (symbols for variables as in Fig. 7)

ables heart rate, cardiac output, and respiratory rate), an intermediate stabilizer (characterized by total peripheral resistance R_0), and a level of local autonomy (characterized by the behavior of renal blood flow Q_{23} and resistance R_{23}). The remaining variables shifted between these variables, depending upon the degree of stress applied to the animal, as indicated in Figure 7.

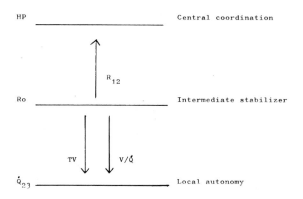

Fig. 7. O_2 transport control hierarchies during stress (arrows indicate changes in dependence of controlled variables with increasing stress levels)

Discussion

In all four series, the results of the analyses were consistent, yielding two major grouping of variables: a supply-demand dimension and a control dimension. Within each of these major groupings, subgroups could be identified representing a spectrum from purely local to more global functions. For example, the separation between local and general supply and demand variables, clearly identified and individually measured in the gracilis experiments (Table 1, Figs. 2 and 3), is also distinguishable in the biceps and blood flow distribution experiments (Figs. 4 and 5) where the global supply variables (cardiac output and flow to the contra-lateral leg; for justification of this choice see [5], are clearly separated from a local supply variable (blood flow to the stimulated leg [Fig. 5]). We interpret the central variables (heart rate, respiratory rate, ventilation, and arterial pressure) as indicators of centrally mediated control. In each instance, at least one of these central variables was always associated with a local variable (pO_2 of venous outflow), indicating some local contribution to centrally mediated control functions. Correspondingly, the change in total O_2 uptake was always larger than the change in local O_2 uptake. Our data also confirm the close correlation between changes in local O_2 consumption and muscle blood flow (Table 1) and support our hypothesis that changes in blood flow distribution account for a large fraction of the increase in blood flow to the stimulated leg and/or muscle. It is for this reason that we chose the ratio of a resistance related to local supply to a resistance related to general supply as an indicator of local control. The results of the flow distribution experiments (column 4 in Table 1 and Figs. 5 and 6) indicate that the ventilation-perfusion ratio assumes a similar role in the pulmonary circulation.

176

The stimulation of the gracilis muscle with its small mass resulted in a significant increase in muscle blood flow, a decrease in the pO_2 of its venous outflow, but had little effect on leg blood flow or the O_2 saturation of the venous outflow from the leg. Yet the effect on the central variables ventilation and arterial pressure was of a similar magnitude as that of the stimulation of the much larger biceps muscle or the entire leg (Table 1). (As already stated, heart rate changes were much smaller than expected, probably because of the preexisting sympathetic tone). In contrast, stimulation of the biceps muscle or the entire leg resulted in a large increase of leg blood flow and a decrease in the O_2 content of the venous outflow from the leg. The pO_2 of the muscle outflow did not change (despite large increases in muscle flow), probably indicating a more homogeneous perfusion, i.e., a reduction in "shunt flow." As the magnitude of the applied stress increases, the local dimensions lose and the more global dimensions increase in importance. This shift in importance occurs both in the supply-demand and the control dimensions and may be mediated by an intermediate control level which in our experiments was characterized by the behavior of the total peripheral resistance (Fig. 7). These results agree well with those of a simulation study carried out earlier [8]. For a three-level hierarchical model combining different degrees of interconnections with different levels of control, the methods correctly identified the two underlying dimensions: interconnection and control. As the connectivity of the system is increased, the two dimensions eventually fuse into one.

The hypothesis that local changes are (at least in part) responsible for changes in heart rate and respiration during exercise was formulated nearly 50 years ago [2, 13]. Stegeman and Kenner described a model that relates the control mechanism of the heart rate during exercise to the exercising muscle itself and postulated metabolic receptors sensitive to a decrease of high energy phosphates [19]. Tibes [20] showed in anesthetized dogs that muscular contraction resulted in significant increases in heart rate, ventilation, and mean arterial pressure. By selectively cooling the sciatic nerve, he found that muscular reflex inputs accounted for the major and humoral drives for the minor portion of total cardiovascular and respiratory responses during onset as well as during steady state of dynamic work, although humoral drives increased with time. He identified group III and IV afferents as the responsible pathways. Tibes' results are very similar to those we have obtained in our biceps preparation using section of the sciatic nerve instead of cold blocks [5]. Thus, the proximal block in Tibes' experiments corresponds to the peripheral stimulation in our experiments, while his distal block corresponds to our proximal stimulation (Table 2 in ref. 11). The reduction in cardiovascular and respiratory responses during a proximal block was larger for the ventilatory variables and much smaller for heart rate and arterial pressure. (In contrast to Tibes, we observed only a small decrease in the response of the blood flow to the leg). For a distal block, on the other hand, the response of heart rate and arterial pressure actually increased while the ventilatory and local blood flow responses were considerably smaller than in the unblocked preparation. For the central variables, the time course of the response was similar in the unblocked and peripherally blocked preparation but much slower in the centrally blocked preparation. The local blood flows, in contrast, responded as fast during a proximal block as in the unblocked state, but considerably slower when the proximal end of the sciatic nerve was stimulated. We conclude that the local input from the contracting muscle is more tightly coupled to respiratory as compared to cardiovascular control. The local input was related to changes in local pO_2 and thus probably of metabolic origin.

Pirnay et al. [17] found that the decrease in the pO_2 of femoral venous blood during muscular exercise is a function of the fraction of inspired O_2 and of the increase in heart rate. They interpreted their data as supporting the hypothesis that maximum O_2 consumption is limited by biochemical factors. Our results suggest that their results can equally well be explained by changes in blood flow distribution.

We have shown earlier [8] that in noise-free systems both cluster and principal component analysis provide identical results with respect to the identification of the contribution of observable variables to systems behavior in terms of underlying (latent) systems dimensions. The finer subdivisions in the cluster analysis, particularly if statistically confirmed, represent useful guides for the interpretation of the physiologic significance of the underlying dimensions. Major discrepancies between the results of the two methods are suggestive of high noise levels. If noise contaminates a system, it first affects the proper identification of lower level components.

Although we were able to identify different hierarchy levels at which various functions interact, the strategy employed in our experiments does not permit one to associate these levels with specific structures. The variability in coupling between the variables as a function of stress also emphasizes the difficulties one encounters in the extrapolation of experimental data obtained in isolated subsystems to overall systems performance.

Summary

In four different sets of experiments, we verified the hypothesis that changes in blood flow distribution represent the most important mechanism for meeting the increase in energy requirements during local muscular activity. Using cluster and principal component analysis we were able to reduce the dimensionality of the oxygen transport system from many observed variables to two intrinsic dimensions: one related to supply and demand, the other to control. Each of the dimensions contained several subclusters representing a spectrum ranging from local to central mechanisms. At low stresses, the local components predominated, but as the level of stress increased, the central components began to dominate. This shift in importance may be mediated by an intermediate, stablizing control level. At each level of stress, part of the overall cardiovascular and ventilatory response was related to an input from the activated muscle. Analysis of the response dynamics further indicated four subgroups in the control dimension relating to 1) local versus central control, 2) magnitude versus rate control, 3) respiratory versus cardiovascular control, and 4) coordination of control (i.e., the stabilizer).

Acknowledgment: The authors are indebted to Messrs. J.M. Adams, J.D. Morrow, D.T. Henry, and D. Ahuja for the development of some of the computer programs and the data processing.

References

1. Adams, J.M., Presto, P.V. del, Anne, A., Attinger, E.O.: Techniques in the consolidation, characterization and expression of physiol. signals in the time domain. Proc. IEEE 65, 689-96 (1977)
2. Alam, M., Smirk, F.H.: Observations in man upon a blood pressure raising reflex arising from the voluntary muscles. J. Physiol. (London) 89, 372-77 (1937)
3. Attinger, E.O., Anne, A.: The use of hybrid computer technology in physiological research. In: Modern Techniques in Physiological Sciences. Gross, J.F., Kaufmann, R., Wetterer, E. (eds.). New York: Acad. Pr. 1973, p. 501
4. Attinger, E.O., Attinger, F.M.: Frequency dynamics of peripheral vascular blood flow. Ann. Rev. Biophys. Biomed. Eng. 2, 7-36 (1973)
5. Attinger, E.O., Attinger, F.M.: Hierarchy levels in the control of blood flow to the hind limb of the dog. Kybernetik 13, 195-214 (1973)
6. Attinger, E.O., Attinger, F.M.: Computers in the care of patients. In: Cardiovascular Systems Dynamics. Noordergraaf, A. (ed.). Cambridge (MA): M.I.T. Pr. 1978, p. 557-562
7. Attinger, E.O., Attinger, F.M.L., Adams, J.M., Morrow, D.: Control hierarchies of the O_2 transport system during multiple stress. (submitted)
8. Attinger, E.O., Henry, D.T., Attinger, F.M.L., Adams, J.M., Anne, A.: Biological control hierarchies. I: Stimulation by a three level, ten component, adaptive model. IEEE Trans. SMC 8; 11-18, 1978
9. Cox, R.H., Peterson, L.H., Detweiler, D.K.: Comparison of arterial hemodynamics in the mongrel dog and the racing greyhound. Am. J. Phys. 230, 211-8 (1976)
10. Gauer, O.H., Henry, J.P.: Circulatory bases of fluid volume control. Physiol. Rev. 43, 423-81 (1963)
11. Guyton, A.C., Coleman, T.C., Granger, H.J.: Circulation; Overall regulation. Ann. Rev. Physiol. 34, 13-46 (1972)
12. Herd. J.A.: Behavior and cardiovascular function. Physiologist 14, 83-89 (1971)
13. Jarisch, A., Gaisboek, F.: Über das Verhalten des Kreislaufes bei postanämische Hyperämie. Arch. Exp. Path. Pharmacol, 13, 159-71 (1929)
14. Noordergraaf, A.: Hemodynamics. In: Biol. Eng. Schwan, H.P. (ed.). New York: McGraw 1969
15. Pennock, B., Attinger, E.O.: Optimization of the O_2 transport system. Biophys. J. 8, 897-896 (1968)
16. Pirkle, J.C., Gann, D.S.: Restitution of blood volume after hemorrhage: Mathematical description. Am. J. Physiol. 228, 821-27 (1975)

17. F. Pirnay, Lamey, M., Dujardin, J., Deroanne, R., Petit, J.M.: Analysis of femoral venous blood during maximum muscular exercise. J. Appl. Physiol, $\underline{33}$, 289-92 (1972)

18. Reeve, E.B., Guyton, A.C. (eds.): Physical Bases of Circulatory Transport; Regulation and Exchange. Philadelphia: Saunders, 1967

19. Stegeman, J., Kenner, Th.: A theory on heart rate control by muscular metabolic receptors. Arch. Kreislaufforsch. $\underline{64}$, 185-214 (1971)

20. Tibes, U.: Reflex inputs to cardiovascular and respiratory centers from dynamically working canine muscles. Circ. Res. $\underline{41}$, 332-41 (1977)

21. Vatner, S.F., Braunwald, E.: Cardiovascular control mechanisms in the conscious state. N. Engl. J. Med. $\underline{293}$, 970-76 (1975)

Optimality Principles Applied to the Design and Control Mechanisms of the Vascular System

M. G. Taylor

Department of Physiology, University of Sydney, Australia

Introduction

The problem of finding the optimum characteristics of a physiologic system is threefold. First, it is necessary to define the system with reasonable accuracy in mathematic form. Secondly, it is necessary to specify the properties or quantities which are to be minimized (maximized). Thirdly, the resulting equations must be solved.

In this paper, we consider two examples in hemodynamics; the first is of the control of a model circulatory system. The second, in a much less complete treatment, of the optimum distribution of elastic properties in a nonuniform system. The mathematic formulations are not particularly complicated, and in each case take the form of sets of differential equations. The quantities to be optimized are treated in detail below, but one may observe at this stage that both examples illustrate the general principle that an "optimal" solution depends on a balance being found between opposing influences. While, for example, the input impedance of the arterial tree may be made very low by making the arterial distensibility very large, thus minimizing the pulsatile work of the heart, such a system would, because it is so distensible, undergo very large changes in volume with changes in mean arterial pressure. This undesirable effect is thus a cost of low input impedance; an optimal design for such a system would, therefore, be one which minimized a weighted combination of the input impedance and the cost. As will be seen below, there are techniques in modern control theory which allow this to be done, but because of their computational difficulty they are very rarely applied to physiologic problems. The solutions here have been obtained by the use of Pontryagin's maximum principle, and an outline of the procedure is given below; but a few preliminary observations may be of use at this point.

When one is dealing with problems of this kind, described by sets of differential equations, the optimal solution is not to be found, as in many simpler cases, by setting the derivative(s) of an equation equal to zero and solving for the value(s) of a variable which produce an extremum. In general, one is dealing here with extremalizing functions, which are themselves solutions of differential equations. This whole field of mathematics is known as the calculus of variations, but in the present examples we use only the maximum principle of Pontryagin. As will be seen, this leads to sets of differential equations with two-point boundary values. These have been solved by the method of quasilinearization, with, in some cases, the additional refinements of continuation and orthogonalization.

The Pontryagin method is described in many works on control theory, but a very illuminating account is that by Pun [3]; the quasilinearization technique was advocated by Bellman and Kalaba [1], and is also well-described by Roberts and Shipman [4], who also give a very clear description of the orthogonalization and continuation procedures. It must be added that the solution of two-point boundary value problems can be sought in other ways [2], but the quasilinearization method has proved quite successful here.

Pontryagin's Maximum Principle

Suppose that a system can be described by n differential equations g_i, involving n state variables, x_i, r control variables u_j, and time t, then we may write

$$\dot{x}_i = g_i (x_i, u_j, t) \qquad \begin{array}{l} i = 1, 2 \ldots \ldots n \\ j = 1, 2 \ldots \ldots r \end{array} \qquad (1)$$

The performance index is defined as

$$S = \sum_{i=1}^{n} c_i \cdot x_i(t_f) \qquad (2)$$

where c_i are known constants, and t_f is the time at which the system reaches its final state. The performance index usually includes nonlinear or quadratic functions of the state variables. For example, where the performance index (cost function) is to include a term such as

$$\int_{0}^{t_f} x^2_k \, dt \qquad (3)$$

this can be accomplished by defining an additional variable

$$\dot{x}_{n+1} = x^2_k \qquad \qquad x_{n+1}(o) = o \qquad (4)$$

The optimizing control function u is to be found such that the performance index is minimized and the differential equations for x are satisfied, with boundary conditions specified:

$$\dot{x}_i = g_i (x_i, u_j, t)$$
$$x_i(o) = \text{given}$$
$$x_{n+1}(o) = o \qquad (5)$$

We now form a function known as the Hamiltonian, which employs $n + 1$ co-state variables, p_i,

$$H = \sum_{i=1}^{n+1} p_i \cdot g_i \tag{6}$$

given that $p_i(t_f) = -c_i$. The equations for p_i are found by

$$\dot{p}_i = \frac{-\partial H}{\partial x_i} \tag{7}$$

while, obviously,

$$\dot{x}_i = \frac{\partial H}{\partial p_i} \tag{8}$$

Where the integration (as here) is over a fixed range, from $t = 0$ to $t = t_f$, the boundary conditions on p_i are in general undetermined where the boundary value of x_i is fixed, and fixed if the corresponding value of x_i is free. Since, in these applications, the only state variable appearing in the performance index is x_{n+1}, $c_i = 0$, except for $c_{n+1} = 1$.
The boundary conditions for $x_i(t_f)$ are in general known, but of course the final value of the performance index is not known. We thus have

$$p_{n+1}(t_f) = -1 \tag{9}$$

and since the variable x_{n+1} does not itself appear in any of the differential equations, we have

$$\dot{p}_{n+1} = \frac{-\partial H}{\partial x_{n+1}} = 0 \tag{10}$$

and hence $p_{n+1} = -1$.

The minimum of the performance index is found by choosing u such that the Hamiltonian H is maximized; thus, with proper attention to the second derivative, and any constraints on u, we find u by solving

$$\frac{\partial H}{\partial u} = 0 \tag{11}$$

As will be seen from the examples which follow, the problem is now reduced to solving a set of $2n$ differential equations, for which some of the boundary conditions are known at one end of the range and some at the other; u, where it appears in the equations, is expressed in terms of the other variables, via the above equation. The solution of this two-point boundary value problem will yield the optimum strategy, but is far from a routine matter. There exist computer routines which are designed to assist the process, but in all cases a good deal depends upon having a good idea of the form of the solution and a good guess at the missing boundary values. All methods begin with guessed values for the missing boundary values, followed by some procedure which improves the estimate and which, one hopes, finally converges to the correct solution.

Quasilinearization

The basis of this method is the Newton-Raphson method of finding the simple root of a scalar equation $f(x) = 0$. In the neighborhood where $f(x)$ is decreasing monotonically, we may write

$$f(x) \cong f(x^0) + (x - x^0)\, \dot{f}(x^0) \tag{12}$$

Thus, where x^0 is an initial approximation, we may find a second one x^1 by solving

$$f(x^1) = 0 = f(x^0) + (x^1 - x^0)\, \dot{f}(x^0) \tag{13}$$

so that

$$x^1 = x^0 - \frac{f(x^0)}{\dot{f}(x^0)} \tag{14}$$

This process can be repeated to give the general expression

$$x^{n+1} = x^n - \frac{f(x^n)}{\dot{f}(x^n)} \tag{15}$$

This is the Newton-Raphson method for improving approximations to the roots of an equation, but of course its success depends upon making an initial estimate of the root in a region where the process can converge. If we are dealing with an n dimensional system, with n simultaneous equations

$$f_i(x_1, x_2, \ldots \ldots x_n) = 0 \qquad i = 1, 2, \ldots . n \tag{16}$$

where x is a vector with components $(x_1, x_2, \ldots \ldots x_n)$, the approximation for the scalar case takes the form

$$f(x) \cong f(x^0) + J(x^0) \cdot (x - x^0) \tag{17}$$

where $J(x^0)$ is the Jacobian matrix

$$
\begin{bmatrix}
\dfrac{\partial f_1}{\partial x_1} & \dfrac{\partial f_1}{\partial x_2} & \cdots & \dfrac{\partial f_1}{\partial x_n} \\[2ex]
\dfrac{\partial f_2}{\partial x_1} & \dfrac{\partial f_2}{\partial x_2} & \cdots & \dfrac{\partial f_2}{\partial x_2} \\[2ex]
\vdots & & & \\[1ex]
\dfrac{\partial f_n}{\partial x_1} & \cdots & & \dfrac{\partial f_n}{\partial x_n}
\end{bmatrix}
\tag{18}
$$

Turning now to the solution of a set of n differential equations, which may in general be nonlinear, we have

$$\dot{x}_i = g_i (x_1, x_2, \ldots \ldots x_n) \tag{19}$$

The boundary conditions are specified at the origin (t_o) and the termination (t_f), thus

$$[x(o), a_i] = b_i \qquad\qquad i = 1, 2, \ldots \ldots k$$
$$[x(t_f), a_i] = b_i \qquad\qquad i = k + 1, \ldots . n \tag{20}$$

where a_i and b_i are n dimensional vectors, and the vector products of the form $[x, a]$ denote $x_1 \cdot a_1 + x_2 \cdot a_2 + \ldots \ldots \ldots \ldots x_n \cdot a_n$

The quasilinearization method generates a sequence of vectors x^n, beginning with an initial guess x^o, using the linear system

$$\dot{x}^{n+1} = g(x^n) + J(x^n) \cdot (x^{n+1} - x^n) \tag{21}$$

with the boundary conditions

$$[x^{n+1}(o), a_i] = b_i \qquad\qquad i = 1, 2, \ldots . . k$$
$$[x^{n+1}(t_f), a_i] = b_i \qquad\qquad i = k + 1, \ldots . n \tag{22}$$

$J(x^n)$ is the Jacobian matrix, where the terms $\partial g_i / \partial x_j$ are evaluated at x^n. The succession of estimates $x^1, x^2, \ldots$ are thus found by solving these sets of linear differential equations, subject to the boundary conditions, as follows. We note that the general solution of

$$\dot{x} = A(t) \cdot x \tag{23}$$

185

is x + Xc, where c is a vector and X is the solution of the matrix equation

$$\dot{X} = A(t) \cdot X \tag{24}$$

subject to the initial condition $X(o) = I$, where I is the identity matrix. The boundary conditions of our linear system of equations may thus be expressed as

$$[X(o) \cdot c, a_i] = b_i \qquad\qquad i = 1, 2, \ldots\ldots k$$
$$[X(o) \cdot c, a_i] = b_i \qquad\qquad i = k+1, \ldots\ldots n \tag{25}$$

whence the components of the vector c may be evaluated.
Where the differential equation has the form encountered in the quasilineariza-tion method, the solution is of the form

$$x = X \cdot c + y \tag{26}$$

where X is the matrix solution of the equation

$$X = J(x^n) \cdot X, \qquad X(o) = I \tag{27}$$

and y is the vector solution of

$$\dot{y} = J(x^n) \cdot y + g(x^n) - J(x^n) \cdot x^n \tag{28}$$

The sequence x^n, x^{n+1} is generated beginning with the guessed vector x^o, of which, of course, some components will be accurately known. At each stage, an improved estimate of x is obtained, unless computational instabilities are encountered.

Computation

Although the methods outlined above, or indeed any methods to be used for these problems, look straightforward, their practical application is not easy. This is principally because numeric problems frequently make the estimation of the vector c very inacurate. The set of simultaneous equations used for the estima-tion of c may easily become singular. There is not space here to go into details, and reference should be made to the excellent and extremely helpful monograph by Roberts and Shipman [4]. Particular attention should be given to the method of continuation, where a solution which is stable for one set of parameters of the system may be used as a starting point for obtaining a solution with a set of parameters which, used directly, would lead to instabilities in the computation. Likewise, attention is directed to the technique of orthogonalization, whereby the vectors of the matrix X are transformed at certain points in the range of integration, so that they are orthogonal. Although the initial value of X, namely I, has orthogonal components, as the integration proceeds, it is not uncommon

186

for a large value of some one variable to come to dominate all the equations, thus making the matrix solution X singular, or nearly so. In suitable cases, this problem can be avoided by reorthogonalizing the matrix at one or more points as the solution proceeds from t = 0. In the example treated below of the control of a model cardiovascular system, orthogonalization was carried out after the third integration step and was effective in avoiding otherwise disastrous instability in the solutions.

All the computations reported here were carried out with programs written in Fortran and employing, where necessary standard library routines for the integration of the differential equations.

Examples

1. Control of a Model Cardiovascular System

The system is illustrated in Figure 1. It consists of an arterial reservoir of capacitance C_1, leading to a "peripheral resistance" which has two components. One

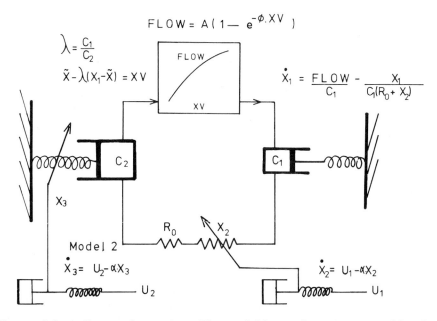

Fig. 1. The model cardiovascular system. The variables and constants are identified in the text

is fixed (R_0) and one is variable (x_2). The variable component is constrained to be greater than zero, and its value is determined by the control variable (u_1) acting through the spring dashpot element with a time constant ($1/a$). This element is to represent the delay between a sympathetic constrictor signal (u_1) and the resulting smooth muscle tone of the resistance vessels (x_2).

187

On the venous side, there is also a reservoir of capacitance (C_2), which is chosen to be 20 times that of the arterial side. Two models of this system were studied; one in which the venous reservoir was unregulated (model 1) and one in which (model 2) it was subject to "venoconstrictor tone" (x_3), regulated by the control signal (u_2), acting, as in the case of the peripheral resistance, through a spring dashpot element of the same time constant ($1/a$). The effect of this venoconstrictor tone was to divide the capacitance by x_3, thus, for any given venous volume, increasing venous pressure in proportion to x_3.

The venous pressure itself (XV) is determined by the arterial pressure (x_1) via a relationship which expresses the fact that the total storage in the two reservoirs is constant; thus,

$$x_1 \cdot C_1 + XV \cdot C_2 = \tilde{x}(C_1 + C_2) \tag{29}$$

where $\tilde{x}$ is a constant, the equilibrium pressure of the system. Rearranging this expression and putting $\lambda = C_1/C_2$, we have

$$XV = \tilde{x} - \lambda(x_1 - \tilde{x})$$

The "heart" in this model is represented by a sort of Frank-Starling relationship between venous "filling pressure" and cardiac output or Flow, such that

$$\text{Flow} = A \cdot (1 - e^{-\phi \cdot XV}) \tag{30}$$

where A and ϕ are constants. There is no attempt in this model to include autonomic influences on the heart. The differential equations describing this system are

$$\dot{x}_1 = \frac{A}{C_1}(1 - e^{-\phi \cdot XV}) - \frac{x_1}{C_1(R_0 + x_2)}$$

$$\dot{x}_2 = u_1 - a\,x_2$$

$$\dot{x}_3 = u_2 - a\,x_3 \quad \dots\dots\dots \text{(model 2 only)} \tag{31}$$

The problem posed here is to find the optimum strategy or time course of the control signal u_1 (and in model 2, of u_2 as well), representing a pattern of sympathetic nervous activity which will take the arterial pressure (x_1) from an initial value of 4.0 units at time $t = 0$ to a final value of 6.0 units at time $t = 15$. This transition is to be accomplished as quickly as possible, during the fixed interval of time, subject to the various "costs" set out below. Deviation of the arterial pressure from its final value

$$W_1 = \int_0^{15} [x_1 - x_1(15)]^2 \, dt \tag{32}$$

188

Deviation of venous pressure (XV); if this deviation is minimized, then naturally the deviations of the cardiac output from its standard value are also minimized (model 2 only)

$$W_2 = \int_0^{15} [XV - XV(0)]^2 \, dt \tag{33}$$

Deviations of the control signals from their final equilibrium values

$$W_3 = \int_0^{15} [u_1 - u_1(15)]^2 \, dt$$

$$W_4 = \int_0^{15} [u_2 - u_2(15)]^2 \, dt \tag{34}$$

These were combined into a cost function or performance index (S) such that

$$\dot{S} = [x_1 - x_1(15)]^2 + \beta[XV - XV(0)]^2 + \gamma[u_1 - u_1(15)]^2 + \kappa[u_2 - u_2(15)]^2 \tag{35}$$

where β, γ, κ, represent weighting constants.

Using the Pontryagin method with quasilinearization as outlined above, the optimum solution for u_1 and, in model 2 u_2 also, was found where the following values of the various constants were used. $A = 2.0$; $\phi = 0.731$; $\tilde{x} = 0.5$; $\lambda = 0.05$; $C_1 = 1.0$; $R_o = 1.0$; $x_1(0) = 4.0$; $x_1(15) = 6.0$; $x_2(0) = 3.1845$; $x_2(15) = 5.2767$; $x_3(0) = 1.0$; $x_3(15) = 1.4444$; $u_1(\text{maximum}) = u_2(\text{maximum}) = 50.0$; $a = 0.2$; $\gamma = 0.2$; $\kappa = 20.0$; $\beta = 400.0$. Two sets of solutions were obtained for the two cases where (model 1) there was no regulation of venous pressure and (model 2) where this was controlled through the second control variable u_2.

The results are shown in Figures 2 and 3; in order not to crowd the Figures, u_2 and x_3 have not been included here. A much more extensive presentation of these results will appear elsewhere.

a) Model 1, (Dotted Lines in the Figures)

It will be observed that the optimal control signal u_1 is one which rises abruptly to a peak value and then declines, slightly undershooting its final equilibrium value. The variable component (x_2) of the peripheral resistance rises more slowly, overshoots its final value, and then settles down. As might be expected, the increase in resistance is reflected in the arterial pressure (x_1) which climbs rapidly from its initial value before leveling off at its final value. In Figure 3, we see the corresponding changes in flow and venous pressure. As the arterial pressure

189

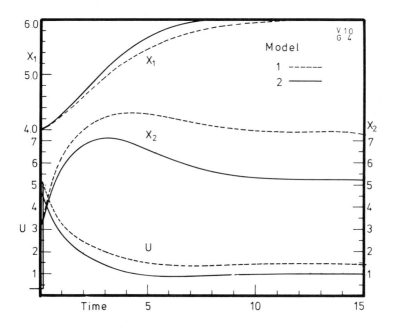

Fig. 2. Response of the system regulated by control signals acting on (model 1) peripheral resistance and (model 2) both peripheral resistance and venous capacitance. The control signal u (u_1) acts on the peripheral resistance (x_2) and is the optimum strategy to take the arterial pressure (x_1) from 4.0 units to 6.0 units, subject to the performance index given in the text. Note that in the case of model 2, where the venous system is also regulated, the desired change in x_1 is brought about more quickly and with smaller changes in u_1 and x_2

rises, the venous reservoir is depleted and the venous pressure (xv) and the flow consequently decrease.

b) Model 2, (Solid Lines in the Figures)

In this model, there is the added influence of a control variable (u_2) acting on the venous reservoir. The performance index, as indicated above, now includes a term expressing the deviation of venous pressure from its standard (initial) value. As can be seen from the Figures, this additional control produces very interesting effects. Because venous pressure, and hence flow, are held more or less constant, the peripheral resistance (x_2) does not have to be increased so much to achieve a given arterial blood pressure. The equilibrium values of both x_2 and u_1 are, therefore, lower than before. In addition, the rise in x_1 toward its final value is faster.

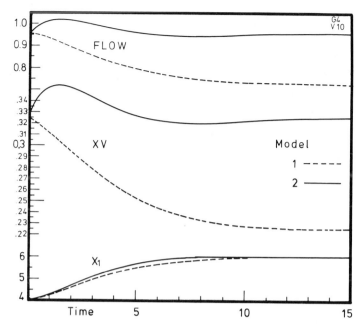

Fig. 3. Arterial flow (Flow), venous pressure (XV), and arterial pressure (x_1) in the two models of the circulatory system (cf. Figs. 1 and 2). Note that for model 1 the venous pressure falls as the arterial pressure rises, with a corresponding fall in flow. When the venous compliance is controlled (model 2), the venous pressure and flow are only subject to small changes

c) Step Change in Peripheral Resistance

In Figure 4 is shown the behavior of the control signal (u_1), the peripheral resistance (x_2), and the arterial pressure (x_1) when in the model 2 system the "fixed" element of the peripheral resistance is increased suddenly from an initial value of 1.0 to 2.0. In an unregulated system, such a change would, of course, lead to a rise in arterial pressure, but in Figure 4 is seen the optimum strategy for u_1 which, in the face of such a disturbance, keeps all variables of the system as near to their initial (control) values as possible. This optimum strategy is seen to be a steep decline in u_1, in fact it goes briefly to zero, followed by a slow rise to a new equilibrium value. The variable component of the peripheral resistance (x_2) falls rather more slowly to its new equilibrium value. The arterial pressure, in the face of a 25% change in peripheral resistance, shows only a brief perturbation of about 2.5%.

2. Optimal Distribution of Elastic Properties

This example follows a different attack on the same problem [5], and although a preliminary result has been obtained, the computation has proved to be partic-

191

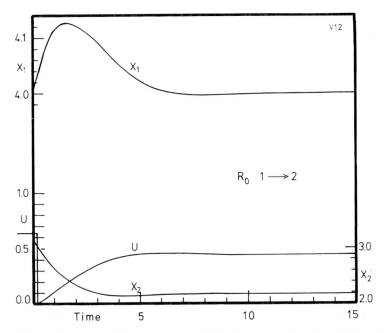

Fig. 4. The arterial pressure (X_1) is shown for the model 2 circulatory system (cf. Fig. 1) when the "fixed" component of the peripheral resistance is changed, stepwise from $R_0 = 1$ to $R_0 = 2$ at $t = 0$. The optimum control strategy (U_1) is shown together with the time course of the resulting change in X_2, the variable component of peripheral resistance

ularly troublesome, and there has not been time, before this Symposium, to overcome all the difficulties. The result must, therefore, be regarded as indicative only. A more satisfactory treatment will, I hope, be forthcoming later on.

The problem is to choose a form for the distribution of elastic properties along a conducting system, in such a way that, for a given terminal impedance, the input impedance is minimized, while the overall distensibility of the system is also minimized. In the earlier treatment, the problem was attacked by expressing the local capacitance $C(x)$ as a quadratic function in x, the distance along the line, and using a search procedure to find the values of the parameters of this quadratic equation which minimized a prescribed cost function. The present optimization procedure, employing Pontryagin's method, allows the optimum form for $C(x)$ to be found directly, given the differential equations of the system and a specified performance index.

In the previous paper, it was shown that if the local impedance of a lossless transmission line is $Z(x) = Z_1 + iZ_2$, then these variables obey the following pair of differential equations

$$\dot{Z}_1 = -\omega \cdot C(x) \cdot Z_1 \cdot Z_2$$
$$\dot{Z}_2 = \omega \left[C(x) \cdot (Z_1{}^2 - Z_2{}^2) - L \right] \tag{36}$$

where C(x) is the local capacitance and L is the (constant) inductance. As boundary conditions, we may choose $Z(x_f) = Z_1(x_f) + i0$, which ensures that at $x = x_f$ the termination of the line $|Z|$ will be smooth, since the condition $Z_2 = 0$ ensures that $\partial|Z|/\partial x = 0$. The performance index includes, as before, the overall distensibility, but here expressed in terms of the square of the local distensibility. However, to bring into account the magnitude and stability of the impedance, which was previously done by averaging over frequency, in this case the performance index includes a term which weights deviations of the local impedance from a constant value (Z_c) integrated along the line

$$S = \int_0^{x_f} (|Z| - Z_c)^2 \, dx + \gamma \int_0^{x_f} C^2(x) \, dx \tag{37}$$

Taking the control variable in this case to be C(x), its optimum form was sought, using Pontryagin's method, as described above. The equations have, however, proved very unstable and so far only one satisfactory solution has been obtained. This is for the rather unimportant case of low frequency oscillations in a short conducting system. The solution, shown in Figure 5, was obtained with the following parameters: $Z_1(x_f) + 3.0$; $Z_c = 1.0$; $L = 1.0$; $\omega = 2.0$; $x_f = 0.05$; $\gamma = 0.1$.

It will be seen that Z(x) is essentially flat over the whole range, but C(x) is large

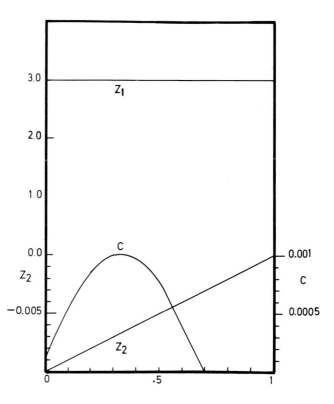

Fig. 5. The form of the optimum distribution of capacitance (C) in a non-uniform lossless transmission line, together with the real (Z_1) and imaginary (Z_2) components of the resulting impedance when the terminal impedance at $x = 1.0$ is 3.0 units. The values of other parameters and the form of the performance index are given in the text

193

over the proximal part of the line and greatly reduced over the distal part. In fact, $C(x)$ is at its limiting value (5×10^{-5}) in that region. This result, while showing the basic feature of the nonuniform arterial system, with distensibility greatest in the proximal region, is otherwise rather disappointing, and much more remains to be done on the problem. It has been presented here, however, to show that the technique under discussion has application to more than one class of problem.

Discussion

The results presented in this paper have demonstrated the successful application of optimal control techniques to the study of the cardiovascular system; we have also discussed some of the computational methods needed to solve the two-point boundary value problems which arise. It is particularly interesting to note the form of the control signal (u_1) in Figures 2 and 4; the steep rise (or fall) followed by a slower settling (with or without overshoot or undershoot) to a new equilibrium value is characteristic of autonomic firing patterns found in animal experiments under circumstances such as those modeled in these calculations. Such patterns arise in these calculations entirely as an expression of the optimum strategy; there are no a priori conditions which prescribe the form to the control signal.

Acknowledgments: It is a privilege to be able to contribute to this Festschrift in honor of my distinguished colleague Professor Wetterer whose friendship I have enjoyed for over 20 years. The work reported here began with my introduction to modern control theory by the late Dr. R. Sridhar of the California Institute of Technology, when I was a visitor to that institution in 1966. The calculations had to await a sabbatical year in 1974, spent as Visiting Fellow of St. Catherine's College, and I wish to acknowledge my indebtedness to the Master and Fellows of that College.

References

1. Bellman, R.E., Kalaba, R.E.: Quasilinearization and Non-Linear Boundary-Value Problems. New York: Am. Elsevier 1965
2. Keller, H.B.: Numerical Methods for Two-Point Boundary Value Problems. Waltham (USA): Blaisdell 1968
3. Pun, L.: Introduction to Optimization Practice. New York: Wiley 1969
4. Roberts, S.M., Shipman, J.S.: Two-Point Boundary Value Problems; shooting methods. New York: Am. Elsevier 1972
5. Taylor, M.G.: Arterial impedance and Distensibility. In: The Pulmonary Circulation and Interstitial space. Fishman, A.P., Hecht, H.H. (eds.). Chicaco: U. Pr. 1969

Autonomic Vascular Responses in the Splanchnic Region

J. Lutz

Physiologisches Institut der Universität Würzburg

The greatest part of cardiac output is known to flow during resting conditions to the splanchnic area. Although the autonomic nervous system plays an eminent role in the distribution of blood flow, there are additional mechanisms of self-regulation in the vasculature itself; these mechanisms will be treated subsequently. The vascular responses can be demonstrated in regions of the circulation which are hemodynamically and nervously isolated. They are independent of the remaining body and its reflexes; furthermore, they appear to be integrated responses of the vascular smooth muscle in a particular organ circulation, different from responses of isolated smooth muscles in vivo, which are often objects of study. A perfusion in situ allows the possibilities of controlled circulatory conditions and registration of the different responses. By increase in perfusion pressure or flow, the phenomenon of autoregulation appears. The increase in vessel resistance contrasts with a pressure-independent behavior, as seen after the administration of calcium antagonists. Even when the vessel resistance remains constant under rising pressures, there is evidence of increasing activation of the vascular muscle. Autoregulation can be quantified by the resistance ratio of two different pressures. However, in this regard, the choice of the pressures used is important, because they influence the ratio, a fact encountered also in the Semple-De Wardener index [13]. When both values are variably grouped in the range of autoregulation, different ratios are obtained. Therefore, we chose mostly the two values 140 and 70 mm Hg and established the quotient

$$Q_A = \frac{R_{140}}{R_{70}} = 2 \cdot \frac{I_{70}}{I_{140}} \tag{1}$$

where Q_A = autoregulation quotient, R = resistance, and I = flow. Values greater than 1 indicate an obvious active response, passive behavior leads to quotients of about 0.75. Between both values, there is a range of latent responses. Increases in the resistance that, instead of being reversible become continuous (e.g., due to edema formation), must be excluded, so that only those values are used which after a pressure reduction again approach control values. Table 1 shows values reached under equal conditions of perfusion. The phenomenon of autoregulation can be shown to be sometimes instable when critically judged in the appropriate manner. There are reports dealing with studies on nearly all organ

Table 1. Quantification of vascular responses in the splanchnic region

| Organ | Autoregulation (n = 21-56) | | Veno-vasomotoric response (n = 80) | | | |
	Q_A	S.E.M.	Q_V	S.E.M.	$\Delta P_A/\Delta P_V$	S.E.M.
Intestine	1.35	± 0.05	1.49	± 0.06	2.78	± 0.21
Spleen	1.13	± 0.05	1.42	± 0.03	2.61	± 0.11
Stomach	1.10	± 0.04	1.25	± 0.03	1.90	± 0.10

circulations in which this response could not be demonstrated. Support of auto-regulation through metabolites or other special organ mechanisms will be discussed below.

Just as from the arterial side, it is also possible that a pressure variation in the veins triggers a response from the vascular muscle: the veno-vasomotoric response. This response is so obvious and strongly triggered that many authors have named it a veno-arterial reflex [3, 5, 6, 16]. This corresponds to the fact that each decrease in the vessel tone, be it due to myotropic anesthetics or strong sympatholytics like dibenzyline, reduces this vessel response or completely abolishes it [2]. Even ganglion blockers, when initially decreasing vascular tone, abolish the response; however, still during the period of nerve block it reappears [8].

Active responses can be judged most easily under constant flow perfusion, since then perfusion pressure increases at a greater extent than venous pressure. Arterial pressure does not increase nearly as much as the venous pressure when calcium antagonists are given. Just as for autoregulation, the resistance ratio can quantify the strength of the reaction. For the intestinal circulation, venous pressure increases of 33 mm Hg prove to be favorable, because at least up to this point the vascular response reveals a progression without the appearance of gross extravasation. The resistance ratio is then defined as

$$Q_V = R_2/R_1 = \frac{P_{A_2} - P_{V_2}}{I_2} \Big/ \frac{P_{A_1} - P_{V_1}}{I_1} \tag{2}$$

These ratios and those of autoregulation are listed in Table 1. Another possibility for quantification is the ratio between arterial and venous pressure increases $\Delta P_A/\Delta P_V$ under constant flow.

Prerequisite for the appearence of this veno-vasomotoric responce is a particular arterial pressure range (Fig. 1). The lines of identity ($\Delta P_A = \Delta P_V$) are plotted in the figure as dashed lines for each step of venous pressure elevation and correspond to the behavior of a rigid tube. The range of active response agrees closely with the pressure range in which autoregulation appears.

It also seemed to be important to investigate the dynamic pattern of the veno-vasomotoric response in situ. Under sinusoidal pressure stimulation at the venous side with increasing duration and decreasing frequency, the extention of the response rises up to a maximum at nearly 1 min or 15 m Hz, respectively (Fig. 2).

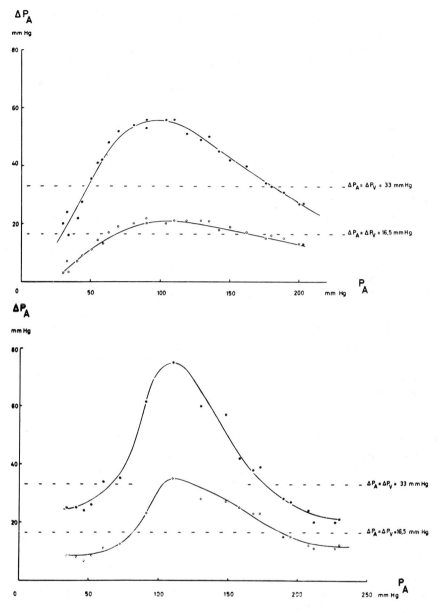

Fig. 1. The dependence of the veno-vasomotoric response on the prevailing arterial blood pressure. The venous pressure was raised in two steps of 16.5 and 33 mm Hg. At the higher pressure step, the active reactions have more than doubled; thus, the responses show a progression

Beyond this value, even with slowest pressure variations, the active response never vanishes [9]. Thus, a static component in the response to continuous pressure stimulations exists. The decrease of amplitude in the range of higher fre-

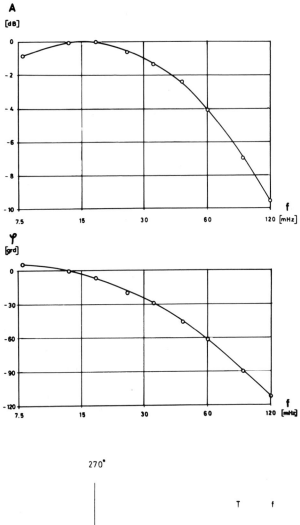

Fig. 2. Response of the intestinal vasculature in situ to rhythmic venous pressure elevations. Bode and Nyquist diagrams

quencies amounts to 5.5 dB/octave. This compares well with other results as reported by Stegemann and Geisen [14] for the baroreceptor system to about 5.7 dB/octave and nearly with those from Penaz and Burianek [12], who found under the stimulation of resistance vessels of the external carotid vascular bed 7.7 dB/octave. In both cases cited, the nerve transmission appears not to be the deciding factor for the slope of amplitude decrease but the vascular muscle itself. Thus, the isolated smooth muscle of taenia coli, as reported by Golenhofen [4], demonstrates a comparable amplitude decrease from 5.2-6.5 dB per octave. The respective phase shift, including a certain delay time, is shown in Figure 2. The resulting Nyquist diagram is plotted on the lower part of the figure. The curve runs across three quadrants until the amplitude only passively follows the pressure increases. The beginning in the first quadrant corresponds with positive phase shifts. They reveal a sensitivity against the derivative of pressure increase and/or a triggering of a quicker response. With this description, considered more closely, we are actually dealing with a simplification since only an average phase shift can be used if the response curve does not exactly equal the stimulus curve. However, a stable behavior can be read from this Nyquist diagram. Positive phase shifts were also seen by Stegemann and Geisen [14] and Basar et al. [1] on arterial vessels. This may be meaningful for a venous triggering because response curves of capacity vessels, as recorded by a plethysmograph, did not show this [11]. Also the integrating behavior and the long delay times of those vessels (up to 33 s) are lacking here, as is the very strong amplitude drop of 14 dB/octave. Apparently by the veno-vasomotoric responses, the venous side only plays the role of a passive transfer. A second response maximum, shown by the isolated smooth muscle (the "element of tetanus," Golenhofen [4], and characterized by a much shorter period of nearly 1.5 s), could not be proved, perhaps because of the strong damping of the venous transfer.

The results with a dependency on initial arterial pressure and the temporal behavior point to the fact that the observed vessel responses originate from a similar myogenic mechanism. The triggering stretch stimulus is effective both from arterial and venous vessels. Venous pressure increases can be brought to bear upon the wall of the responding resistance vessels in greater amounts. This is explained by the following schema. Under increased venous pressure, the flow is reduced passively, and combined with this, a decrease in the pressure along the vessels appears which lets a greater part of the pressure change become effective. During an increased arterial pressure, the flow becomes at first greater, the flow-related pressure gradient is increased, and in addition, a reduction in the stretch stimulus results. Pressure measurements in small intestinal arteries under either arterial or venous pressure increases confirm this. From the arteries (as compared to the veins under equal pressure increases) a smaller pressure stimulus reaches the measuring point. Thus, the veno-vasomotoric response shows greater resistance quotients than autoregulation (Table 1) and is partly easier to prove, especially if autoregulation is only latently evident. This applies, at least, to the abdominal organs. In the kidney, renin release is an auxiliary mechanism for autoregulation; the veno-vasomotoric response is present but weaker. The liver sinusoids provide the best conditions, the kidney glomerula the worst, for the propagation of the pressure stimulus from the venous system [10]. Against the hypothesis of autoregulation, in which the variation of transmural pressure in the form of different wall tensions is the triggering mechanism of the myogenic response, objections have been raised [15]. If wall tension should remain constant, then according to the LaPlace relationship, the vessel radius should decrease nearly proportional to the internal pressure increase. That would, however, mean that under twice the pressure and half the radius, the flow would be reduced to nearly 1/16 th, which of course has never been seen. (The "nearly" applies to the fact that transmural pressure is not as high as the increase in internal pressure and that vessel wall thickness increases with a smaller radius).

If one were to consider, besides the actively reacting vessels, the always present passive vasculature which is partly serially, partly parallelly connected, then a satisfactory autoregulatory behavior can be explained with a simple model (Fig. 3). The related "law of flow" might be stated as

$$I = P \cfrac{1}{R_s + \cfrac{1}{r_2{}^4 + 1/R_p}} \quad \text{with} \quad r_2 = \frac{r_1 \cdot P_1}{P_2} \cdot \frac{d_2}{d_1} \tag{3}$$

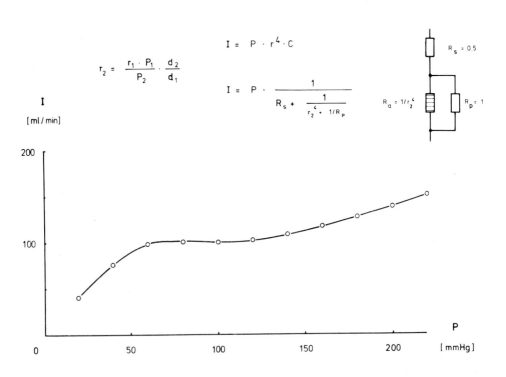

Fig. 3. Effect of a pressure-sensitive vessel resistance together with a passive serial and parallel resistance on the IP curve (symbols are explained in the text)

200

R_a	= actively responding resistance
R_s	= serial resistance with a constant value of $0.5\,R_a$ at 100 mm Hg
R_p	= parallel resistance with a constant value of $1\,R_a$ at 100 mm Hg
P_1	= control pressure (= 100 mm Hg)
P_2	= variable pressure
r_1	= control radius (when P_1 = 100 mm Hg)
r_2	= variable radius
d_1, d_2	= wall thickness (the quotient d_2/d_1 is neglected, because it is nearly 1)

Johnson and Intaglietta [7] also have used the regulation of wall tension to explain control of autoregulation. They applied a gain factor < 1 in the control system which resulted in sections of IP curves with very different increase or decrease of flow.
If autoregulation is regarded as a process to maintain constant blood flow, it functions as an antagonist to the veno-vasomotoric response, because the latter causes a further reduction of the already diminished blood flow. The action of metabolites is also different in both responses. Autoregulation is supported by metabolites which are released in an increased quantity during decreased pressure; the veno-vasomotoric response, however, will be diminished by metabolites.

If, however, autoregulation is considered to have the function of controlling the normal capillary and filtration pressure, both responses work parallel. In the veno-vasomotoric response, an increased capillary pressure is regulated after venous pressure elevations in metarterioles and perhaps precapillary sphincters, in the autoregulation the same happens by constriction of more proximal arterioles. Both responses triggered in a different way thus reveal the same protecting mechanism.

References

1. Basar, E., Tischner, H., Weiss, Ch.: Untersuchungen zur Dynamik druckinduzierter Änderungen des Strömungswiderstandes der autoregulierenden, isolierten Rattenniere. Pflügers Arch. 299, 191-213 (1968)
2. Benitez, D., Baez, S.: Venous-arteriolar response in striated cremaster muscle in the rat. Microvasc. Res. 11, 115-116 (1976)
3. Girling, F.: Critical closing pressure and venous pressure. Am. J. Physiol. 171, 204-207 (1952)
4. Golenhofen, K.: Rhythmische Dehnung der glatten Muskulatur vom Blinddarm des Meerschweinchens. Pflügers Arch. 284, 327-346 (1965)
5. Haddy, F.J., Gilbert, R.P.: The relation of a venous-arteriolar reflex to transmural pressure and resistance in small and large systemic vessels. Circ. Res. 4, 25-32 (1956)
6. Henricksen, O., Sejrsen, P.: Local reflex in microcirculation in human skeletal muscle. Acta Physiol. Scand. 99, 19-26 (1977)
7. Johnson, P.C., Intaglietta, M.: Contributions of pressure and flow sensitivity to autoregulation in mesenteric arterioles. Am. J. Physiol. 231, 1686-1698 (1976)

8. Lutz, J.: Über veno-vasomotorische Gefäßreaktionen im Mesenterialkreis-lauf der Katze. Pflügers Arch. 287, 330-344 (1966)

9. Lutz, J.: Die Reaktion der Gefäßmuskulatur in situ auf rhythmische Dehnungsreize. Pflügers Arch. 291, R 22 (1966)

10. Lutz, J., Biester, J.: Comparison of veno-vasomotoric reactions in the ab-dominal circulatory systems of intestine, stomach, spleen, liver and of the kidney. In: Vascular Smooth Muscle. Betz, E. (ed.). New York –Heidelberg-Berlin: Springer 1972, p. 139

11. Penaz, J.: Frequenzgang der vasomotorischen Reaktionen der kapazitiven Gefäße des Kaninchenohres; ein Beitrag zur Deutung des Plethysmogrammes. Pflügers Arch. 276, 636-651 (1963)

12. Penaz, J., Burianek, P.: Dynamic performance of vasomotor responses of the resistance vessels of the carotid vascular bed in the rabbit. Arch. Int. Physiol. Biochem. 71, 499-517 (1963)

13. Semple, S.J.C., Wardener, H.E. de: Effect of increased renal venous pressure on circulatory "autoregulation" of isolated dog kidney. Circ. Res. 7, 643-648 (1959)

14. Stegemann, J., Geisen, K.: Zur regeltheoretischen Analyse des Blutkreis-laufes. IV Phasen- und Amplitudenverhalten der Druck-Stromstärke-Bezie-hung des arteriellen Systems auf sinusförmige Druckänderungen im isolier-ten Carotissinus des Hundes. Pflügers Arch. 287, 276-285 (1966)

15. Thurau, K.: Niere. In: Physiologie des Kreislaufs. Bauereisen, E. (ed.). Berlin-Heidelberg-New York: Springer 1971, p. 293

16. Yamada, S. Burton, A.C.: Effect of reduced tissue pressure on blood flow of the finger: the veni-vasomotor reflex. J. Appl. Physiol. 6, 501-505 (1954)

Response of Renal Blood Flow and Renal Sympathetic Nerve Activity to Baroreceptor and Emotional Stimuli in the Conscious Dog

H. R. Kirchheim and R. Gross

I. Physiologisches Institut der Universität Heidelberg,
D-69 Heidelberg 1, Im Neuenheimer Feld 326

Introduction

With respect to the nervous control of kidney blood flow, a traditional discrepancy is evident in the literature when the results of electrophysiologic studies are compared with those applying hemodynamic measurements [1]. Undoubtedly, there is efferent pulse-synchronous activity in the renal nerves in cats, dogs, and rabbits under various types of anesthesia at a normal blood pressure. Recent recordings by Kirchner [8] and by Schad and Seller [12] in conscious cats have shown, however, that renal sympathetic nerve activity is increased by general anesthesia. This might explain that in the anesthetized animal some authors still find an increase of renal blood flow upon elimination of nervous tone [5, 11]. The majority of hemodynamic studies have demonstrated that denervation or adrenergic blockade fails to induce a significant change in renal blood flow [1]. There is still good reason to agree with Smith [14] that under basal conditions the renal nervous activity is too low to have appreciable influence on total renal blood flow.

Some disagreement between electrophysiologic and hemodynamic studies also exists with regard to the reflex adjustment of renal vascular tone by the arterial and low pressure system receptors. While the arterial baroreceptors effectively control renal sympathetic nerve discharge [9, 16], their effect on renal blood flow is surprisingly small [7]. The activation or unloading of the low pressure system receptors by a 10%-15% change in blood volume decreases or increases renal sympathetic nerve activity by 30%-40% of control [4, 13]; however, a nonhypotensive hemorrhage of 17% of blood volume fails to reduce renal blood flow in conscious dogs or baboons [15].

The strongest renal vascular responses have been reported to occur with emotional stress in cats, dogs, and monkeys [3, 6, 10, 17]. This correlates well with the observation that sympathetic activity rises by 200% of control during a stressful stimulus in the conscious cat [8].

Since up to now successful recordings of renal sympathetic activity have not been reported in the conscious dog, it was considered important to perform neurophysiologic and hemodynamic measurements under comparable conditions. The effects of common carotid occlusion, nonhypotensive hemorrhage, and emotional stress on renal blood flow and of common carotid occlusion and emotional stress on renal sympathetic nerve activity were, therefore, studied in six trained conscious foxhounds.

203

Material and Methods

The dogs received a standard diet (5 g Na/kg food); the aortic baroreceptors were left intact. Blood pressure was measured with a solid-state miniature pressure transducer (Konigsberg Instruments, type P-19) or an indwelling catheter chronically implanted into the abdominal aorta. A small pneumatic cuff implanted around the common carotid artery on either side was used to induce carotid sinus hypotension. Carotid sinus pressure was recorded with another catheter implanted downstream of one of the carotid cuffs. Renal blood flow was measured with an electromagnetic flow meter (Zepeda Instruments) or a directional doppler flow meter (L & M Instruments) on the left renal artery. Another pneumatic cuff was implanted around the abdominal aorta proximal to the renal artery; it served to reduce kidney perfusion pressure back to its control level when systemic hypertension was induced by bilateral common carotid occlusion. Blood was withdrawn and reinfused from a catheter which was placed into the inferior vena cava close to the right atrium; this catheter was also used to measure central venous pressure. Blood volume was determined using Evans blue. In two of the dogs, we succeeded in recording renal sympathetic nerve activity for 3 postoperative days. Except for minor modifications, the technique for recording nerve activity with an implanted electrode was identical to that described by Schad and Seller [12].

Results

Common carotid occlusion reduces carotid sinus pulse pressure from 40-50 mm Hg to less than 5 mm Hg (Fig. 2). Mean blood pressure at the sinus initially drops to 50 mm Hg but gradually recovers to reach a steady-state level between 65 and 80 mm Hg (Fig. 1 and 2). In the conscious dog, this procedure does not change tidal volume or respiratory rate since sinus perfusion pressure remains well above the threshold pressure which induces a chemoreceptor discharge [2].

Figure 1 shows that under normovolemia the reflex rise in arterial blood pressure is not associated with a significant change in kidney blood flow. This is also observed when kidney perfusion pressure is reduced to its control level (aortic compression) during common carotid occlusion. In order to increase resting sympathetic discharge to the kidney, blood volume was reduced by 13.3 ml/kg corresponding to 16.7%. This reduced the central venous pressure by 2 mm Hg, increased the heart rate by 12 beats/min, but caused no significant change in renal blood flow. Since hemorrhage caused a small decrease only in mean aortic blood pressure (5 mm Hg), it was considered "nonhypotensive." Carotid sinus hypotension during hypovolemia also failed to induce a statistically significant decrease in kidney blood flow (Fig. 1).

Figure 2 demonstrates pulse-synchronous sympathetic discharge in a resting conscious dog on the 2nd postoperative day. Carotid sinus hypotension reflexly elevated systemic blood pressure by 50 mm Hg and during the steady state increased renal sympathetic nerve activity by 40% of control. The step increase in

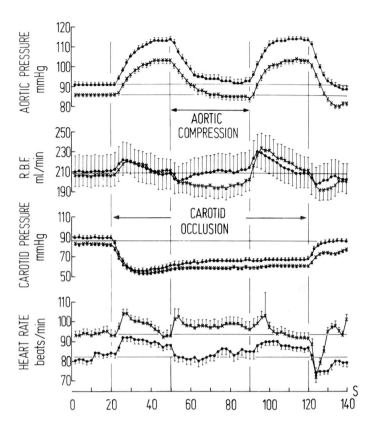

Fig. 1. Effect of common carotid occlusion on kidney blood flow before (—o—)
and 60 min after a nonhypotensive hemorrhage (—x—; blood loss: 13.3 ml/kg
= 16.7% of measured blood volume). Aortic compression: reduction of kidney
perfusion pressure back to its control level. Depicted are averages ± SE of 58
(—o—) and 73 (—x—) experiments in two healthy conscious dogs

sinus pressure due to the release of the carotid cuffs immediately reduced sympathetic discharge to the noise level for 3 s.

Figure 3 shows that emotional stress associated with slight head and leg movements induced a decrease in renal blood flow from 250 to 100 ml/min (see phasic
record) while arterial blood pressure simultaneously increased. The increase in
renal vascular resistance is of short onset and duration (5 s); it is followed regu-
larly by a secondary delayed rise in renal vascular resistance after approximately
6-10 s. The vasoconstrictor response is blocked by 5 mg/kg phenoxybenzamine.

The cardiovascular responses to emotional stress shown in Figure 4 were associated
with slight head movements only. The heart rate rose by 30-40 beats/min, blood
pressure increased by 10-15 mm Hg. Renal sympathetic nerve discharge demonstrates a regular pulse-synchronous activity under resting conditions. During the
short bursts of activation (4 s duration) elicited by each emotional stimulus, renal
sympathetic activity rises by 200%-280% of control.

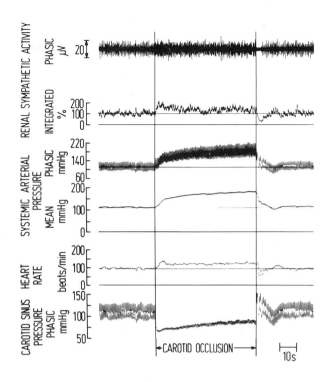

Fig. 2. Effect of common carotid occlusion on systemic arterial pressure, carotid sinus pressure, heart rate, and renal sympathetic nerve activity in a conscious dog (2nd postoperative day)

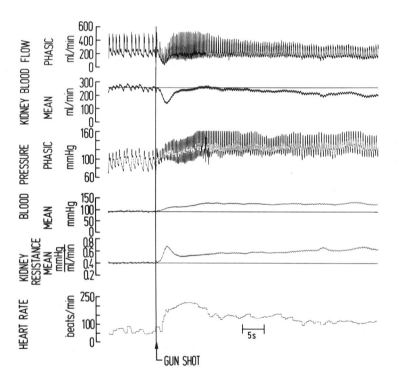

Fig. 3. Cardiovascular changes in a conscious dog (4th postoperative week) occurring with the emotional response to an unexpected loud noise (gun shot). Note intense renal vasoconstriction with short latency followed by a second wave of delayed vasoconstriction

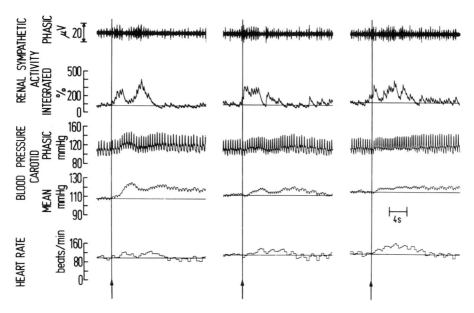

Fig. 4. Changes in blood pressure (recorded in common carotid artery), heart rate, and renal sympathetic nerve activity during emotional responses (startling, orienting reaction) elicited by (arrows from left to right): 1) shouting, 2) whistling, 3) approaching and scolding the dog (2nd postoperative day)

Summary and Conclusions

Our experiments have demonstrated that carotid sinus hypotension — with intact aortic baroreceptors — is not associated with a sympathetic adrenergic vasoconstriction in the kidney, although under comparable experimental conditions, renal sympathetic nerve activity was increased by 40% of control. As far as total renal blood flow is concerned, neither nonhypotensive hemorrhage nor carotid sinus hypotension during hypovolemia induce renal vasoconstriction. In contrast, emotional stress elicited a remarkable sympathetic a-adrenergic vasoconstriction of short duration which was obviously brought about by short bursts of sympathetic activation by 200%-280% of control. The secondary phase of renal vasoconstriction due to emotional stress is probably related to a hormonal component.

It is concluded that the increase in sympathetic discharge elicited by carotid sinus hypotension and probably also the activation observed after nonhypotensive hemorrhage is too weak to induce a reduction in total blood flow to the kidney. Therefore, we should like to suggest that moderate changes in sympathetic discharge to the kidney mainly serve to trigger the release of renin-angiotensin and/or prostaglandins or other intrarenal mechanisms associated with the control of blood volume. The tremendous sensitivity of those central structures responsible for renal sympathetic discharge to emotional stress may well play a role in the pathogenesis of hypertension.

Acknowledgment: This study was supported by the Deutsche Forschungsgemeinschaft (S.F.B. 90 Kardiovaskuläres System, Heidelberg).

References

1. Aukland, K.: Renal blood flow. In: Thurau, K. (ed.). International Review of Physiology, Kidney and Urinary Tract Physiology II. Baltimore: U. Park Pr. 1976, Vol. 11, p. 302-348
2. Biscoe, T.J., Bradley, G.W., Purves, M.J.: The relation between carotid body chemoreceptor discharge, carotid sinus pressure and carotid body venous flow. J. Physiol. 208, 99-120 (1970)
3. Caraffa-Braga, E., Granata, L., Pinotti, O.: Changes in blood flow distribution during emotional stress in dogs. Pflügers Arch. 339, 203-216 (1973)
4. Clement, D.L., Pelletier, C.L., Shepherd, J.T.: Role of vagal afferents in the control of renal sympathetic nerve activity in the rabbit. Circ. Res. 31, 824-830 (1972)
5. Kendrick, E., Öberg, B., Wennergren, G.: Vasoconstrictor fibre discharge to skeletal muscle, kidney, intestine and skin at varying levels of arterial baroreceptor activity in the cat. Acta Physiol. Scand. 85, 464-476 (1972)
6. Kirchheim, H.: Effect of common carotid occlusion on arterial blood pressure and on kidney blood flow in unanesthetized dogs. Pflügers Arch. 306, 119-134 (1969)
7. Kirchheim, H.: Systemic arterial baroreceptor reflexes. Physiol. Rev. 56, 100-176 (1976)
8. Kirchner, F.: Correlations between changes of activity of the renal sympathetic nerve and behavioural events in unrestrained cats. Basic Res. Cardiol. 69, 243-256 (1974)
9. Kezdi, P., Geller, E.: Baroreceptor control of postganglionic sympathetic nerve discharge. Am. J. Physiol. 214, 427-435 (1968)
10. Mancia, G., Baccelli, G., Zanchetti, A.: Regulation of renal circulation during behavioral changes in the cat. Am. J. Physiol. 227, 536-542 (1974)
11. Pelletier, C.L., Shepherd, J.T.: Relative influence of carotid baroreceptors and muscle receptors in the control of renal and hindlimb circulations. Can. J. Physiol. Pharmacol. 53, 1042-1049 (1975)
12. Schad, H., Seller, H.: A method for recording autonomic nerve activity in unanesthetized, freely moving cats. Brain. Res. 100, 425-430 (1975)
13. Schad, H., Seller, H.: Reduction of renal nerve activity by volume expansion in conscious cats. Pflügers Arch. 363, 155-159 (1976)
14. Smith, H.W.: The Kidney, Structure and Function in Health and Disease. New York: Oxford U. Pr. 1951
15. Vatner, S.F.: Effects of hemorrhage on regional blood flow distribution in dogs and primates. J. Clin. Invest. 54, 225-235 (1974)
16. Wilson, M.F., Ninomiya, I., Franz, G.N., Judy, W.V.: Hypothalamic stimulation and baroreceptor reflex interaction on renal nerve activity. Am. J. Physiol. 221, 1768-1773 (1971)
17. Zbrożyna, A.W.: Renal vasoconstriction in naturally elicited fear and its habituation in baboons. Cardiovasc. Res. 10, 295-300 (1976)

Cerebral Blood Flow Regulation Under the Conditions of Arterial Hypoxia

J. Grote

Institute of Physiology, Department of Applied Physiology. University of Mainz, D-65 Mainz

Pronounced arterial hypoxia induces a decrease of cerebrovascular resistance and an increase of total and regional cerebral blood flow. Under the conditions of normal arterial blood pressure and normal acid base status, the changes of both parameters commence when the oxygen tension in the arterial blood decreases below approximately 50 mm Hg. At the same time, the oxygen tension in the cerebral venous blood reaches values below approximately 28 mm Hg. Different authors [23, 28, 30, 31, 33] reported that cerebral blood flow responses to PaO_2 decrease are threshold at these oxygen tensions. The threshold oxygen tension of cerebral venous blood was accorded a special significance because Noell and Schneider [30, 31] observed that, under the conditions of insufficient oxygen supply in the brain tissue induced by different causes, an increase of the total cerebral blood flow always occurred when cerebral venous oxygen tension values were nearly constant between 25-28 mm Hg.

The general validity of these threshold blood oxygen tensions for blood flow regulation in brain tissue must be called into question. Under the conditions of nonrespiratory acidosis, normocapnia, and normal blood pressure, the stepwise decrease of arterial oxygen tension caused the typical hypoxic reactions of cerebrovascular resistance and total cerebral blood flow before the "reaction threshold" values were reached.

The experiments were performed on nine mongrel dogs during nitrous oxide anesthesia, muscle relaxation, and artificial ventilation. Blood acidosis was caused by an increase in lactate concentration. Total cerebral blood flow was measured using a dye dilution technique [24]. In two cases, regional cortical blood flow was measured by means of the [85]Kr clearance method. As can be seen from Figure 1, cerebrovascular resistance decreased and total cerebral blood flow increased when the oxygen tension in the cerebral venous blood reached a mean value of 35 mm Hg. The corresponding mean arterial oxygen tension was 53 mm Hg. The response of regional cortical blood flow to arterial hypoxia was nonuniform. Areas with increased flow rates were found adjacent to those with unchanged or decreased regional blood flow.

Our results are comparable to findings obtained under the conditions of normal acid-base status as well as during respiratory acidosis. Betz and Wünnenberg [4] observed an increase of regional cerebral flood flow in cats when ventilating the animals with gas mixtures containing 16 vol % O_2; Borgström and co-workers [9] measured increased total cerebral blood flow in rats after decreasing the ar-

209

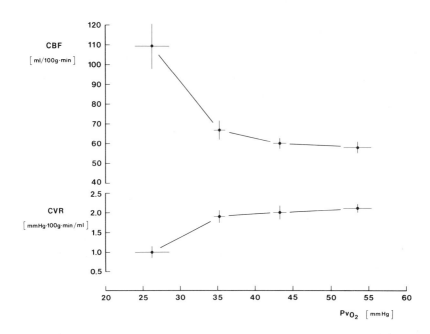

Fig. 1. Relations of cerebral venous oxygen tension to cerebral blood flow (CBF) and cerebrovascular resistance (CVR) under the conditions of arterial hypoxia, nonrespiratory acidosis, and normal blood pressure in dogs. $PaCO_2$: 38.4-41.4 mm Hg; pHa: 7.134-7.168; CPP: 107-119 mm Hg

terial oxygen tension to 75-85 mm Hg. Flohr et al. [13] as well as our group [16] found that, under respiratory acidosis and arterial hypoxia, response of total cerebral blood flow occurred before the oxygen tension values of the reaction threshold were reached. Similar inhomogeneous blood flow changes in brain tissue during arterial hypoxia were found by Leniger-Follert et al. [27] in cats and by Fujihuma et al. [14] in dogs. It is assumed that local mechanisms cause vasodilatation and blood flow increase in brain circulation under hypoxia. The increase of hydrogen ion concentration in the perivascular space and in the smooth muscle cells of the brain vessels is thought to be of great importance. The results of numerous investigations could be summarized in a "metabolic hypothesis" of cerebral blood flow regulation under the conditions of insufficient brain oxygen supply [2, 28, 38]. According to this concept, tissue hypoxia leads to increased lactate production and to acidosis, which in turn induces vasodilatation, and with sufficient perfusion pressure, leads to an increase in cerebral blood flow. The hypothesis is supported by the finding that, during arterial hypoxia occurring simultaneously with increased cerebral blood flow, an increase of brain tissue lactate concentration [19, 39] was observed. Additionally, it was found during hypoglycemia that arterial oxygen tensions below 50 mm Hg had no influence on cerebral blood flow [23]. Through theoretic investigations of O_2 diffusion in brain tissue [15, 42] and through tissue oxygen tension measurements in brain cortex [18], we could show that anoxia occurs in brain areas with high oxygen need when arterial oxygen tension falls below 50 mm Hg.

Further factors which may influence cerebral blood flow during arterial hypoxia are the concentrations of different ions such as Ca^{2+} and K^+ as well as of cate-cholamines in the perivascular space [2, 3, 6, 7, 21, 25]. The question of whether the increase of cerebral blood flow under hypoxia conditions is influenced by changes of adenosine concentration in brain tissue is still open [35, 44, 45].

Quite recently, the metabolic hypothesis describing the interrelation between brain tissue hypoxia and cerebral blood flow regulation was questioned. Under nonsteady-state conditions, Siesjö et al. [9, 40] found that, during arterial hypoxia, an increase in cerebral blood flow occurred before brain tissue lactate concentration rose. Additionally, this group could not substantiate the results of investigations on hypoglycemic animals. Direct measurements of the H^+ and K^+ activity in brain extracellular space showed that both increased with delay after arterial oxygen tension had been reduced [5, 8, 11, 21, 41]. The increase of H^+ activity is frequently preceded by a decrease of short duration. In many cases, distinct changes of both parameters could be observed only after several minutes of continuous hypoxia. Since Leniger-Follert and co-workers [27, 43] in their investigations on cats found that, after N_2 ventilation, H^+ and K^+ activity in brain extracellular space increased, brain oxygen tension decreased, and micro-flow changed, all occurring simultaneously, it is currently questionable whether these findings contradict the metabolic hypothesis.

The results presented here do not allow a direct conclusion concerning the cause of cerebral blood flow increase in hypoxia. During nonrespiratory acidosis and arterial hypoxia, however, the increase in total cerebral blood flow occurred simultaneously with a more than 100% rise in brain lactate output (1.1 mg/100 g min). Since the blood-brain barrier does not essentially hinder lactate exchange, it must be concluded that lactate acidosis in the perivascular space of the brain vessels was present under these conditions. According to latest investigations cerebral blood flow regulation does not appear to be influenced by carotid chemo- and baroreceptor stimulation [1, 12, 20, 34].

The regulation of cerebral blood flow during arterial hypoxia is impaired or abolished in brain tissue areas with increased water content. During experiments on 16 cats in which local brain edema was induced in the right frontal cortex by a cryolesion according to Klatzo [22], stepwise reduction of arterial oxygen tension led to a progressive and significant increase in regional blood flow in the undamaged hemisphere, while the flow rate of the perifocal edematous tissue zones remained unaffected (Fig. 2). The animals were anesthetized with sodium pentobarbital (Nembutal, 30 mg/kg body weight) and, after tracheotomy and complete relaxation, artificially ventilated. Regional cerebral blood flow measurements were performed using the ^{85}Kr clearance technique. In all experiments, blood pressure and arterial CO_2 tension remained within the normal range. Simultaneously, with increased tissue water content, increased tissue lactate concentrations but decreased regional flow rates were measured under the conditions of arterial normoxia as well as of arterial hypoxia. For tissue oxygen tension, low values reaching 0 were measured during normoxic and hypoxic states in the

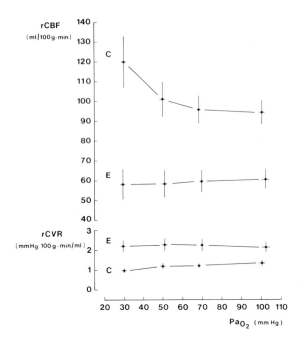

Fig. 2. Influence of arterial hypoxia on regional cerebral blood flow (rCBF) and regional cerebrovascular resistance (rCVR) in unaffected (C) and edematous (E) cortical brain tissue of cats during arterial normocapnia and normal blood pressure. $PaCO_2$: 28.5-29.6 mm Hg. Pm_a: 106-120 mm Hg

edematous areas as well as in the unaffected brain tissue zones. The results indicate that, with decreasing extracellular pH and decreasing tissue oxygen tension, the normal behavior of cerebrovascular resistance and cerebral blood flow is locally counteracted in edematous brain tissue. This may be explained by the increase in tissue pressure [36, 27] following increased water content.

References

1. Bates, D., Chir, B., Sundt, T.M.: The relevance of peripheral baroreceptors and chemoreceptors to regulation of cerebral blood flow in the cat. Circ. Res. 38, 488-492 (1976)
2. Betz, E.: Cerebral blood flow: Its measurement and regulation. Physiol. Rev. 52, 595-630 (1972)
3. Betz, E.: Experimental production of cerebral vascular disorders. In: Handbuch der experimentellen Pharmakologie. Vol. 16/3: Experimental Production of Diseases. Schmier, J., Eichler, O. (eds.). Berlin-Heidelberg-New York, Springer 1975, p. 183
4. Betz, E., Wünnenberg, E.: Anpassung der Gehirndurchblutung an Sauerstoffmangel. Arch. Physik. Therapie 16, 45-55 (1964)
5. Betz, E., Heuser, D.: Cerebral cortical blood flow during changes of acid-base equilibrium of the brain. J. Appl. Physiol. 23, 726-733 (1967)
6. Betz, E., Brandt, H., Csornai, M., Heuser, D.: The role of ions in the regulation of pial arterial diameters. Arzneim.-Forsch. 26, 12-13 (1976)

7. Bicher, H.: Brain Oxygen Autoregulation: A protective reflex to hypoxia? Microvasc. Res. $\underline{8}$, 291-313 (1974)

8. Bito, L.Z., Myers, R.E.: On the physiological response of the cerebral cortex to acute stress (reversible asphyxia). J. Physiol. $\underline{221}$, 349-370 (1972)

9. Borgström, L., Johannsson, H., Siesjö, B.K.: The relationship between arterial Po_2 and cerebral blood flow in hypoxic hypoxia. Acta Physiol. Scand. $\underline{93}$, 423-432 (1975)

10. Crone, C., Sorensen, S.C.: The permeability of the blood-brain barrier to lactate and pyruvate. Acta Physiol. Scand. $\underline{80}$, 47-A (1970)

11. Dora, E., Zeuthen, T.: Brain metabolism and ion movements in the brain cortex of the rat during anoxia. In: Ion and Enzyme Electrodes in Biology and Medicine. Kessler, M., Clark, L.C., Lübbers, D.W., Silver, I.A., Simon, W. (eds.). München-Berlin-Wien: Urban und Schwarzenberg 1976 p. 294

12. Eidelman, B.H., McCalden, T.A., Rosendorff, C.: The role of the carotid body in mediating the cerebravascular response to altered arterial carbon dioxide tension. Stroke $\underline{7}$, 72-76 (1976)

13. Flohr, H., Pöll, W., Brock, M.: Effect of arterial oxygen tension on cerebral blood flow at different levels of arterial P_{CO_2}. Experientia (Basel) $\underline{26}$, 615 (1970)

14. Fujishima, M., Scheinberg, P., Busto, R.: Cerebral cortical blood flow. Variable effects of hypoxia in the dog. Arch. Neurol. $\underline{25}$, 160-167 (1971)

15. Grote, J.: Die Sauerstoffspannung im Gehirngewebe. In: Hydrodynamik, Elektrolyt- und Säure-Basen-Haushalt im Liquor und Nervensystem. Kienle, G. (ed.). Stuttgart: Thieme 1967, p. 41

16. Grote, J., Kreuscher, H., Schubert, R., Russ, H.J.: New studies on the influence of PaO_2 and $PaCO_2$ on regional and total cerebral blood flow. In: 6th Europ. Conf. Micorcirculation, Aalborg 1970. Ditzel, J., Lewis, D.H. (eds.). Basel: Karger 1971, p. 294

17. Grote, J., Kreuscher, H., Vaupel, P., Günther, H.: The influence of reduced Pa_{O_2} during respiratory and nonrespiratory acidosis on cerebral oxygen supply and cerebral metabolism. In: Cerebral blood flow and intracranial pressure. Fiesci, C. (ed.). Europ. Neurol. $\underline{6}$, 335-339 (1971/72)

18. Grote, J., Schubert, R.: The effect of brain edema on cortical oxygen supply during arterial normoxia and arterial hypoxia. Bibl. Anat. $\underline{15}$, 355-358 (1977)

19. Gardjian, E.S. Stone, W.E., Webster, J.E.: Cerebral metabolism in hypoxia. Arch. Neurol. Psychiat. $\underline{51}$, 472-477 (1944)

20. Heistad, D.D., Marcus, M.L., Ehrhardt, J.C., Abbond, F.M.: Effect of stimulation of carotid chemoreceptors on total and regional cerebral blood flow. Circ. Res. $\underline{38}$, 20-25 (1976)

21. Heuser, D., Astrup, J., Lassen, N.A., Nilsson, B., Norberg, K., Siesjö, B.K.: Are H^+ and K^+ factors for the adjustment of cerebral blood flow to changes in functional state: a microelectrode study. In: Cerebral Function, Metabolism and Circulation. Ingvar, D.V., Lassen, N.A. (eds.). Acta Neurol. Scand. (Suppl. 64) $\underline{56}$, 216 (1977)

22. Klatzo, I., Wiesniewski, H., Steinwall, O., Streicher, E.: Dynamics of cold injury edema. In: Brain Edema. Klatzo, I., Seitelberger, F. (eds.). Wien-New York: Springer 1967, p. 554

23. Kogure, K., Scheinberg, P., Reinmutz, O.M., Fujishima, M., Busto, R.: Mechanisms of cerebral vasodilatation in hypoxia. J. Appl. Physiol. 29, 223-229 (1970)

24. Kreuscher, H.: Die Hirndurchblutung unter Neuroleptanaesthesie. Anaesthesiologie und Wiederbelebung. Berlin-Heidelberg-New York: Springer 1967, Vol. 21

25. Kuschinsky, W., Wahl, M.: Alpha-receptor stimulation by endogenous and exogenous norepinephrine and blockade by phentolamine in pial arteries of cats. Circ. Res. 37, 168-174 (1975)

26. Lassen, N.A.: Brain extracellular pH: the main factor controlling cerebral blood flow. Scand. J. Clin. Lab. Invest. 22, 247-251 (1968)

27. Leniger-Follert, E., Wrabetz, W., Lübbers, D.W.: Local tissue PO_2 and microflow of the brain cortex under varying arterial oxygen pressure. In: Oxygen Transport to Tissue — II. Grote, J., Reneau, D., Thews, G. (eds.). Adv. Exp. Med. Biol. 75, 361-367 (1976)

28. McDowall, D.G.: Interrelationships between blood oxygen tension and cerebral blood flow. In: A Symposium on Oxygen Measurements in Blood and Tissues and their Significance. Payne, J.P., Hill, D.W. (eds.). London: Churchill 1966, p. 215

29. Nemeto, E.M., Severinghaus, J.W.: The stereospecific influx permeability of rat blood brain barrier (BBB) to lactic acid (LA). Clin. Res. 19, 146 (1971)

30. Noell, W.: Über die Durchblutung und die Sauerstoffversorgung des Gehirns. VI-Einfluß der Hypoxämie und Anämie. Pflügers Arch. 247, 553-575 (1944)

31. Noell, W., Schneider, M.: Über die Durchblutung und die Sauerstoffversorgung des Gehirns im akuten Sauerstoffmangel. III. Die arteriovenöse Sauerstoff- und Kohlensäuredifferenz. Pflügers Arch. 246, 207-249 (1942)

32. Oldendorf, W.H.: Blood brain barrier permeability to lactate. In: Cerebral Blood Flow and Intracranial Pressure, Fieschi, C. (ed.). Europ. Neurol. 6, 49-55 (1971/72)

33. Opitz, E., Schneider, M.: Über die Sauerstoffversorgung des Gehirns und den Mechanismus von Mangelwirkungen. Erg. Physiol. 46, 126-260 (1950)

34. Ponte, J., Purves, M.J.: The role of the carotid body chemoreceptors and carotid sinus baroreceptors in the control of cerebral blood vessels. J. Physiol. 237, 315-340 (1974)

35. Rehncrona, S., Nordstrom, C.-H., Siesjö, B.K., Westerberg, E.: Adenosine in rat cerebral cortex during hypoxia and bicuculline-induced seizures. In: Cerebral Function, Metabolism and Circulation. Ingvar, D.V., Lassen, L.A. (eds.). Acta Neurol. Scand. (Suppl. 64) 56, 220 (1977)

36. Reulen, H.J., Kreysch, H.G.: Measurement of brain tissue pressure in cold induced cerebral oedema. Acta Neurochir. 29, 29-40 (1973)

37. Reulen, H.J., Graham, R., Klatzo, I.: Development of pressure gradients within brain tissue during the formation of vasogenic brain edema. In: Intracranial Pressure II. Lundberg, N., Ponten, U., Brock, M. (eds.). Berlin-Heidelberg-New York: Springer 1975, p. 233

38. Siesjö, B.K., Kjällquist, A., Ponten, U., Zwetnow, N.: Extracellular pH in the brain and cerebral blood flow. In: Cerebral Circulation, Luyendijk, W. (ed.). Progress in Brain. Research 30, 93-98, Amsterdam: Elsevier 1968

39. Siesjö, B.K., Nilsson, L.: The influence of arterial hypoxemia upon labile phosphates and upon extracellular and intracellular lactate and pyruvate concentration in the rat brain. Scand. J. Clin. Lab. Invest. 27, 83-96 (1971)

40. Siesjö, B.K., Borgström, L., Johannsson, H., Nilsson, B., Norberg, K., Quistorff, B.: Cerebral oxygenation in arterial hypoxia. In: Oxygen Transport to Tissue-II. Grote, J., Reneau, D., Thews, G. (eds.). Adv. Exp. Med. Biol. 75, 335-342 (1976)

41. Silver, I.A.: Tissue responses to hypoxia, shock and stroke. In: Oxygen Transport to Tissue-II. Grote, J., Reneau, D., Thews, G. (eds.). Adv. Exp. Med. Biol. 75, 325-333 (1976)

42. Thews, G.: Die Sauerstoffdiffusion im Gehirn. Ein Beitrag zur Frage der Sauerstoffversorgung der Organe. Pflügers Arch. 271, 197-226 (1960)

43. Urbanics, R., Leniger-Follert, E., Lübbers, D.W.: Extracellular K^+ and H^+ activity of the brain cortex during and after a short period of ischemia and arterial hypoxia. In: Oxygen Transport to Tissue-III. Adv. Exp. Med. Biol. (in press)

44. Wahl, M., Kuschinsky, W.: The dilatatory action of adenosine on pial arteries of cats and its inhibition by theophylline. Pflügers Arch. 362, 55-59 (1976)

45. Wahl, M., Kuschinsky, W.: Dependency of the dilatatory action of adenosine on the perivascular H^+ and K^+ at pial arteries of cats. In: Cerebral Function, Metabolism and Circulation. Ingvar, D.V., Lassen, L.A. (eds.). Acta Neurol. Scand. (Suppl. 64) 56, 218 (1977)

Minimization of the External Work of the Left Ventricle and Optimization of Flow and Pressure Pulses

K. P. Pfeiffer and T. Kenner

Physiologisches Institut der Universität Graz, Graz/Österreich

Introduction

The problem of optimization of the action of the heart was first discussed by Broemser [1] in 1935. He assumed that there is an optimal relationship between heart frequency and stroke volume. During the last several years, Yamashiro and Grodins [8], Kenner and Estelberger [5], and Estelberger [3] have taken up this problem from a new point of view. The statement of the problem can be summarized as follows. The time course of the aortic root flow should be determind in such a way that the heart has to do a minimum amount of stroke work for the ejection of a fixed stroke volume (V_s) in a given systolic period (S). With the aid of an improved windkessel model, the optimal course of the aortic root flow was calculated using variational calculus. In the following study, we shall summarize this question and discuss the problem as to how much evidence exists im support of such an optimization in vivo.

Description of the Model and the Optimal Pulse Shapes

The electric analogue model of the arterial system is shown in Figure 1. It consists of a longitudinal resistance (Z), an aortic compliance (C), and a peripheral resistance (R). Between the flow [q(t)] through the resistance (Z) and the flow [x(t)] through the peripheral resistance (R), the following relation during the systole is valid

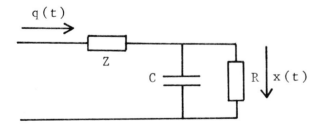

Fig. 1. Electric analog model of the arterial system. a(t) inflow, x(t) outflow, Z longitudinal resistance representing the characteristic impedance of the aorta, R peripheral resistance, C compliance

$$q(t) = x(t) + RC\dot{x}(t)$$

$$q(t) = x(t) + \tau \dot{x}(t)$$

$$0 \leqslant t \leqslant S \qquad \tag{1}$$

$$\tau = CR$$

It was assumed that the systolic duration (S) and the total cycle duration (T) of the periodic pulses are known. Beside this, $[q(t)]$ must fulfil the following condition

$$\int_0^S q(t)\, dt = V_s, \qquad \tag{2}$$

which means that during the systole a given stroke volume V_s must be ejected. During the systole, the following conditions are valid

$$q(t) = 0 \qquad\qquad S \leqslant t \leqslant T \qquad \tag{3}$$

$$x(t) = x(0)\, e^{\frac{T-t}{\tau}} \qquad S \leqslant t \leqslant T \qquad \tag{4}$$

As mentioned above, it is assumed that the pulses are periodic. Consequently

$$x(0) = x(T) \qquad \tag{5}$$

The criterion of optimality for our model is

$$A = Z \int_0^S q^2(t)\, dt + R \int_0^S x^2(t)\, dt + R \int_S^T x^2(t)\, dt \rightarrow min. \qquad \tag{6}$$

Here the total external stroke work is divided into a systolic and a diastolic part. With the aid of the calculus of variations, we (2, 7) look for an optimal solution of this equation. For this reason the functional

$$F(x, \dot{x}, t) = Z(x + \tau \dot{x})^2 + R\, x^2 + \mu(x + \tau \dot{x}) \qquad \tag{7}$$

must be a solution of the Euler-Lagrange equation

$$\frac{\partial F}{\partial x} - \frac{d}{dt}\left[\frac{\partial F}{\partial \dot{x}}\right] = 0 \qquad \tag{8}$$

μ is a Lagrange multiplier. The Euler-Lagrange equation for Eq. 7 has the following form

$$\ddot{x}(t) - \frac{Z + R}{Z_\tau{}^2}\, x(t) = \frac{\mu}{Z_\tau{}^2} \qquad \tag{9}$$

where $\mu/Z_\tau{}^2$ is an integration constant, which is determined after the solution of Eq. 8, whose common solution is

$$x(t) = A e^{nt} + B e^{-nt} + C \qquad (10)$$

A necessary condition for the integral to become a minimum on an extremal is the Legendre condition

$$\frac{\partial^2 F}{\partial x^2} \geqslant 0 \quad . \qquad (11)$$

Because $\partial^2 F / \partial x^2 = 2 Z_\tau^2 \geqslant 0$, this condition is also satisfied. By inserting Eq. 10 in Eq. 1, we get

$$q(t) = A e^{nt} (1 + \tau n) + B e^{-nt} (1 - \tau n) + C \qquad (12)$$

Considering all boundary conditions and all constraints (Eqs. 2, 3, and 5), we get a system of three equations for the three unknown variables A, B and C.

The solution of the system of equations and the iteration for the calculation of $x(0)$ were implemented on a HP 2100A digital computer. Figure 2 show the calculated optimal time course of the aortic root flow and of the aortic pressure for different values of the peripheral resistance (R) and of the aortic compliance (C). Longitudinal resistance (Z), systolic duration (S), cycle duration (T), and stroke volume (V_s) are assumed constant. It can be seen that the basic course of the optimal aortic root flow is triangular. With decreasing peripheral resistance (R) and decreasing aortic compliance (C), the optimal time course of flow differs more and more from a triangular course for a small Z and shows a "late systolic nose," which disappears with increasing Z.

Calculation of the Pulse Shape and the Stroke Work for Triangular Flow

For the calculation of the nonoptimal pressure course in the aorta and the appropriate heart work, triangular aortic root flow was assumed. The systolic peak of these triangles with constant area (V_s) was shifted in [O, S] (Fig. 3a). Figure 3b shows the shape of calculated pressure pulses for differnt assumed flow pulses.

Estimation of the Efficiency of Optimization

To find out the magnitude of the energetic advantage of an optimal flow course as compared with a triangular flow course, we compared the necessary external stroke work for the ejection of a given stroke volume (V_s) within a systole of duration (S) for an optimal flow course with the external stroke work of non-optimal flow shapes. The latter was calculated as a function of the position of the flow peak. Figure 4 shows the position of the peak of the triangle within the systole on the abscissa and the stroke work for the corresponding triangular pulse

218

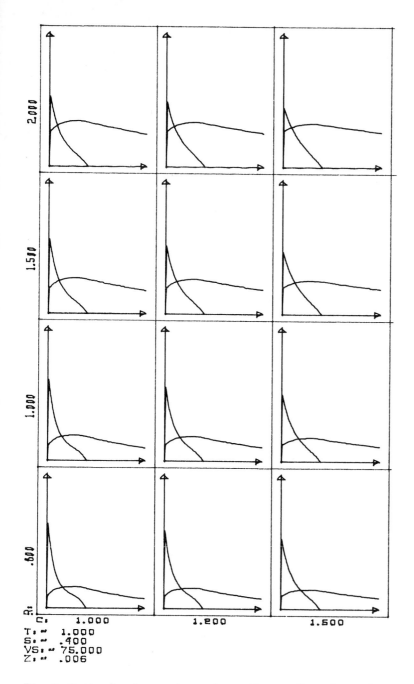

Fig. 2. Optimal pulse contours depending on the values of the resistances Z and R (mm Hg sec/ml) and compliance C (ml/mm Hg). T pulse perid (sec), S duration of the systole (sec), VS stroke volume (ml)

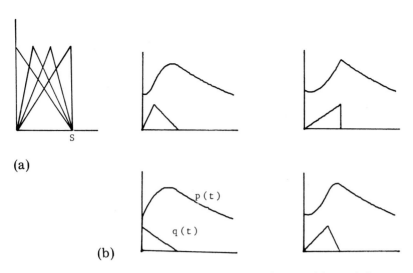

(a)

(b)

Fig. 3. (a) Triangular flow pulses with varying position of the systolic peak
(b) Pressure pulses p(t) generated by triangular flow pulses q(t) with varying position of the systolic peak

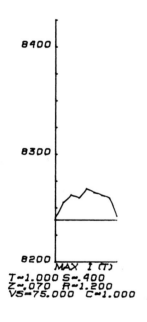

MAX I (T)
$T\sim1.000$ $S\sim.400$
$Z\sim.070$ $R\sim1.200$
$VS\sim75.000$ $C\sim1.000$

Fig. 4. Stroke work (ordinate, mm Hg. ml) of triangular flow pulses depending on the position of the systolic peak within the systole (abscissa, sec). The straight line indicates the stroke work of the corresponding optimal pulse shape. Symbols as in Fig. 2

on the ordinate. The horizontal line marks the stroke of the optimal pulse shape with systolic duration (S) and stroke volume (V_S). The result of this computation shows that the gain of energy by optimization of the flow course is only very small.

220

Further Developments

This kind of model shows that the optimal pulse shape improves the economy of the heart work only by a very small extent in comparison with triangular non-optimal flow courses. Furthermore, the agreement between calculated and normal physiologic pulse shapes is deficient; the infinitely steep pressure rise at the beginning of the systole is in particular incorrect. Therefore, it is questionable if this kind of a model is qualified as a basis for a parameter estimation procedure, especially one aiming at the estimation of the stroke volume, as proposed by Estelberger [3]. The question of whether the stroke work in vivo is in fact minimized or whether there are other factors of importance leads to possible further criteria of optimization. In a recent paper by Noldus [6], the following criterion was suggested

$$J = \int_0^S \left| p^2(t) + ap(t) x(t) \right| dt , \qquad a \geqslant 0$$

Besides mechanical work, this criterion also takes the ventricular pressure into consideration. Another aspect we examined was the question of the necessary supply of the heart by the coronary flow. With decreasing systolic duration, the work necessary to eject some given stroke volume increases considerably. On the other hand, the volume which flows through the coronary vessels during the diastole is approximately proportional to the diastolic duration. A sufficient supply of the myocardium depends very much on the ratio of systolic to diastolic duration, when the duration of the pulse period is fixed. This proportion must be considered as a very important constraint of every optimization. Figure 5 shows the steep increase of stroke work with shortening diastolic duration, which can be compared with the rather small increase of diastolic coronary flow. The assumed requirement of minimization of coronary flow yields as limiting case a systolic duration which is derivable from the point of contact of the two curves. Therefore, taking into account coronary flow, any solution of the problem also yields a certain systolic duration as a result of the optimization procedure.

Conclusion and Summary

In this analysis, pressure and flow pulse shapes were derived assuming an energetic optimization of the external heart work. Characteristic for these pulse shapes is their triangular shape, the presence of a "late systolic nose," and the steep pressure rise at the beginning of the systole. Furthermore, we could demonstrate that the gain of energy by the optimal solution compared with the nonoptimal solution is surprisingly small. In our team, we tried to apply the concept of optimization within a parameter estimation method. Estelberger [3] proposed an estimation of the stroke volume. The possibility of an estimation of the contractility with the aid of a model also seems important to us. But in the current version, it is nearly impossible to apply this model for practical purposes because of the

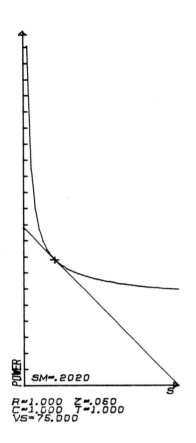

POWER

SM≈.2020

R≈1.000 Z≈.050
C≈1.000 T≈1.000
VS≈75.000

Fig. 5. Energy supply by coronary flow (lower straight line) and energy expenditure of the ventricle (hyperbolic line) depending on the duration of the systole (abscissa). The duration of the pulse period is considered fixed (T = 1 sec). An optimal systolic duration is indicated by the point where the two curves touch (x).
Symbols as in Fig. 2

uncertainty of the agreement between computed and real physiologic pulses. Therefore, it is necessary for further development to take other criteria like ventricular pressure or the energy supply of the myocardium into account. It would also be interesting to extend the question of optimality to the whole pulse period including the filling of the ventricle.

Acknowledgment: This work was supported by the Austrian research fund.

References

1. Broemser, Ph.: Über die optimalen Beziehungen zwischen Herztätigkeit und physikalischen Konstanten des Gefäßsystems. Z. Biol. 96, 1-10 (1935)
2. Elsgolc, L.E.: Calculus of Variations. Reading Massachusetts: Addison-Wesley 1962
3. Estelberger, W.: Eine neue nichtinvasive Pulskontur-Schlagvolumsbestimmungs-methode aufgrund eines Optimierungsmodells der Herzarbeit. Biomed. Technik, 22, 212-217 (1977)

4. Kenner, Th.: Physical and Mathematical Modeling in Cardiovascular Systems. In: Engineering Principles in Cardiovascular Research. N.H.C. Hwang (ed.). Univ. Park. Pr., Baltimore-London-Tokio (1978) (in press)
5. Kenner, T.H., Estelberger, W.: Zur Frage der optimalen Abstimmung der Herzkontraktion an die Eigenschaften des Arteriensystems. Verh. Dtsch. Ges. Kreislaufforsch. 42, 132-135 (1976)
6. Noldus, E.J.: Optimal control aspects of left ventricular ejection dynamics. J. Theor. Biology, 63, 275-309 (1976)
7. Schultz, D.G., Melsa, J.L.: State Functions and Linear Control Systems. New York: McGraw 1967
8. Yamashiro, S.M., Daubenspeck, J.A., Bennett, F.M., Edelmann, S.K., Grodins, F.S.: Optimal Control Analysis of Left Ventricular Ejection. In: J. Baan, A. Noordergraaf, J. Raines (eds.), Cardiovascular System Dynamics, MIT-Press, Cambridge, Mass. 1978

Cardiovascular Dynamics and Coronary Arteries

Influence of Arterial Impedance on Ventricular Function*

W. R. Milnor

The Johns Hopkins University, Department of Physiology, Baltimore MD/USA

The input impedance of the aorta is a measure of the extent to which the arterial system opposes the ejection of blood by the left ventricle, and the same is true for the pulmonary artery and right ventricle. Arterial impedance, therefore, represents the load on the heart [4] and influences the ventricles in two ways: by affecting ventricular work and by determining the relationships between pressure and flow. The input impedance of an artery is calculated experimentally from the frequency components of observed pressure and flow waves and is expressed as a complex frequency spectrum.

Figure 1 shows, for example, the average pulmonary input impedance spectrum in a group of 29 anesthetized dogs studied in our laboratory [2]. The abscissa of the graph is frequency, and the ordinate is impedance modulus in the upper portion and impedance phase in the lower portion. The impedance modulus is the ratio of pressure to flow modulus at each frequency. Impedance phase is the difference between pressure and flow phase angles. By convention, we designate impedance angles as negative when flow leads pressure.

The contours of the impedance spectrum are very similar in the pulmonary artery and aorta in man and dog. At zero frequency, the pulmonary input impedance is simply mean pressure divided by mean flow and is, therefore, very similar to the conventional pulmonary vascular resistance, except that here we use the pulmonary arterial input pressure not the gradient of pressure across the whole pulmonary bed. Impedance is relatively high at zero frequency, falls very steeply in the lower frequency range, reaches a minimum at about 3 Hz, rises to a maximum at about 6 Hz, and is fairly constant at higher frequencies. Impedance phase is initially negative, rises to cross the zero line at about the same frequency as the minimum modulus, and is usually somewhat positive thereafter. Arterial impedance is determined first of all by the physical properties of the artery (the elasticity of its wall, the dimensions of the vessel, the viscosity of blood and the wall, and other factors) and secondly by reflections, i.e., waves reflected back from peripheral sites [1]. The physical properties determine what is called the characteristic impedance (shown in Fig. 1 by the broken line that is almost constant with frequency above 0.5 Hz). Because of reflections, the observed impedance moduli oscillate around this characteristic impedance with frequency,

---

* The experimental work reported here was a collaborative effort of Drs. C.R. Conti, W.W. Nichols, P. Sipkema, W.E. Walker, and W.R. Milnor.

227

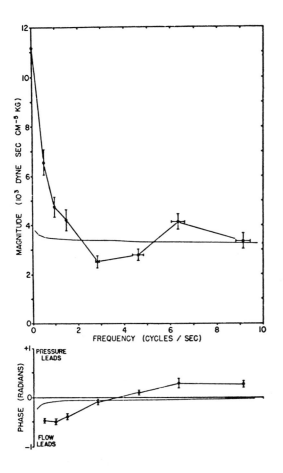

Fig. 1. Pulmonary arterial input impedance spectrum in anesthetized dogs, average from 29 animals, including four animals with complete atrioventricular block and very slow heart rates. Bars represent ± 1 SEM. Impedance moduli were normalized for body size by using flow per kg weight in the computations. Broken lines are estimates of characteristic impedance from the observations and are equivalent to the theoretic (Womersley) impedance of a constrained elastic tube with a diameter of 1.4 cm and wave velocity of 2.0 m/s (from data in Milnor et al. [2])

producing a minimum and maximum as shown. Characteristic impedance in large arteries can be estimated approximately by averaging the observed moduli between 2 and 10 Hz.

The influence of impedance on pressure-flow relations is implicit in the definition of impedance

$$Z(\omega) = \frac{P(\omega)}{Q(\omega)} \tag{1}$$

where $Z(\omega)$ is the impedance, $P(\omega)$ the pressure, and $Q(\omega)$ the flow, all at radial frequency ω. All three variables are complex numbers, usually expressed as a modulus, or amplitude, and a phase angle. Since arterial impedance depends on the physical properties of the arteries, the physiologic significance of this equation is that for any given arterial state, the ventricle must deliver pressure and flow waves whose ratio matches the arterial input impedance. As far as impedance is concerned, the ventricle is free to produce any pressure and flow combination it chooses, as long as their ratio equals the arterial impedance.

The relation between ventricular work per unit time ($\dot{W}$) and the arterial input impedance is

$$\dot{W} = (\overline{Q}^2 R) + \left[\frac{1}{2} \sum_{n=1}^{\infty} |Q_n|^2 \cdot |Z_n| \cos \theta_n \right] \qquad (2)$$

where $\overline{Q}$ is mean flow, R is input resistance, or mean pressure/mean flow, $|Q_n|$ the flow modulus at frequency n, $|Z_n|$ the impedance modulus, and θ_n the impedance phase at the same frequency. Total ventricular work per unit time is thus the sum of the work at all relevant frequencies, including zero. Almost all (95%) of the energy of pulsations in vivo appears at frequencies below 8 Hz. As Eq. 2 indicates, the higher the input resistance, the greater the ventricular power for a given flow. The higher an impedance modulus, or the smaller its phase angle, the greater the power. The first term in Eq. 2 has been called the "steady-flow" power, because it depends on the average, or nonpulsatile flow. The second component, which contains the pulsatile flow and impedance terms, has been called the "pulsatile power" [2]. Separating power into these two components has a physiologic significance, for the steady-flow term depends mainly on the arterioles and microcirculation, where most of the DC resistance is located, whereas the pulsatile power depends mainly on the state of the aorta, which determines the rest of the impedance spectrum.

I will present examples of both of these kinds of interaction between the heart and arteries, beginning with the influence of impedance on ventricular work and then going on to consider the interaction between myocardial force and velocity and arterial impedance, which I think has some implications about the basic mechanics of muscle contraction.

Some observations we have made on human subjects will serve to illustrate the influence of impedance on cardiac work and power. The average aortic input impedance spectra and other hemodynamic data in three groups of human subjects that we have studied [5] are listed in Table 1. The subjects in group A had

Table 1. Hemodynamic data, human ascending aorta[a] (averages, $\pm$ 1 SEM)

Variable	Group A	Group B	Group C
Number of subjects	5	7	4
Mean flow (ml/s)	114 ($\pm$ 17)	82 ($\pm$ 7)	119 ($\pm$ 5)
Mean pressure (mm Hg)	97 ($\pm$ 4)	85 ($\pm$ 1)	120 ($\pm$ 5)
Input resistance[b]	1218 ($\pm$147)	1390 ($\pm$163)	1344 ($\pm$49)
Characteristic impedance[b]	53 ($\pm$ 4)	95 ($\pm$ 12)	202 ($\pm$32)
Total power[c](W)	1.71 ($\pm$ .24)	1.12 ($\pm$ .09)	2.37 ($\pm$.15)
Pulsatile/total power (%)	13 ($\pm$ 1)	17 ($\pm$ 1)	19 ($\pm$ 2)

[a] From data of Nichols et al. [5].   [c] External, kinetic energy omitted.
[b] Units, dyn s/cm^5.

normal cardiovascular systems, those in group B had coronary arterial disease and normal mean aortic pressures, and those in group C had coronary disease and moderately elevated mean pressures. In the normal group, the aortic input impedance spectrum was qualitatively similar to the one shown in Figure 1. Impedance was relatively high at zero frequency, fell steeply at low frequencies to a minimum, then rose to a maximum. Impedance phase was negative at low frequencies, then rose to become positive above 4 Hz. The characteristic impedance was estimated to be 53 dyn s/cm^5 in that group. Input resistances in groups B and C were slightly higher than in A. Characteristic impedance moduli, however, were strikingly different in the three groups, averaging about twice the normal level in group B, and four times normal in group C.

We do not know with certainty the cause of these increased impedances, but age is probably one factor. The normal subjects were all less than 40 years of age, the patients with coronary disease (groups B and C) were all over 40, and it has been clearly established that arteries become stiffer with age, which would tend to raise the impedance. The difference between groups B and C, which had the same average age, is attributable (at least in part) to distention of the aorta by the higher pressures in group C, since it is also well-known that the elastic modulus of the arterial wall increases as a vessel is distended. We have found very similar changes in pumonary input impedance in patients with pulmonary vascular disease and hypertension [3]. At present, however, we are not concerned with the mechanism for these impedance changes but with the effects on ventricular work.

In group A, input resistance was about 24 times as great as the characteristic impedance. On first thought, this suggests a similar proportion between steady-flow and pulsatile power, but that is not the case. The power components also depend on the relative magnitudes of mean flow and pulsations, which is determined by the heart. As a result, the actual ratio of steady-flow to pulsatile power in group A was about 8:1. In group B, the fact that the characteristic impedance (and all individual impedance moduli) were higher than in group A might lead one to expect that ventricular power would be higher than normal, but that again be an error. Mean and pulsatile flow, and hence ventricular power, were lower in group B than in group A. Although impedance is one determinant of ventricular power, the particular flow generated by the heart is also an important factor and a powerful one because power is proportional to the square of the flow moduli.

In group C, the cardiac output and flow pulses were not significantly different from the normals, but the results demonstrate still another factor that plays a part in cardiac work. Ventricular power is not proportional to the impedance modulus alone, but rather to the real part of the complex impedance, the product of impedance modulus and the cosine of the impedance phase (Eq. 2). The larger the phase angle, the smaller the real part of impedance and the smaller the power per unit flow. Although the low frequency impedance phases in group C were only a few tenths of a radian more negative than in group A, that was enough to make the power in group C only 40% greater than in group A, in spite of the fourfold difference in impedance moduli. Each one of the variables in the power equation, in other words, can change significantly in vivo.

The difference in cardiac power between groups B and C (see Table 1) tells us something about the state of the myocardium in the two groups. In both groups, the left ventricle faced an abnormally high impedance, but group C was still able to produce a normal cardiac output and more than normal power, while group B was not. This and other considerations led us to investigate the way in which the normal ventricle responds when faced with a high impedance. As is well-known, many questions about ventricular function remain unanswered. Investigators cannot even agree on a definition of myocardial contractility, much less measure it, and we thought that some new and useful information about myocardial contraction might be found by studying the changes in ventricular performance brought about by changes in impedance. The experiments we did were very simple in concept — we changed the aortic input impedance suddenly between two heartbeats [6]. Several others have used the same general technique, but for different purposes.

Figure 2 is part of a record from one such experiment, showing blood flow in the ascending aorta and pressure in the left ventricle. We also measured pressure in

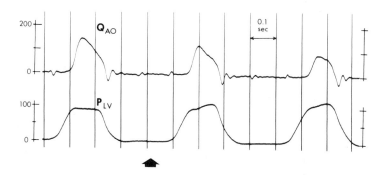

Fig. 2. Record from an experiment to measure the effects of altered impedance on ventricular performance. Q_{ao}: blood flow in ascending aorta, measured by perivascular cuff and electromagnetic flowmeter; P_{LV}: left ventricular pressure, determined by Millar catheter tip strain gauge transducer. At time indicated by arrow, input impedance was altered by inflating an occluding cuff placed around the aorta just beyond the arch

the ascending aorta (not shown here) so that we could calculate aortic input impedance and measured the end diastolic volume of the ventricle by a thermodilution method. Knowing the end diastolic volume and having a continuous record of outflow, we then knew the volume of the ventricle at every instant. After a control period, we suddenly changed the impedance (arrow in Fig. 2) by inflating an occluding cuff placed around the aorta just beyond the arch. We could control the degree of occlusion and hence the change in impedance. Pressure and flow waves changed in the next beat, and while the occluding cuff was kept on, pressure continued to rise and flow slowly decreased. We were not concerned with these later chronic adaptations to increased impedance, however. We simply compared the first and second beats in Figure 2 because we could safely assume that the end diastolic volumes and pressure were the same in both, that the neural input was the same, and that the chemical environment was the same. The only difference between the two beats was that when the aortic valve opened, the ventricle faced a different, known impedance in each case. Comparison of the two should show us the intrinsic response of the myocardium when faced with a higher impedance.

A tracing comparing two such beats is shown on the left in Figure 3. The unbroken line is the control beat. The broken line is the beat immediately after occluding the aorta to 30% of its previous cross-sectional area, which raised the

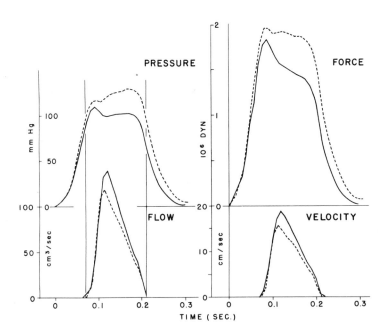

Fig. 3. Data replotted from an experiment like that shown in Figure 2. Left: intraventricular pressure (above) and aortic flow (below). Right: circumferential force (above) and velocity of circumferential shortening (below), computed from data at left, assuming a thin-walled sphere as a ventricular model. Continuous line: control beat; broken line: beat immediately after partial aortic occlusion

impedance modulus by a factor of 2, made the impedance phase more negative by 0.2 radians, and increased the input resistance by 50%. The pressures are exactly the same in the two beats until the aortic valve opens, as they should be. The ventricle after all does not know until then what the aortic impedance is. During ejection, the pressure was higher and altered in shape, with a late peak. The flow was lower after the occlusion, but the shape of the pulse scarcely changed. Now this is such a familiar response — any impedance to outflow from the ventricle produces a rise in pressure and a drop in flow — that we tend not to think about it. But remember that an increased impedance modulus means only that the ratio of pressure and flow must increase. That condition would be met if flow remained constant and pressure rose even higher. It would be met if the pressure stayed constant and the flow decreased markedly or by an infinite number of other combinations. The fact that the heart chooses this particular response tells us, I think, something basic about myocardial function if only we knew how to decode the message.

In considering myocardial function, we should look at the force exerted by muscle fibers instead of ventricular pressure and at the changing fiber length instead of blood flow. To do that, we need to know (or assume) the shape of the ventricle. For the present purpose, we have assumed that the ventricle acts like a thin-walled sphere. One could assume more realistic models, an ellipsoidal shape for example, but the results are qualitatively (though not quantitatively) the same. The right side of Figure 3 shows the circumferential force and velocity of shortening calculated from the pressures and flow on the left in the same Figure, assuming the simple spheric model. Increased impedance raises the force curve just as it does the pressure, but there is a significant difference in shape. The force curve does not show the delayed peak seen in the pressure. Instead, the force curve peaks early and then falls throughout the remainder of the ejection period. This characteristic was observed in all of our experiments, and the lower the impedance, the more rapidly the force declined. The velocity curve, on the other hand, was always similar in shape to the flow curve.

One point worth noting is that force and velocity are both rising during early ejection, contrary to the conventional concept that there is an inverse relation between force and velocity. Some investigators would say that one cannot study the relationships during normal ejection because the "load" is continually changing. I would suggest instead that the load is perfectly constant, but that it is a viscoelastic load, and can be described by a complex frequency spectrum, i.e., the arterial input impedance.

Two other interventions are shown in Figure 4, where the change in circumference is shown in place of shortening velocity. The continuous line represents a control beat, the dotted line represents the beat after altering impedance to the same extent as in Figure 3. The occlusion was then removed, and after an interval during which ventricular performance returned to approximately the previous control state, an "infinite impedance," so to speak, was applied by clamping the aorta shut just beyond the coronary ostia. The dashed line indicates the force developed in the subsequent isovolumic (or almost isovolumic) beat. In a truly isovolumic beat, of course, there would be no change in ventricular circumference. Again, the force developed in all these beats is about the same until the aortic valve opens. Then, during ejection, the higher the impedance, the greater the force, and the smaller the amount and velocity of shortening.

The simplest hypothesis that would explain these changes with increasing impedance is that they depend predominantly on fiber length. In other words, force would always rise up to the peak of the appropriate isovolumic curve were it not for the shortening of muscle fibers as the ventricle ejects blood. The dependence of force on end diastolic fiber length is familiar , of course, in the form of Starling's Law. What I am suggesting is that the relationship to length applies

233

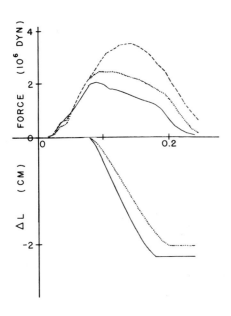

Fig. 4. Circumferential force (above) and shortening of circumference (below). Abscissa: time in s; continuous line: control beat; dotted line: beat following an increase in aortic input impedance similar to that shown in Figure 3; dashed line: isovolumic beat

throughout myocardial contraction. This is a concept that fits very well with the current idea that force is a function of the degree of overlap of actin and myosin filaments in the muscle cells. To put the hypothesis in another way, in any given neurochemical state, force depends only on fiber length and time. Force and impedance together determine velocity of shortening and thus determine fiber length at every instant.

The three-dimensional graph in Figure 5 expresses this theory. The force-length-time surface is a continuum of isovolumic curves, and the shorter the fiber length, the lower the peak force. The surface represents the ability of the ventricle to perform in one particular neurochemical environment and could be used as an operational definition of "myocardial contractility." The path taken over the surface in any beat depends on the initial, or end diastolic, fiber length and the artertial impedance. The trajectory indicated by the dashed line in Figure 5 is a control beat. Contraction begins at a certain fiber length, the trajectory first rises along an isovolumic curve until the aortic valve opens, and then travels over the surface in accordance with the shortening fiber length at every instant. When the aortic valve closes, it falls down along another isovolumic curve. The dotted line represents a beat against a moderately increased impedance, like the one shown in Figure 4, and the fibers do not shorten as fast or as much as in the control beat. An isovolumic beat, against an infinitely high impedance, would follow one of the isovolumic curves that make up the surface. Arterial impedance thus influences ventricular performance by determining the specific path taken by each beat out of all the paths made possible by the myocardial state.

One disadvantage of this hypothesis, which it shares with all others so far, is the difficulty of stating it in a comprehensive analytic equation. Aortic impedance is expressed in the frequency domain and vetricular function in the time domain. Mathematic transformations from one to the other are possible, but we have not

234

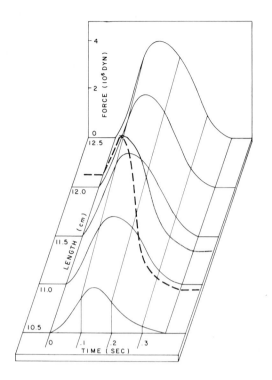

Fig. 5. Hypothetic relation between myocardial force-length-time properties and aortic input impedance. Vertical axis: circumferential force; horizontal axis: time; third axis: circumference. Surface represents functional ability of left ventricular myocardium in a given, constant neurochemical state. Trajectory of any given beat over this surface depends on initial (end diastolic) circumference and aortic input impedance. Dashed line: control beat; dotted line: beat with increased impedance

found a practical way of applying them to this problem. Experimental data that define "contractility" in terms of this surface, together with measurements of the arterial input impedance, would uniquely determine the trajectory of a beat from any initial length, but the only way to calculate the specific trajectory is by trial and error or, to use a more dignified term, by iterative computation. The theory does, however, give some conceptual insight into the relation between arterial impedance and vetricular function.

References

1. McDonald, D.A.: Blood Flow in Arteries. 2nd edition, London: Arnold 1974
2. Milnor, W.R., Bergel, D.H., Bargainer, J.D.: Hydraulic power associated with pulmonary blood flow and its relation to heart rate. Circ. Res. 19, 467-480 (1966)
3. Milnor, W.R., Conti, C.R., Lewis, K.B., O'Rourke, M.R.: Pulmonary arterial pulse wave velocity and impedance in man. Circ. Res. 25, 637-649 (1969)
4. Milnor, W.R.: Arterial impedance as ventricular afterload. Circ. Res. 36, 565-570 (1975)
5. Nichols, W.W., Conti, C.R., Walker, W.E., Milnor, W.R.: Input impedance of the systemic circulation in man. Circ. Res. 40, 451-458 (1977)
6. Walker, W.E.: The influence of changes of aortic input impedance on the dynamics of left ventricular performance. Ph.D. Dissertation, Johns Hopkins University 1975

The Effect of Systolic Rise in Arterial Pressure on Stroke Volume and Aortic Flow *

H. Reichel and K. Baumann

Physiologisches Institut der Universität Hamburg, D-2000 Hamburg

Introduction

In many papers, the effect of arterial end diastolic pressure (afterload) on ventricular function has been studied [4, 5, 8, 17, 28]. In all these experiments, afterload was varied b e f o r e systole. Under conditions in situ, however, the heart encounters changes in pressure which occur d u r i n g systole. Shortly after the onset of the primary pulse resulting from aortic flow [31], superimposed reflected pulse waves determine the further rise and time course of systolic aortic pressure. Such waves might depress flow and diminish stroke volume. The extent of this effect must depend on the properties of the heart, as far as its pumping function is concerned.

Broemser [3] suggested the existence of minima and maxima of cardiac output in dependence on the conditions for wave reflections in the arterial beam. He supposed that in the normal cardiovascular system the conditions of wave reflections are adjusted to the time relations of systole and diastole. The conception of such an adjustment presumes a pump which responds to any changes in pressure induced during systole with an opposite change in stroke volume. Preliminary studies on a frog's heart [24], however, have shown that transient changes in pressure during auxotonic contractions have only a small effect on stroke volume as far as they have finished before the end of systole. In later experiments, the same problem was studied more quantitatively on isotonic contractions of a turtle's heart [15]. From both series of experiments, the following conclusions are to be drawn:

1. A rise in pressure of a magnitude comparable to wave reflections in the human body does not reduce stroke volume more than 15%.

2. Transient changes in pressure are only effective in later stages of ejection.

From the view point of muscle physiology, the response of heart muscle to sudden changes in pressure has two components [22, 23]:

1. An instantaneous passive lengthening or shortening of series elastic structures

2. A delayed adjustment in speed of active shortening to the new load [9].

For evaluation of the former and elimination of the latter, the interventions (length changes in isometric contractions, load changes in isotonic contractions) have to be much faster than velocity of contraction. For this purpose, sinusoidal

---

*Supported by Deutsche Forschungsgemeinschaft.

length changes of high frequency have been applied to slowly contracting heart preparations during isometric contractions [20, 25]. In such experiments, the normal time course of contraction is not perturbed by superimposed changes in length. In a rapidly contracting mammalian heart muscle perturbations cannot be avoided, but they can be eliminated by Fourier analysis as successfully done by Templeton et al. [29] on isovolumetric contraction cycles of canine hearts on which sinusoidal small changes in volume are imposed. The results of all these experiments agree in the finding that viscoelastic stiffness is a linear function of force or pressure. This means that under physiologic conditions, i.e., during auxo-tonic contractions, stiffness increases with rise of pressure from end diastolic ventricular to systolic pressure. During ejection, stiffness determinations are complicated by a concomitant decrease of volume.

The reduction in stroke volume by transient changes, however, does not imply elastic components when they are completed within the ejection period, as elastic distension by loading is compensated by elastic constriction by the following unloading. Therefore, the effect of transient changes as studied in earlier experiments [15, 24] must be caused predominantly by changes in the speed of shortening. Any loading reduces and any unloading enhances the speed of shortening [9]. The latter may counterbalance the former completely when time for recovery is available. As this time is shortened with proceeding ejection, stroke volume is affected only in later stages of systole. Pulse wave reflections, however, overlast ejection time. For simplification, they may be compared with a rise in pressure which is induced at an early stage of ejection and persists during its whole duration. Under such conditions, recovery from preceding loading is excluded and stroke volume must be reduced. The extent of this reduction, however, might depend on the inotropic state (i.e., contractility in terms of maximal isovolumetric pressure development or its maximal rate), because, with increasing contractility, the speed of shortening at a given load rises during ejection [27]. The following experiments are described with the purpose of revealing the possible effect of a variation in inotropic state on the response to a sudden rise in pressure induced during ejection.

Methods

1. Material and Instrumentation

Eight mongrel dogs (weight 15-20 kg) were anesthetized with pentobarbital (12 mg/kg) and L-Polamidon (0.5 mg/kg). After thoracotomy, artificial ventilation was applied. The left intraventricular pressure was taken with a tipmanometer (Millar PC 350) inserted into the left ventricular cavity through the left atrium and the aortic pressure with a second tipmanometer of the same type inserted into the root of the aorta ascendens. Aortic flow was measured with an electromagnetic flow meter (Hellige/Speth) located in the root of the aorta ascendens; pressure and flow were recorded by an ultraviolet optical recorder (Siemens). Integration and evaluation of records were performed by a curve digitizer and an appropriate computer technique (Wissenschaftliche Datenverarbeitung, Garching).

2. Experimental Procedure

For a sudden rise in pressure, the counterpulsation method was applied by means of a balloon inserted into the abdominal aorta. Inflation was triggered by the artificial heart stimulus. The delay between stimulus and inflation was adjusted to various experimental conditions in such a way that the rise in aortic pressure was initiated a few milliseconds later, after the opening of the aortic valve. The balloon remained inflated about 250 ms, i.e., during the whole ejection time. For variation of the inotropic state, the heart rate was changed from 60/min to 220/min, by means of two bipolar stimulus electrodes, one of each located on the right atrium for supraventricular stimulation, the other on the apex of the heart for ventricular stimulation. During pacemaking, the peripheral trunk of the right n. vagus was stimulated continuously. When the heart was in a steady state at a certain rate, stimulation was interrupted during 1 s. The interruption has the following advantages:

1. The potentiating effect of a rise in rate is augmented by the pause ("pause potentation"). The first contraction after the pause ("pause contraction") reveals the greatest variations in the inotropic state at various rates of preceding rhythmic stimulation [12, 16, 26].
2. During the long resting period end diastolic ventricular pressure rises to almost the same value (7-9 mm Hg), independently of the rate of the preceding stimuli. The same holds true for end diastolic aortic pressure which falls during the pause to about 50 mm Hg at all rates.
3. Ejection time, which is highly affected by rate during rhythmic stimulation, varies only little in pause contractions.

Results

Figure 1 shows original records at two different rates (80/min and 180/min). In the steady state of rhythmic stimulation, aortic flow, aortic pressure, and intraventricular pressure change with rate as described in many previous studies [21, 10, 19]. The potentiating effect of the rise in rate from 80/min to 180/min is obvious in the first contraction after a resting period of 1 s. It is mostly pronounced in peak flow which, in the mean, increases from 107 ($\pm$ 13) to 156 ($\pm$ 23 ml/s). In the range of 60/min 240/min, peak flow is a linear function of maximal rate of isovolumetric pressure development, which rises from 1400 ($\pm$ 200) mm Hg/s to 5900 ($\pm$ 400) mm Hg/s (Fig. 2).

Figure 3 shows the effect of counterpulsation induced during auxotonic pause contractions shortly after the opening of the aortic valve. The records are taken at various rates of preceding stimuli (80/min, 160/min, and 180/min). Control curves (without counterpulsation) and curves with counterpulsation are drawn upon each other. The black area corresponds to the rise in pressure induced by counterpulsation (lower records) and to the corresponding decrease in flow (upper records). The rise in pressure (difference between counterpulsation peak and control peak) is almost the same at all rates (30 mm Hg), in spite of some differences in its time course at low and high rates. The differences in flow,

238

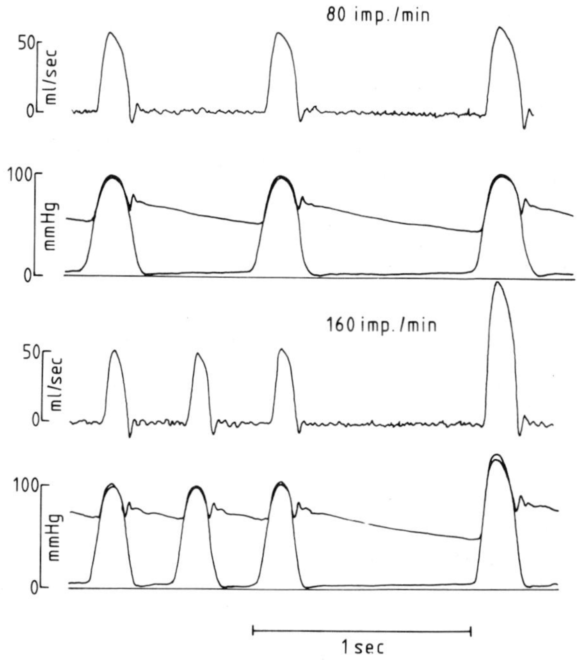

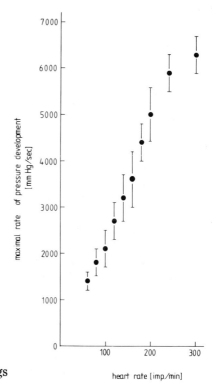

80 imp./min

160 imp./min

1 sec

Fig. 1. Original records of aortic flow (above) and aortic and left ventricular pressure (below) at two rates of supraventricular stimulation. Rhythmic stimulation is interrupted during 1 s. The following contraction is a pause contraction

maximal rate of pressure development [mm Hg/sec]

heart rate [imp/min]

Fig. 2. Dependence of maximal rate of isovolumetric pressure development of pause contractions on rate of preceding supraventricular stimulation. Mean ± SD of eight dogs

239

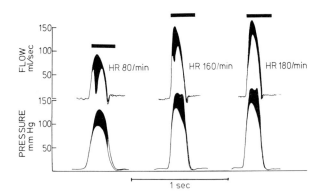

Fig. 3. Original records of flow (above) and left ventricular pressure (below) of pause contractions at three different rates of preceding supraventricular stimulation. Control and counterpulsation curves are drawn upon each other. Black area corresponds to depression in flow and to elevation in pressure. Black bar indicates time of counterpulsation

however, are more striking. At a rate of 80/min, flow is greatly reduced immediately after the onset of counterpulsation but recovers quickly when pressure falls. At a rate of 160/min, a dip in the flow record is still present, but less pronounced than at 80/min. At a rate of 180/min, the flow curve maintains its normal contour during counterpulsation, in spite of a certain depression of peak flow. Flow is also reduced in later stages of ejection, because ejection time is shortened.

In Figure 4, the stroke volume of pause contraction is plotted against the systolic left ventricular peak pressure. At any rate of foregoing stimulation, stimulus is

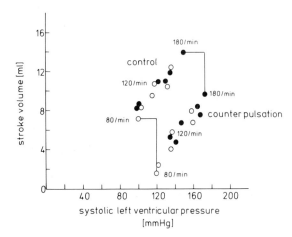

Fig. 4. Stroke volume related to left ventricular pressure of pause contractions at various rates of preceding supraventricular (closed circles) and ventricular stimulation (open circles). Each value represents the mean of three pause contractions on one dog

switched from a supraventricular (atrial) to a ventricular (apical) location. In the control, systolic left ventricular pressure rises with stroke volume, both increasing with the rate of preceding rhythm. At the same rate, stroke volume is larger and pressure is higher at supraventricular stimulation than at ventricular stimulation. The smallest stroke volumes are obtained at ventricular stimulation of a low rate (80/min), the largest at a supraventricular stimulation at a high rate (180/min). The same holds true for counterpulsation experiments. Comparable

240

changes in pressure induced by counterpulsation reduce stroke volume mostly at a low rate of ventricular stimulation and much less at a high rate of supraventricular stimulation.

Figure 5 shows the dependence of stroke volume of pause contractions (as percentage of control) on the rate of preceding stimulation. The values are the mean of all counterpulsation experiments with ventricular stimulation. At the lowest rate (60/min), counterpulsation reduces stroke volume to 20%, at the highest rate (180/min) to 85% of control.

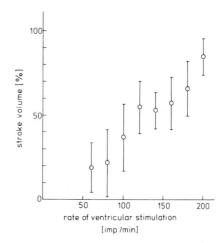

Fig. 5., Stroke volume of pause contractions with counterpulsation (in percentage of the control value at each rate) plotted against rate of ventricular stimulation. Mean ± SD of four dogs

Discussion

The hearts used in these experiments are hypodynamic at physiologic rates, probably because of anesthesia, surgical interventions, and vagal stimulation. During rhythmic contractions with a rate of 80/min, peak flow amounts to 50 ml/s and systolic peak pressure to 100 mm Hg (Fig. 1; [for comparison, see, e.g., 1]) at a rate of 120/min, flow reaches 180 ml/s and systolic pressure 135 mm Hg. However, as the potentiating effect of a rise in stimulation rate is much more pronounced in a hypodynamic heart than under physiologic conditions [2], its inotropic state can vary within a wide range as is shown by the change in maximal rate of isovolumetric pressure development from very low to normal values due to the combination of frequency and pause potentiation (Fig. 2).

The counterpulsation method is not suited for well-defined or even rectangular rises in pressure. The time course of pressure is modified by shift of volume into the vascular system and by a change in the conditions of wave reflections. In spite of these uncertainties, mean absolute pressure rise is almost the same in all experiments and at all rates. The mean response of stroke volume, however, appears to be different — at least if one compares the values obtained at the highest and lowest rates. For interpretation of this finding, one has to consider the following possibilites:

241

1. A change in the relation between outflow resistance (R_o) and source resistance (R_i), as a determinant of pump characteristics [7, 14, 31]. Source resistance, as revealed from instantaneous flow-pressure relations during pause contractions with and without counterpulsation and from isovolumetric pressure [13], amounts to about 1000 dyn $\cdot$ s $\cdot$ cm^{-5} at supraventricular stimulation and to 800 dyn $\cdot$ s $\cdot$ cm^{-5} at ventricular stimulation. Outflow resistance as calculated from integrated pressure and flow values during systole [18, 32] amounts to about 1800 dyn $\cdot$ s $\cdot$ cm^{-5}. Both resistances do not depend on the rate of preceding stimulation. Thus, only the difference between the values obtained at supraventricular and ventricular stimulation may be explained by an increase of R_o/R_i.
2. A change in viscoelastic stiffness. During the pause contractions of these experiments, counterpulsation is induced on about the same pressure level at all rates of preceding stimulation (about 60 mm Hg, Fig. 3). As viscoelastic stiffness depends only on pressure but not on a variation in inotropic state [6], it cannot be responsible for the striking difference in the instantaneous response of flow to the onset of counterpulsation at a rate of 80/min and 180/min (Fig. 3).
3. A change in the speed of shortening force relationship. Little is known on this relationship in the case of variations in the inotropic state of pause contractions. However, if one assumes that the potentiating effect of the resting pause is caused by an increase in available Ca^{2+} [11, 26, 30], the effect of high Ca^{2+} on the velocity-force relation may serve for comparison. As shown by Sonnenblick [27], a rise of Ca^{2+} raises isometric force more than maximal velocity of shortening at small loads. This means that a given rise in load slows down shortening to a lesser extent when contractility is enhanced.

Certainly, this explanation also lacks direct evidence. Nevertheless, our findings show clearly, that the heart — in a state of contractility enhanced by frequency and pause potentiation — is able to maintain the contour of flow curve even against counterpressures which exceed the half of normal pulse pressure. If this ability is thought to be a criterion for characterization of the heart as a pump [7], the heart may be considered as a flow source, at least in the range of physiologic systolic pressures. This property appears to be impaired severely in the hypodynamic or failing heart.

Summary

A general survey is given on the conditions which favor a possible effect of reflected waves, i.e., of a rise in pressure induced during systole, on stroke volume, and aortic flow. The response to transient pressure changes as studied in previous experiments was determined by ventricular viscoelastic stiffness and force-velocity relation. The latter depends on the inotropic state ("contractility"). In experiments on eight anesthetized thoracotomized mongrel dogs, the inotropic state was changed by combined frequency-pause potentiation. In pause contractions, elicited 1 s after rhythmic stimulation at rates varying from 60-240/min, the maximal rate of isovolumetric pressure development rose from 1400 mm Hg/s to 6000 mm Hg/s. A rise in pressure of about 30 mm Hg, induced shortly after the opening of aortic valve by counterpulsation, led to a strong instantaneous reduction in aortif flow at a low rate of stimulation but has only a small effect at higher rates. Stroke volume also appears to be more affected at lower than at higher rates. Source resistance and outflow resistance do not depend on rate, but the former is lowered by switching from supraventricular to ventricular stimulation.

References

1. Bauer, R.D., Busse, R., Schabert, A., Summa, Y., Wetterer, E.: Methoden der Blutströmungsmessung in Physiologie und Klinik. Wiener Med. Wochenschr. 126, 225-260 (1976)
2. Baumann, Kl., Reichel, H.: Time and rate dependence of the inotropic action of noradrenaline in the isolated guinea pig's atrium. Pflügers Arch. 354, 339-348 (1975)
3. Broemser, Ph.: Über die optimalen Beziehungen zwischen Herztätigkeit und physikalischen Konstanten des Gefäßsystems. Z. Biol. 96, 1-10 (1935)
4. Bugge-Asperheim, B., Kill, F.: Cardiac response to increased aortic pressure. Scand. J. Clin. Lab. Invest. 24, 345-360 (1969)
5. Bugge-Asperheim, B., Kill, F.: Preloads contractility and afterload as determinants of stroke volume during elevation of aortic blood pressure in dogs. Cardiovasc. Res. 7, 528-541 (1973)
6. Covell, J.W., Taylor, R.R., Sonnenblick, E.H., Ross, J. (Jr.): Series elasticity in the intact heart. Pflügers Arch. 357, 225-236 (1975)
7. Elzinga, G., Westerhof, N.: Pressure and flow generated by the left ventricle against different impedances. Circ. Res. 32, 178-186 (1973)
8. Goodjer, A.V.N., Goodkind, M.J., Landry, A.B.: Ventricular response to a pressure load. Circ. Res. 10, 885-896 (1962)
9. Hill, A.V.: The heat of shortening and the dynamic constants of muscle. Proc. R. Soc. Lónd. [Biol.] B 126, 136-169 (1938)
10. Jacob, R., Kissling, G., Ohnhaus, E.E., Peiper, U., Segarra-Domenech, J.: Die „Kontraktilität" des suffizienten Herzens unter rechtsventrikulärem Schrittmacherantrieb. Arch. Kreislaufforsch. 54, 192-215 (1967)
11. Kaufmann, R., Bayer, R., Fürniss, T., Krause, H., Tritthart, H.: Calcium-Movement controlling cardiac contractility II. Analog computation of cardiac excitation-contraction coupling on the basis of calcium kinetics in a multicompartment model. J. Mol. Cell. Cardiol. 6, 543-559 (1974)
12. Kedem, J., Mahler, Y., Rogel, S.: The effect of heart rate on myocardial contractility during single and paired pulse stimulation in vivo. Arch. Int. Physiol. Biochim. 77, 880-892 (1969)
13. Kenner, Th.: Zur Frage der Optimierung in der Abstimmung zwischen Herztätigkeit und Kreislauf. Pacemaker Digest 13, 51-82 (1977)
14. Kenner, Th., Estelberger, W.: Zur Frage der optimalen Abstimmung der Herzkontraktion an die Eigenschaften des Arteriensystems. Verh. Dtsch. Ges. Kreislaufforsch. 42, 132-135 (1976)

15. Kiwull, P., Rueadas, G., Reichel, H., Bleichert, A.: Der Einfluß definierter Druckstöße auf die Dynamik des Schildkrötenherzens. Pflügers Arch. 279, 228-238 (1964)
16. Koch-Weser, J., Blinks, J.R.: The influence of interval between beats on myocardial contractility. Pharmacol. Rev. 15, 601-657 (1963)
17. Levine, H.J., Forwand, St.A., McIntyre, K.M., Schechter, E.: Effect of afterload on force velocity relations and contractile element work in the intact dog heart. Cir. Res. 18, 729-744 (1966)
18. Liedtke, A.J., Buoncristiani, J.F., Kirk, E.S., Sonnenblick, E.H., Urschel, Ch.W.: Regulation of cardiac output after administration of isoproterenol and ouabain: interactions of systolic impedance and contractility. Cardiovasc. Res. 6, 325-332 (1972)
19. Limbourg, P., Wende, W., Henrich, H., Peiper, U.: Frequenz-inotropie und Frank-Starling-Mechanismus am Hundeherzen in situ unter natürlichem und künstlichem Herzantrieb. Pflügers Arch. 322, 250-263 (1971)
20. Lundin, G.: Mechanical properties of cardiac muscle. Act. Physiol. Scand. 7 [Suppl. 20] 7-84 (1944)
21. Noble, M.I.N., Trenchard, D., Guz, A.: Effect of changing heart rate on cardiovascular function in the conscious dog. Circ. Res. 19, 206-213 (1966)
22. Reichel, H.: Kontraktilität und Elastizität des Herzmuskels als Modellvorstellung. Verh. Dtsch. Ges. Kreislaufforsch. 16, 13-15 (1950)
23. Reichel, H.: Muskelphysiologie. Berlin-Heidelberg-New York: Springer 1960
24. Reichel, H., Kapal. E.: Die Mechanik des Herzens bei Änderug des arteriellen Drucks. Z. Biol. 99, 581-589 (1939)
25. Reichel, H., Zimmer, F., Bleichert, A.: Die elastichen Eigenschaften des Skelett- und Herzmuskels in verschiedenen Phasen der Einzelzuckung. Z. Biol. 108, 188-195 (1956)
26. Rumberger, E., Reichel, H.: The force-frequency relationship; a comparative study between warm- and cold blooded animals. Pflügers Arch. 332, 206-217 (1972)
27. Sonnenblick, E.H.: Force-velocity relation in mammalian heart muscle. Am. J. Physiol. 202, 931-939 (1962)
28. Sonnenblick, E.H., Downing, S.V.: Afterload as a primary determinant of ventricular performance. Am. J. Physiol. 204, 604-610 (1963)
29. Templeton, G.H., Nardizzi, L.R.: Elastic and viscous stiffness of the canine left ventricle. J. Appl. Physiol. 36, 123-127 (1974)
30. Tritthart, H., Kaufmann, R., Volkmer, H.P., Bayer, R., Krause, H.: Ca-movement controlling myocardial contractility I. Voltage, current- and time-dependence of mechanical activity under voltage clamp conditions (cat papillary muscles and trabeculae). Pflügers Arch. 338, 207-231 (1973)
31. Wetterer, E., Kenner, Th.: Grundlagen der Dynamik des Arterienpulses. Berlin-Heidelberg-New York: Springer 1968
32. Wilcken, D.E.L., Charlier, A.A., Hoffman, J.I.E., Guz, A.: Effects of alteration in aortic impedance on the performance of the ventricles. Circ. Res. 14, 283-293 (1964)

Effect of Ventricular Pacing on Systolic Blood Pressure of Patients With Hypertension

M. Schöttler and J. Schaefer

Abteilung für Spezielle Kardiologie der Universität Kiel, D-2300 Kiel 1,
Schittenhelmstr. 12

Patients with bradycardia often suffer from high systolic blood pressure. Generally, this hypertension is thought to be the result of a high stroke volume [1, 3, 8, 10, 13, 14]. It is known that hypertension with bradycardia drops when heart rate is normalized by artificial pacing; on the other hand, we know that there are patients with bradycardia without hypertension and others with hypertension without bradycardia. The effects of artificial ventricular pacing on blood pressure have not yet been examined systematically. In particular, we have no information about the role of increasing heart rate and the importance of ventricular pacing itself on the decrease of systolic pressure. Therefore, we studied the effects of ventricular pacing on arterial blood pressure in 150 patients with bradycardia, 38-87 years old, and in nine patients with hypertension without bradycardia, 58-77 years old. Blood pressure was measured by the method of Riva-Rocci-Korotkow. The criteria of this method correspond to the advice proffered by a committee of the German Society for Cardiovascular Research in 1971.

In our study, we calculated the mean values of the systolic and diastolic arterial pressures of each patient for the time before and after pacemaker insertion. In each case, the time of observation after pacemaker implantation was longer than 1 year. Systolic pressure before pacemaking ranges from 110-280 mm Hg. There is no clear maximum in the distribution. We did not find any correlation between the level of systolic pressure and the age of the patients, the heart rate, and the heart size. After pacemaker insertion, there is a significant change in the distribution of systolic pressure to smaller values. There is a clear maximum at 140 mm Hg. In more than 90%, systolic pressure does not exceed 160 mm Hg. After implantation of an artificial pacemaker, the pressure amplitude decreases. Only in some cases does the pressure amplitude remain unchanged. We never observed any increase in amplitude. Changes of diastolic pressure are usually small. Therefore, the decrease in pressure amplitude is mainly due to the decrease in systolic pressure.

Figure 1 shows the correlation between the changes of systolic pressure after pacemaker insertion and the level of the systolic pressures before pacemaking. The fall in systolic pressure increases with the value which was measured before pacemaker implantation. Patients with a low pressure before implantation show only a small if any reduction. All symbols to the left of the dashed line represent cases with normal systolic pressures during pacing, i.e., systolic pressure is not

245

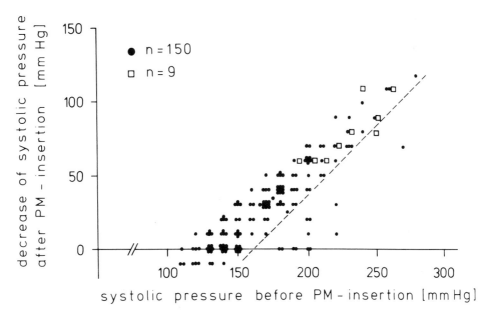

Figur. 1. Correlation between the systolic pressure before and after pacemaker insertion. The closed circles represent the values of the 150 patients with brady-cardia and the open squares those of the 9 patients with hypertension without bradycardia

higher than 160 mm Hg. Systolic hypertension itself persisted in only 12 cases, although the systolic pressure also dropped in six cases. The open squares represent the values of those nine patients who had hypertension without brady-cardia. In all cases, systolic pressure shifted to normal values during pacing.

Figure 2 shows the correlation between the amount of the decrease in systolic pressure and the increase in heart rate produced by the artificial pacemaker. The stimulation rate of the pacemaker was 70/min throughout. Before pacemaker insertion, the heart rate of the 150 patients with bradycardia varied between 28 and 60 beats/min. Therefore, the increase in heart rate during pacing was 10-42/min. The open squares represent those patients who had hypertension without bradycardia. In these cases, the increase in heart rate amounts to only 4-10 beats/min. There is no significant correlation between the change in systolic pressure and the increase in heart rate.

In several cases, we recorded the time course of aortic pressure by means of a tipmanometer. Figure 3 shows an example of such a record of a 65-year-old man who suffered from intermittent bradycardia. During examination and implantation, the patient had an atrioventricular dissociation in the electrocardiogram. Spontaneous heart rate was 75 beats/min. Before implantation, systolic pressure rose to nearly 200 mm Hg, diastolic pressure was about 115 mm Hg, and mean aortic pressure was 145 mm Hg. After transvenous implantation of an unipolar

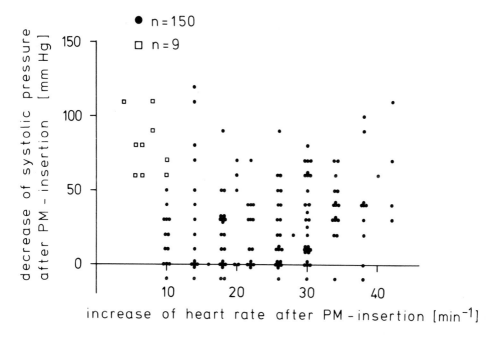

Fig. 2. Correlation between the decrease in systolic pressure after pacemaker insertion and the increase in heart rate produced by the artificial pacemaker. The closed circles represent the values of the 150 patients with bradycardia and the open squares those of the 9 patients with hypertension without bradycardia

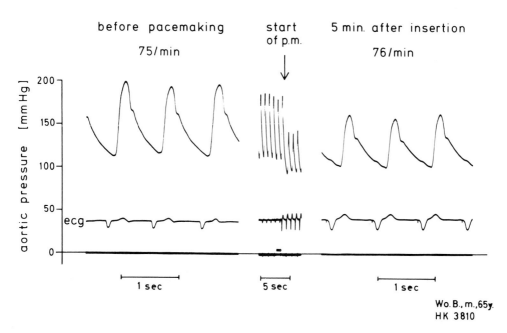

Wo. B., m.,65y.
HK 3810

Fig. 3. Time course of aortic pressure before and after pacemaker insertion

electrode to the right ventricle, we started ventricular pacing with an external pacemaker. The stimulation rate was 76/min. Immediately after the onset of pacing, aortic pressure decreased. Five minutes later, a new steady state was reached. Although there was practically no increase in heart rate, systolic pressure remained at a rather low level of about 160 mm Hg. The main effect of the pacemaker appears to be the reduction in the steep peak systolic pressure after treatment. It has only a minor effect on the mean pressure, which only decreases about 15 mm Hg to 130 mm Hg. The ejection time is somewhat shorter than during spontaneous heart rate.

The explanation of our results is based on several points:

1. It is a well-known fact that the main hemodynamic effect of raising heart rate is the decrease in stroke volume [1, 2, 3, 5, 6, 8, 10]. Thus, systolic pressure and pressure amplitude become smaller.

2. We could show that there may be a tremendous decrease in systolic pressure with only very small changes in heart rate produced by the artificial pacemaker. Therefore, ventricular pacing itself may cause a reduction in stroke volume. It is known that ventricular pacing slows down ventricular contraction and particular ejection velocity and lowers stroke volume to a certain degree [4, 7, 9, 11]. In some patients, the loss of a coordinated action of atrial and ventricular contraction may decrease the stroke volume.

3. Other factors could be important, e.g., alterations in the properties of the windkessel and changes in the total peripheral resistance by regulative mechanisms.

Our study cannot answer all questions, because up to now we have not systematically measured cardiac index, pulse wave velocity, or other parameters which may be of importance. From a clinical point of view, the reduction of an increased arterial pressure solely by ventricular pacing is a new aspect in the therapy of hypertension [12].

References

1. Benchimol, A., Li, Y.B., Dimond, E.G.: Cardiovascular dynamics in complete heart block at various heart rates. Effect of exercise at a fixed heart rate. Circulation 30, 542-553 (1964)

2. Bevegård, S., Jonsson, B., Karlöf, I., Lagergren, H., Sowton, E.: Effect of changes in ventricular rate on cardiac output and central pressures at rest and during exercise in patients with artificial pacemakers. Cardiovasc. Res. 1, 21-33 (1967)

3. Büchner, Ch., Gebhardt, W., Amat y Leon, F., Reindell, H.: Befunde hämodynamischer Untersuchungen vor und nach Implantation eines elektrischen Schrittmachers. Therapiewoche 15, 710 (1964)

4. Daggett, W.M., Bianco, J.A., Powell, W.J., Austen, W.G.: Relative contributions of the atrial systole — ventricular systole interval and of patterns of ventricular activation to ventricular function during electrical pacing of the dog heart. Circ. Res. 27, 69-79 (1970)

5. Gattenlöhner, W., Schneider, K.W.: Schrittmachertherapie und Hämodynamik. Münch. Med. Wochenschr. 115, 2137-2142 (1973)

6. Gerhardt, W., v. Smekal, P., Grosser, K.D.: Kreislaufdynamik bei totalem atrioventrikulärem Block vor und nach Anwendung eines elektrischen Schrittmachers unter verschiedenen Frequenzen. Dtsch. Med. Wochenschr. 92, 1488-1493 (1967)
7. Gilmore, J.P., Sarnoff, S.J., Mitchell, J.H., Linden, R.J.: Synchronicity of ventricular contraction: observations comparing hemodynamic effects of atrial and ventricular pacing. Br. Heart J. 25, 299-307 (1963)
8. Gobel, F.L., Jorgensen, C.R., Kitamura, K., Yang Wang: Acute changes in left ventricular volume and contractility during ventricular pacing in patients with complete heart block. Circulation 44, 771-781 (1971)
9. Jacob, R., Kissling, G., Ohnhaus, E.E., Peiper, U., Segarra-Domenech, J.: Die „Kontraktilität" des suffizienten Herzens unter rechtsventrikulärem Schrittmacherantrieb. Arch. Kreislaufforsch. 54, 192-215 (1967)
10. Nager, F.: Hämodynamik nach Implantation eines Schrittmachers. Schweiz. Med. Wochenschr. 96, 331-332 (1966)
11. Samet, P., Castillo, C., Bernstein, W.H.: Hemodynamic consequences of sequential atrio-ventricular pacing: subjects with normal hearts. Am. J. Cardiol. 21, 207-212 (1968)
12. Schaefer, J., Schwarzkopf, H.J., Pape, C., Schöttler, M.: Permanent cardiac pacing as a possible adjunct for the treatment of hypertensive heart disease with bradycardia. Johns Hopkins Med. J. 135, 143-151 (1974)
13. Scheppokat, K.D., Rodewald, G., Saborowski, F., Westermann, K.W.: Die schweren bradykarden Störungen. Internist 9, 280-289 (1968)
14. Vogel, H.C., Terhaag, B., Rikirsch, P., Schäbitz, J., Teichmann, W.: Untersuchungen über das Blutdruckverhalten bei Patienten mit bradykarden Rhythmusstörungen vor und nach Schrittmacherimplantation. Ber. Ges. Inn. Med. 28, 292-294 (1973)

Dependence of Peripheral Resistance on Heart Rate *

E. Rumberger, K. Baumann, and M. Schöttler

Physiologisches Institut der Universität Hamburg, Martinistr. 52, D-2000 Hamburg 20 und
I. Medizinische Klinik der Universität Kiel, Schittenhelmstr. 12, D-23 Kiel

The input impedance of the arterial system depends on the heart rate [3, 7, 10, 11] and is calculated only with data on the pulsatile action. The pressure level of the pulse depends on the peripheral resistance. Two questions arise. Is the total peripheral resistance also dependent on the heart rate? To what extent is the heart confronted with impedance and resistance during the ejection phase? In conjunction with other problems we studied these questions on anesthetized (fentanyl and dehydrobenzperidol as premedication, 1-Polamidon and pentobarbital) and thoracotomized dogs. The flow was measured electromagnetically on the root of the aorta and the pressure by means of catheter tipmanometers, also positioned in the root of the aorta (other measurement devices are not important for the question under consideration). The heart was artificially driven with different stimulation rates. One couple of electrodes was sewn on the right atrium, another couple on the right ventricle. Thus, it was possible to stimulate either the atrium or the ventricle. Pressure and flow signals were registered with an UV multichannel recorder (Oscillofil, Siemens). The curves obtained in the steady state of rhythmic stimulation at various rates in a range of 40-240 impulses/min were evaluated by means of a graphic table and a process computer (WDV/Interdata).

As has already been shown by many authors [2, 6, 9] , we also observed that the stroke volume (SV) decreases with increasing stimulation rate (F, beats/min). The relationship is $SV = 17.5 - 0.0515 \cdot F$ (ml) for atrial stimulation and $SV = 16.0 - 0.0515 \cdot F$ (ml) for ventricular stimulation. Accordingly, the equation for the cardiac output (CO) is $CO = 17.5 - 0.0515 \cdot F^2$ (ml/min) and $CO = 16.6 - 0.0515 \cdot F^2$ (ml/min), respectively.

At atrial stimulation, the cardiac output is maximum at a stimulation rate of 170 impulses/min and at ventricular stimulation at 155 impulses/min. The mean aortic pressure depends on the stimulation rate in nearly the same way as the cardiac output does. In Figure 1 the cardiac output is plotted against the mean aortic pressure. All values at all rates can be connected by one straight line irrespective of the site of stimulation. The reciprocal slope of the line gives the differential resistance of the arterial system. It seems to be independent of the stimulation rate. The quotient between mean aortic pressure and cardiac output as a usual measure of total peripheral resistance increases with decreasing mean

---

* Supported by a grant of the Deutsche Forschungsgemeinschaft.

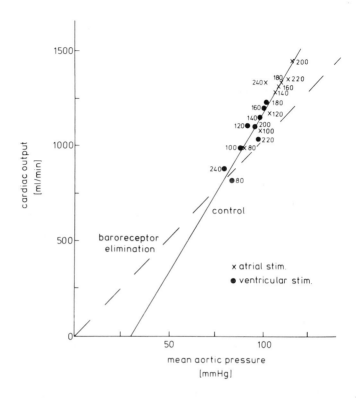

Fig. 1. Cardiac output is plotted against mean aortic pressure for one dog. The numbers next to the symbols indicate the heart rate in beats/ min. The solid connecting line is extrapolated to the pressure axis. The broken line connects the values obtained after baroreceptor elimination and is also extrapolated. After baroreceptor elimination, cardiac output lies in the same range as before (control). Single values are not shown for reasons of clarity

aortic pressure because the connecting line intersects the abscissa at positive pressures, as already shown by Wetterer and Pieper [14]. Therefore, the total peripheral resistance is pressure dependent, and because the pressure is rate dependent, the total peripheral resistance also becomes rate dependent as it is shown in Figure 2.

The slope and the intersection of the cardiac output pressure curve are changed by partial elimination of baroreceptors done by cutting the N. vagi and occlusion of both A. carotides [see also 5]. This is shown by the broken line in Figure 1 (for clarity's sake, the values are not presented singly). The connecting line after baroreceptor elimination is less steeper than before, indicating that both the differential and the total peripheral resistance are increased. However, the connecting line now intersects the abscissa at pressure values nearly at zero. Thus, the quotient between mean aortic pressure and cardiac output becomes almost independent of pressure, and the rate dependence of total peripheral resistance disappears (Fig. 2).

Our results demonstrate that under the conditions of anesthesia total peripheral resistance does not show any specific rate dependence and that the baroreceptor reflex is not influenced by heart rate. This is in agreement with findings by Stegemann and Tibes [13], who found that in the range of physiologic heart rates the rate does not influence the reflex response. Thus, it is not amazing that the rate of aortic pressure decline during diastole is independent of heart rate [12].

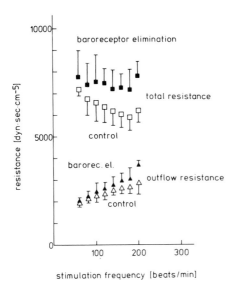

Fig. 2. Total peripheral resistance (squares) and outflow resistance (triangles) as function of stimulation rate. Mean values of four dogs. White symbols: before baroreceptor elimination (control); black symbols: after baroreceptor elimination

The next question is to what extent the rate-dependent input impedance influences the working heart. The heart is connected with the arterial system only during the ejection phase. Therefore, it seems to be a worthwhile attempt to evaluate the rate dependence of that resistance whose effect is limited to the ejection phase. It is known as outflow impedance or outflow resistance [1, 4, 15] and is calculated as the ratio between mean systolic pressure and mean systolic flow in the root of the aorta.

In Figure 2, systolic outflow resistance is plotted against heart rate. While the total peripheral resistance decreases with rate, the outflow resistance increases. Under the conditions of partial baroreceptor elimination, this increase is steeper. The ratio between outflow resistance and total peripheral resistance increases with rate but is not altered after baroreceptor elimination (Table 1). The ratio

Table 1. Ratio between outflow resistance and total peripheral resistance before and after baroreceptor elimination (mean values)

Heart rate (beats/min)	Before	After
60	0.26	0.26
80	0.3	0.3
100	0.33	0.31
120	0.36	0.34
140	0.40	0.38
160	0.42	0.41
180	0.45	0.43
200	0.46	0.47

between outflow resistance and total peripheral resistance indicates the extent to which the heart is confronted with the peripheral resistance during the ejection phase. Thus, the higher the rate, the more the heart must work against total peripheral resistance. The pressure-dependent decrease of total peripheral resistance with rise in rate (Fig. 2) is not sufficient to counterbalance the increasing ratio and, therefore, external cardiac work which is necessary to eject a given pulsatile flow increases with rate. This assertion is contrary to the interpretation of the well-known rate dependence of input impedance, according to which, the external cardiac work needed to eject a given pulsatile flow increases with decreasing rate, particularly in the range below about 120 impulses/min [8]. This discrepancy may result from a difference in interpretation of the heart as flow and pressure source. In our opinion, the heart has to be seen as a pump generating an interrupted direct current rather than an alternating current. Switch-on processes must also be taken into account to describe the resistance against which the heart ejects stroke volume. These processes are better borne in mind by using the outflow resistance rather than the input impedance because the latter is calculated with pressure and flow values obtained also during diastole.

References

1. Imperial, E.S., Levy, M.N., Zieske, H. (jr.): Outflow resistance as an independent determinal of cardiac performance. Circ. Res. 9, 1148-1155 (1961)
2. Jacob, R., Kissling, G., Ohnhaus, E.E., Pieper, U., Segassa-Domenech, J.: Die „Kontraktilität" des suffizienten Herzens unter rechtsventrikulärem Schrittmacherantrieb. Arch. Kreislaufforsch. 54, 192-215 (1967)
3. Kenner, Th.: Der Eingangswiderstand des Arteriensystems. Z. Biol. 111, 178-188 (1959)
4. Liedtke, Buoncristiani, J.F., Kirk, E.S., Sonnenblick, E.H., Urschel, Ch.W.: Regulation of cardiac output after administration of isoproterenol and ouabain: interactions of systolic impedance and contractility. Cardiovasc. Res. 6, 325-332 (1972)
5. Liedtke, A.J., Urschel, Ch.W., Kirk, E.S.: Total systemic autoregulation in the dog and its inhibition by baroreceptor reflexes. Circ. Res. 32, 673-677 (1973)
6. Limbourg, P., Wende, W., Henrich, H., Peiper, U.: Frequenzinotropie und Frank-Starling-Mechanismus am Hundeherzen in situ unter natürlichem und künstlichem Herzantrieb. Pflügers Arch. 322, 250-263 (1971)
7. McDonald, O.A.: The relation of pulsatile pressure to flow in arteries. J. Physiol. (London) 127, 533-552 (1955)
8. Nichols, W.W., Conti, C.R., Walker, W.E., Milnor, W.R.: Input impedance of the systemic circulation in man. Circ. Res. 40, 451-458 (1977)
9. Noble, M.I.M., Trenchard, D., Guz, A.: Effect of changing heart rate on cardiovascular function in the conscious dog. Circ. Res. 19, 206-213 (1966)
10. O'Rourke, M.F., Taylor, M.G.: Input impedance of the systemic circulation. Circ. Res. 20, 365-380 (1967)

11. O'Rourke, M.F.: Steady and pulsatile energy losses in the systemic circulation under normal conditions and in simulated arterial disease. Cardiovasc. Res. 1, 313-326 (1967)
12. Rumberger, E., Schaefer, J., Reichel, H., Schwarzkopf, H.J., Baumann, K., Schöttler, M.: Strömungswiderstand und diastolischer Abfall des arteriellen Druckes beim Hund unter dem Einfluß künstlich induzierter Herzfrequenzänderungen. Verh. Dtsch. Ges. Kreislaufforsch. 40, 159-162 (1974)
13. Stegemann, J., Tibes, U.: Der Einfluß von Amplitude, Frequenz und Mittelwert sinusförmiger Reizdrucke an den Pressorezeptoren auf den arteriellen Mitteldruck des Hundes. Pflügers Arch. 305, 219-228 (1969)
14. Wetterer, E., Pieper, H.: Ein indirektes Verfahren zur Bestimmung des diastolischen Abstroms aus dem Arteriensystem und seine Anwendung zum Studium der Druck-Stromstärke-Beziehungen in vivo. Verh. Dtsch. Ges. Kreislaufforsch. 21, 430-439 (1955)
15. Wilcken, D.E.L., Charlier, A.A., Hoffman, J.I.E., Guz, A.: Effects of alterations in aortic impedance on the performance of the ventricles. Circ. Res. 14, 283-293 (1964)

Instantaneous Blood Flow Velocity Profiles After Aortic Valve Replacement

S. Hagl, H. Meisner, W. Heimisch, E. Gams, E. Struck, and F. Sebening

Deutsches Herzzentrum München, Klinik für Herz- und Gefäßchirurgie (Direktor: Prof. Dr. F. Sebening) D-8000 München 2, Lothstraße 11

Modern artificial heart valves show good hydrodynamic characteristics when evaluated under in vitro conditions [14, 17, 18, 19, 32]. In vivo, however, after implantation in man — independent of whether they were inserted in a tricuspid, mitral, or aortic position — the hemodynamic properties of heart valve prostheses are less satisfying. Despite sufficiently large geometric orifice areas, important transvalvular pressure gradients were measured, especially during exercise [5, 9, 10]. The "effective orifice area" calculated from the hemodynamic data according to Gorlin's formula [8] was shown to be only 50%-70% of the geometric value [5, 6, 12, 27]. Aside from the discussion of whether the constant in the Gorlin formula is appropriate for the different types of artificial valves [26], the presence of pressure gradients indicates a hemodynamically effective stenosis, which cannot be explained on the basis of a small geometric opening area alone. According to the results of in vitro studies in the pulse duplicator system, this energy loss across the valve is most probably caused by eddies, splitting vortices, and turbulence, which originate from the sharp edges of the valve ring, the flat disc, the cage or struts or by heavy distortion of flow by a centrally moving obstacle [1, 3, 14, 17, 28, 33]. This fact is further supported by the clinical observation that in patients with heart valve prostheses even small pressure gradients at rest can increase sharply during exercise despite only modestly elevated transvalvular flows [5, 9]. This indicates a break in the linear pressure-flow relation demonstrating the occurrence of turbulence. Turbulent flow requires a larger pressure gradient than the equivalent laminar flow [21, 30].

Incomplete opening of tilting disc valves — often observed in high-speed angiographic studies [7, 12, 27] — may be caused by eddies and vortices, which by this mechanism further augment transvalvular impedance. Aside from the hemodynamic data, there is additional evidence for turbulence beyond artificial heart valves. An indirect anatomic indicator for turbulence is the proliferation of fibrous tissue in the immediate vicinity of implanted prostheses. In necropsy studies, Roberts and co-workers [25] observed thickening of the endocardium and the aortic wall including coronary ostia distal of mitral and aortic valve prostheses. In some cases, the anatomic changes were so pronounced that ventricular relaxation was inhibited or coronary perfusion was critically reduced.
When flow through a prosthetic heart valve is turbulent, blood cell damage may arise and intravascular hemolysis is the consequence [4, 13]. Furthermore,

thrombosis may occur in regions of stasis and turbulence [29]. Subsequently, the hemodynamic performance of a prosthetic heart valve is an important factor, determining not only the effectiveness of hemodynamic repair but also the incidence of secondary complications, which seem highly related to transvalvular flow characteristics. The purpose of the present paper was to evaluate blood flow velocity profiles in the human ascending aorta beyond artificial heart valves and central flow substitutes.

Methods

The studies were performed intraoperatively in a total of 22 patients who underwent aortic valve replacement because of aortic stenosis and/or regurgitation. The diseased aortic valve was substituted by ball (Starr-Edwards 1260) and tilting-disc valves (Björk-Shiley, Lillehei-Kaster) or by porcine xenografts (Hancock). The outer diameters of the implanted prostheses were in the range of 23-29 mm. Measurements of volume flow, phasic and mean velocity, and velocity distribution in the ascending aorta were performed before and after aortic valve replacement utilizing a pulsed doppler ultrasonic flowmeter (Peronneau et al. [23, 15]. Three piezoelectric crystals (8 mHz) embedded at a 60° angle in plastic shoes were inserted in a hinged lucite ring (Fig. 1). The diameter of this perivascular ring was chosen 10% less than the diameter of the ascending aorta at the site of measurement. This probe was placed 50 mm distal to the valve ring around the aorta and turned in such a way that the tranducers faced the bases of the three leaflets.

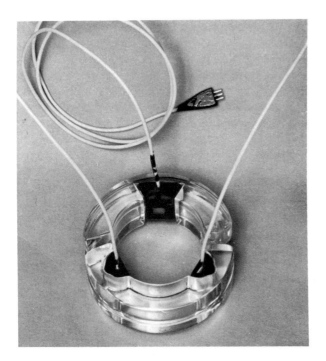

Fig. 1. Perivascular ultrasonic probe: three piezoelectric crystals embedded in plastic shoes (60° angle) are mounted 120° apart on a hinged lucite ring

By activation of the piezoceramic transducers, pulses of ultrasound (f_o = 8 mHz) with a repetition rate of 15 KHz and duration of 1 μs were emitted (Fig. 2). The direction of sound propagation is given by the 60° angle of the transducer in respect to the longitudinal axis of the aorta. According to the doppler principle, a frequency shift directly related to the velocity of the moving erythrocytes occurs. Sampling the mean velocity along the entire oblique diameter and calculating the inner radius of the aorta, volume flow was computed.

On the other hand, by reducing the receiver gate width to 1 μs peak velocity (V) and mean velocity ($\overline{Vm}$) components with a resolution given by the gate width can be detected in any depth inside the aorta. To record the velocity distribution along the sound axis — defined by the position and direction of the ultrasonic crystals — an automatic electronically controlled delay timer was developed. The gate width was fixed at 1 μs and the gate progressively shifted by a rate of 0.5 mm/s. This slow rate was chosen to assure correct mean velocity computation by an analogue averager. To detect inhomogenous distribution of velocities across the cross-sectional area of the aorta and to exhibit flow abnormalities and hemo-dynamic irregularities, three velocity profiles were recorded along three diameters shifted by 120°. Mean velocity profiles were mapped one after the other assuring constant hemodynamic conditions by pressure and ECG monitoring. For peak velocity registration, a multiplexer was used sampling signals alternatively from the three diameters during continuous gate shift. To analyze the dynamic changes of the velocity distribution within the heart cycle, actual velocity profiles were computed in steps of 30 ms after aortic valve opening from high-speed UV recordings. In addition, pressures in the left ventricle and the ascending aorta were determined using Millar microtip transducers. The pressure in the radial artery was measured by a Statham P 23 Db transducer and a Siemens amplifier. The electrocardiogram was monitored to control heart rate and to detect arrythmias.

Results and Comments

The upper panel of Figure 3 shows the peak blood flow velocity distribution as it was generally found in the ascending aorta of human subjects with normal aortic valves. The velocity profile is constructed out of 25 single measurements. In this case, the peak velocity was 105 cm/s, the mean value 76 cm/s. The peak systolic profile appears flat and was similar along the three different diameters. This statement, however, is only valid if the measurement within the critical zone close to the oscillating vessel walls is accurate. In earlier studies [11], we could demonstrate that out of a distance of one to two wave lengths from the vessel wall the measurement is highly reliable. Even if we consider the first value on each side as an outlier, the profile does not change significantly.

A flat velocity profile in the ascending aorta of dogs was found by Lynch and Bove [20] who used high-speed cineangiography. These authors suggested that the flat profile results from the directly observed radial and axial movement of fluid. In contrast to this direct visualization, the ultrasound method shows only the net effect of eddies and vortices on velocity components directed forward and backward. Using a thin film anemometer, Bergel et al. [2] also showed flat

257

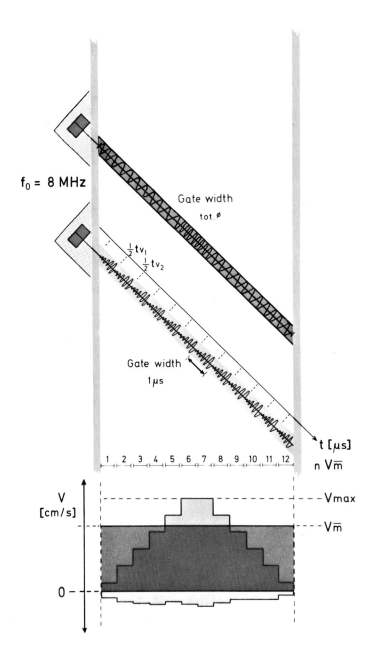

$f_0 = 8$ MHz

Gate width

tot. ∅

$\frac{1}{2} tv_1$
$\frac{1}{2} tv_2$

Gate width
1 μs

t [μs]

1 2 3 4 5 6 7 8 9 10 11 12

n V$\overline{m}$

V
[cm/s]

Vmax

V$\overline{m}$

0 –

Fig. 2. Schematic representation of the pulsed doppler ultrasonic method used for measurement of velocity profiles in the human ascending aorta. The 8 mHz sound pulse travels through the aorta along an oblique diameter defined by the 60° angle of the crystal in respect to the longitudinal axis of the aorta. Extending the receiver gate width across the entire oblique diameter, phasic blood velocity in the aortic root averaged along the given section was determined. Volume flow was computed from the mean velocity (V$\overline{m}$) and the calculated transversal diameter. Reducing the gate width to 1 μs, maximal and mean velocity components within this space could be detected in any depth of the aorta corresponding to the chosen delay (tv). The velocity distribution was recorded by shifting the gate automatically along the oblique diameter at a constant speed of 0.5 mm/s. The resolution of velocity components was given by the gate width of 1 μs

258

normal aortic valve

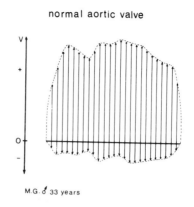

M.G. ♂ 33 years

aortic stenosis

aortic stenosis
and insufficiency

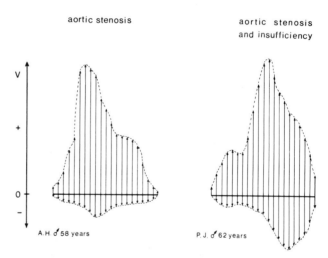

A.H. ♂ 58 years

P.J. ♂ 62 years

Fig. 3. Normal and pathologic velocity profiles in the human ascending aorta: forward and backward peak velocities are depicted. Every arrow defines the average value of the velocity distribution within the space of 1 μs given by the fixed gate width. The profiles were drawn from 25 and 21 single measurements

velocity profiles near the normal aortic and pulmonary valve. In the lower thoracic aorta, however, they found almost parabolic profiles. Reuben et al. [24] performed velocity mappings in the main pulmonary artery of dogs and man using thin film resistance anemometry. The profiles they found were flat. The peak velocities in the pulmonary artery averaged 70 cm/s.
A flat velocity distribution across the sectional area of the aorta suggests turbulence. The definition of turbulence under pulsatile flow conditions, however, is crucial. The critical Reynold's number 2000 is only applicable to steady flow.

Calculations in subjects with normal aortic valves in this study showed values exceeding 3000 in every case. According to McDonald [21], the Reynold's number in oscillatory arterial flow, where acceleration and deceleration is very marked, has no significance. Bergel et al. [2] demonstrated that the flow profile in the aorta of dogs can remain laminar even with peak velocities as high as 200 cm/s which correspond to a Reynold's number of ~ 11,500. On the other hand, eddies and turbulence may occur at a Reynold's number as low as 800 according to Meisner and Rushmer [22].

In contrast to the normal velocity distribution in the ascending aorta, anomalous profiles from two patients with severe aortic stenosis and regurgitation are depicted in the lower part of Figure 3. In both cases, the velocity profiles were extremely flat along one diameter but show high velocity jets along the other axes. The maximal velocity within the jet reached over 200 cm/s. The negative velocity vectors were very pronounced, particulary in the patient with aortic regurgitation. These findings are in agreement with the everyday observations in the cardiac catheter laboratories, where turbulence and eddies are consistently found distal to diseased valves. The turbulent flow appears during acceleration but disturbed flow remains during deceleration and may persist in diastole [2, 1].

The phasic and mean velocity distribution along three aortic diameters are displayed in Figure 4. This patient suffered from a predominant aortic insufficiency. The posterior leaflet was extremely shrunk; hence, the positive and negative velocity vectors at this site were highest and fell slightly to the opposite wall. The distribution along the other axes was almost symmetric with the highest velocity component in the axial stream. These profile mappings were performed one after the other. Simultaneous ECG and pressure recordings demonstrate fair stability of the circulatory situation during the period of measurement.

In Figure 5, velocity profiles beyond different heart valve prostheses are depicted. The velocity distribution along the diameter, exhibiting the most typical pattern, is shown. At first sight, each profile reflects the specific architecture of the prosthesis. Independent of the type of valve used, the profiles appeared flat, which agrees with the in vitro findings of Wieting et al. [32]. In a pulse-duplicator system, the authors observed extreme turbulence immediately distal to several types of artifical heart valves. In contrast, Björk and Olin [3] reported laminar profiles beyond larger Björk-Shiley valves. According to own preliminary studies, the flat velocity profiles in the ascending aorta tend to become more parabolic as the distance from the valve increases.

Generally, the peak velocities beyond artificial valves were about 30% higher compared to normal aortic valves. There were also higher retrograde velocities during early diastole, which may reflect — aside from coronary flow — some valvular regurgitation which is necessary to produce drag on the moving element so that it will open or close [16, 18].

Distal to tilting disc valves, a profile was consistently found which is determined by the preference of high flow velocities at the site of the large opening area. In contrast to Huhmann et al. [12], who suggested from angiographic studies that flow exclusively passes the large valve orifice, high velocity components can also be demonstrated immediately behind the small orifice area. The delved velocity profile behind Starr-Edwards ball valves corresponds perfectly with the shape

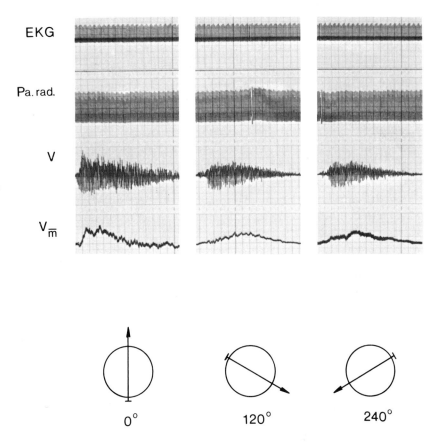

Fig. 4. Blood velocity distribution in the ascending aorta along three diameters obtained from a patient with severe aortic insufficiency. EKG: electrocardiogram; $P_{a.\ rad.}$: pressure in the radial artery; V: phasic velocity; $V_{\overline{m}}$: mean velocity

found in in vitro studies [23]. High velocities on both sides of the central obstacle and relatively small net forward vectors behind the ball characterize the velocity distribution distal to this prosthesis. With increasing distance from the valve, the typical delved shape disappeared and the profile became increasingly flat. Surprisingly, the velocity distribution beyond Hancock's xenograft was similar to the profiles found distal to artificial valves. The profile exhibited in some cases an oblique irregular front with lower velocities at the sector of the muscular leaflet of the porcine valve. Compared to the other prostheses, the peak forward velocities were lower suggesting larger effective orifice areas in this central flow substitute. Despite this fact, the velocity profile was extremely flat and showed an irregular disturbed front. As sources of turbulence, the struts of the valve which project into the stream and the muscle-bearing leaflets with its reduced mobility must be considered. The rigidity of glutaraldehyde-fixed valvular tissue may further contribute to this effect. It appears that the velocity profiles found beyond artificial valves are similar to those recorded distally of normal aortic valves.

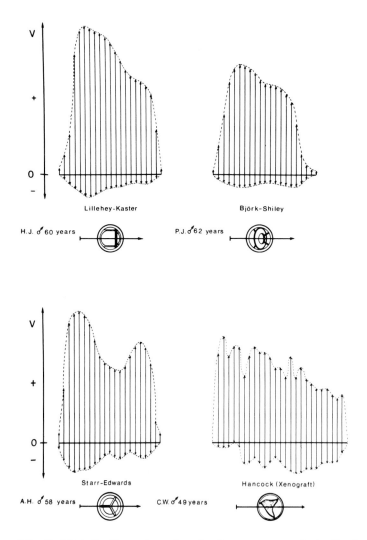

Fig. 5. Distribution of peak velocity components in the human ascending aorta after aortic valve replacement with different types of prostheses. Lillehei-Kaster, Björk-Shiley: tilting disc valves; Starr-Edwards: ball valve; Hancock xenograft: central flow valve. The inserts show the direction of the depicted velocity profile in respect to the moving element of the valve. The profiles reflect the specific hydraulic configuration of the prosthetic heart valve

From this result, one may deduce that the flow distribution beyond heart valve prostheses reflects physiologic conditions. However, in contrast to normal valves, negative net velocity components were detected beyond each artificial mechanical prosthesis, at least during limited periods of the ejection phase.

Figure 6a shows the velocity profile beyond a Björk-Shiley valve during different periods after aortic valve opening. Lower velocities were recorded at the site of

262

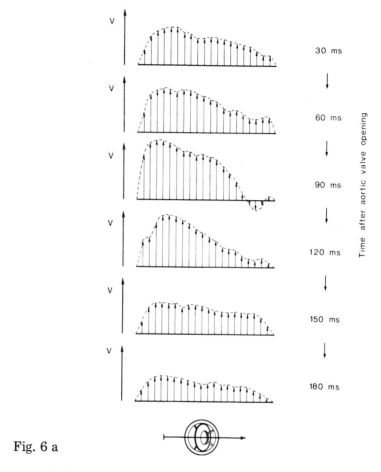

Fig. 6 a

Fig. 6. The development of velocity profiles in the human ascending aorta 5 cm distal to different types of artificial valves. The profiles were drawn from high-speed recordings in steps of 30 ms after aortic valve opening. Velocity distribution beyond a
A: Björk-Shiley valve; B: Lillehei-Kaster valve; C: Starr-Edwards valve; D: Hancock xenograft valve

the small opening area 90 ms after aortic valve opening; negative net velocity components appear distal to the disc suggesting the presence of eddies or vortices. Similar patterns were observed distal to a Lillehei-Kaster valve (Fig. 6b). The negative velocity vectors which can be demonstrated after 60 ms and which persist up to 100 ms seem to be even more pronounced. Figure 6c demonstrates the development of the profiles beyond a Starr ball valve: the negative velocity

263

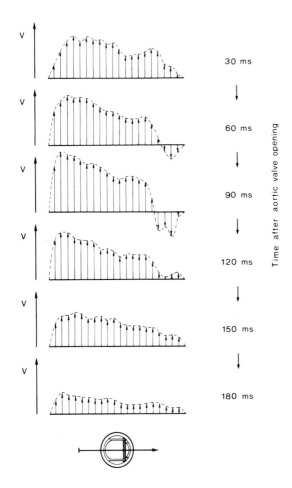

Velocity profiles
beyond a Lillehei- Kaster aortic valve

30 ms

60 ms

90 ms

120 ms

150 ms

180 ms

Time after aortic valve opening

Fig. 6 b

components can be shown immediately behind the ball. In contrast, distal to central flow substitutes (Hancock valve, Fig. 6d), no negative net velocities were recorded, suggesting that eddies are less compared to mechanical valves. The disturbed irregular front, however, indicates the presence of turbulence also distal to this type of valve.

The measurement of blood flow velocity distribution in the human ascending aorta demonstrated flat velocity profiles and negative velocity components during ejection distal to artificial heart valves. This suggests the presence of highly turbulent flow. The interruption in the linear pressure-flow relationship, occurring with turbulence contributes — besides the reduced geometric opening area of the prostheses — to the known energy loss which is measured across artificial heart valves. The flat velocity profile observed beyond normal aortic valves may not be compared with this very special hemodynamic condition after valve re-

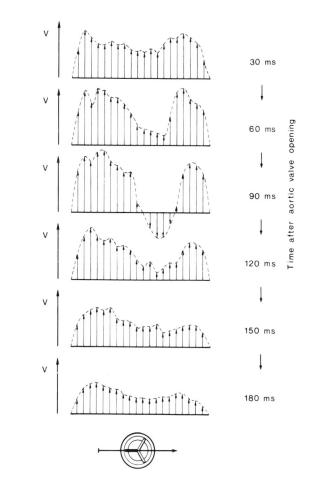

Velocity profiles

beyond a Starr-Edwards aortic valve

30 ms

60 ms

90 ms

120 ms

150 ms

180 ms

Time after aortic valve opening

Fig. 6 c

placement. The additional distortion of flow by mechanical obstacles such as the valvular ring, the struts, or the moving parts and the presence of areas of stasis may be considered the cause of energy loss and may favor the origin of hemolysis or thrombosis. The fact that even under normal conditions turbulence is present in the ascending aorta ought to stimulate engineering efforts to develop valves which further reduce the additional flow disturbance by mechanical features of the valve itself.

Summary

Blood velocity profiles in the ascending aorta were analyzed before and after aortic valve replacement (Starr-Edwards, Björk-Shiley, Lillehei-Kaster, Hancock

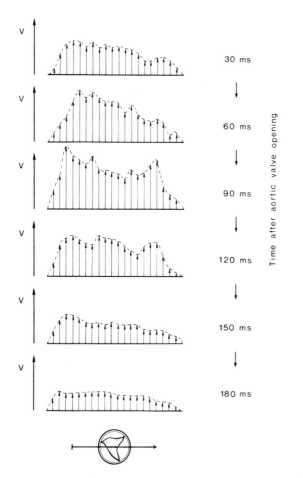

Velocity profiles

beyond a Hancock porcine aortic valve

30 ms

60 ms

90 ms

120 ms

150 ms

180 ms

Time after aortic valve opening

Fig. 6 d

xenografts) in 22 patients. Three piezoceramics, mounted on a lucite ring 120°
apart, were placed around the ascending aorta. By successive activation of the
crystals, three velocity profiles were detected shifting the gate automatically
across the diameter. Every artificial valve revealed a typical profile, reflecting
the specific construction characteristics of the prostheses. All profiles distal to
the artificial heart valves were flat, suggesting the presence of eddies and turbulent flow. Porcine xenografts revealed a flow profile most likely approaching the
physiologic conditions of normal aortic flow.

References

1. Affeld, K., Mohnhaupt, R.: Turbulenzuntersuchung an Herzklappen. Biomed. Tech. (Berlin) $\underline{20}$ [Suppl.] 73 (1975)
2. Bergel, D., Clark, C., Schultz, D.L., Tunstall Pedoe, D.S.: Measurement of instantaneous blood flow velocity in major vessels using a thin film anemometer. J. Physiol. (London) $\underline{204}$, 72 (1969)
3. Björk, V.O., Colin, C.: A hydrodynamic comparison between the new tilting disc aortic valve prosthesis (Björk-Shiley) and the corresponding prostheses of Starr-Edwards, Kay-Shiley, Smelloff-Cutter and Wada-Cutter in the pulse duplicator. Scand. I. Thorac. Cardiovasc. Surg. $\underline{4}$, 31 (1970)
4. Blackshear, P.L., Forstrom, R., Watters, C., Dorman, F.D.: Effect of flow and turbulence on the formed elements of blood. In: Heart Valves. Brewer, L.A. (ed.). Springfield (Illinois): Thomas 1969 p. 52
5. Both, A., Haerten, K., Credner, Chr., Fischer, G., Herzer, J., Loogen, F., Lück, J.: Hämodynamische Untersuchungen nach Mitralklappenersatz in einem randomisierten Krankengut. Z. Kardiol. [Suppl.] $\underline{3}$, 30 (1976)
6. Dalichau, H., Huhmann, W., Lichtlen, P., Borst, H.G.: Klinische und hämodynamische Untersuchungen über die Brauchbarkeit der Starr-Edwards Diskusklappen in Mitralposition. Thoraxchirurgie $\underline{24}$, 401 (1976)
7. Gleichmann, U.,Schmidt, H., Sigwart, U., Mertens, H.M., Dalichau, H., Leitz, K., Borst, H.G.: Björk-Shiley oder Lillehei-Kaster Klappe? Vergleichende hämodynamische Untersuchungen zweier Aortenklappenprothesen. Z. Kardiol. [Suppl.] $\underline{3}$, 26 (1976)
8. Gorlin, R., Gorlin, S.G.: Hydraulic formula for calculation of the area of the stenotic mitral valve, other cardiac valves and central circulatory shunts. Am. Heart J. $\underline{41}$, 1 (1951)
9. Grosse, G., Rutsch, W., Krais, T., Michel, U.S., Michel, U., Paeprer, H., Schmutzler, H.: Vergleich hämodynamischer und angiographischer Parameter vor und nach Klappenersatz. Z. Kardiol. [Suppl.] $\underline{3}$, 23 (1976)
10. Hagl, S.: Hämodynamik nach Mitral- und Aortenklappenersatz. Herz $\underline{2}$, 299 (1977)
11. Hagl, S., Messmer, K., Pfau, B., Meisner, H.: Influence of stenosis on the velocity profile analyzed by a pulsed Doppler ultrasonic flowmeter. In: Cardiovascular Application of Ultrasound. Reneman, R.S. (ed.). Amsterdam-London: North Holland 1974 p. 216
12. Huhmann, W., Dalichau, H., Lichtlen, P., Borst, H.G.: Zur Funktionsfähigkeit der Lillehei-Kaster-Klappe in Aortenposition. Thoraxchirurgie $\underline{24}$, 390 (1976)
13. Indeglia, R.A., Shea, M.A., Varco, R.L.: Erythrocyte destruction by prosthetic heart valves. Circulation $\underline{37/38}$ [Suppl. II], 86 (1968)
14. Kaster, R.L., Bonnabeau, R.C., Tanaka, S., Lillehei, C.W.: Comparative analysis of in vitro flow characteristic heart valves. In: Heart Valves. Brewer, L.A. (ed.). Springfield (Illinois): Thomas 1969, p. 137
15. Knutti, J.W., Gill, R.W., Meindl, J.D., Brody, W.R., Angell, W.W.: Intraoperative blood flow measurements using the pulsed Doppler ultrasonic blood flowmete r. Proc. $\underline{26}$th ACEMB $\underline{15}$, 9.2 (1973)

16. Köhler, J., Kramer, C.: Zum Schließvorgang künstlicher Herzklappen. Acta Medicotechnica 20, 36 (1972)
17. Köhler, J., Kurz, W.: Modelluntersuchung des Druckverlustes der Björk-Shiley und Lillehei-Kaster Klappen in Aortenposition. Biomed. Techn. (Berlin) 20, [Suppl. 1], 71 (1975)
18 Kramer, C., Naumann, A., Bleifeld, W., Effert, S.: Über die Durchströmung künstlicher Herzklappen. Thoraxchirurgie 16, 529 (1968)
19. Lillehei, C.W., Kaster, R.L., Colemann, M., Block, J.H.: Heart valve replacement with Lillehei-Kaster pivoting disc prosthesis. N.Y. State J. Med. 74, 1426 (1974)
20. Lynch, P.R., Bove, A.A.: Patterns of blood flow through the intact heart and its valves. In: Heart Valves. Brewer, L.A. (ed.). Springfield (Illinois): Thomas 1969, p. 24
21. McDonald, D.A.: The velocity profiles in pulsatile blood flow. In: Flow Properties of Blood and Other Biological Systems. Copley, A.L., Stainsby, G. (ed.). London, New York: Pergamon Press 1960, p. 84
22. Meisner, H., Rushmer, R.F.: Eddy formation and turbulence in flowing liquids. Circ. Res. 12, 455 (1963)
23. Peronneau, P., Hinglais, J., Pellet, M., Leger, F.: Vélocimètre sanguin par effet Doppler à émission ultra-sonore pulsée. L'onde Electrique 50, 3 (1970)
24. Reuben, S.R., Swalding, J.P., DeLee, G.J.: Velocity profiles in the main pulmonary artery of dogs and man, measured with a thin film resistance anemometer. Circ. Res. 27, 995 (1970)
25. Roberts, W.C., Fishbein, M.C., Golden, A.: Cardiac pathology after valve replacement by disc prosthesis: A study of 61 necropsy patients. Am. J. Cardiol. 35, 740 (1975)
26. Shepherd, R.L., Glancy, D.L., Reis, R.L., Epstein, St.E., Morrow, A.G.: Hemodynamic function of the Kay-Shiley prosthetic cardiac valve. Chest 63, 323 (1973)
27. Sigwart, U., Gleichmann, U., Schmidt, H., Borst, H.G.: Die Lillehei Klappenprothese: Bemerkungen zur Hämodynamik und -mechanik in vivo. Thoraxchirurgie 24, 397 (1976)
28. Smelloff, E.A., Davey, T.B., Kaufman, B.: Patterns of blood flow through artificial valves. In: Heart Valves. Brewer, L.A. (ed.). Springfield (Illinois): Thomas 1969 p. 70
29. Smith, R.L., Blick, E.F., Coalson, J., Stein, P.D.: Thrombus production by turbulence. J. Appl. Physiol. 32, 261 (1972)
30. Wetterer, E., Kenner, Th.: Grundlagen der Dynamik des Arterienpulses. Berlin-Heidelberg-New York: Springer Verlag 1968
31. Wieting, E.W., Hall, C.W., Liotta, D., DeBakey, M.E.: Dynamic Flow behavior of the natural human aortic valve. Proc. 21th ACEMB, 10, 9-B1 (1968)
32. Wieting, D.W. Hall, C.W., Liotta, D., DeBakey, M.E.: Dynamic flow behavior of artificial heart valves. In: Heart Valves. Brewer, L.A. (ed.). Springfield (Illinois): Thomas 1969, p. 34
33. Yellin, E.L.: Laminar-turbulent transition process in pulsatile flow. Circ. Res. 19, 791 (1966)

Fluid Mechanics of Natural Cardiac Valves

N. Talukder* and H. Reul

Helmholtz-Institut für Biomedizinische Technik an der RWTH, Aachen

Introduction

Natural cardiac valves are believed to open and close in a passive way under the forces exerted by the adjacent blood on the valve leaflets. Many attempts were made in the past by different investigators to explain the fluid mechanics of these valves — especially the closure mechanism of the aortic valve and that of the mitral valve. There are still some misinterpretations of the flow phenomena associated with the valve motion, leading to confusion and controversies about the roles of the different factors involved.

Henderson and Johnson [7], performing simple model experiments to study cardiac valve behavior, found that in a pulsatile flow a valve moves gradually toward closure during flow deceleration to finally close without regurgitation. But the reasons behind these interesting phenomena were not clearly understood, and the importance of these early findings were not fully appreciated by later investigators of the problem. It was generally believed that the valves, in order to minimize regurgitation, somehow move to a partially closed position prior to flow reversal. The controversies c o n c e r n e d the mechanism of this early partial valve closure. According to Bellhouse and Bellhouse [2, 4], vortices behind the valve leaflets play the crucial role of bringing the valve to a partial closure before the flow through the valve is reversed, so that only a little regurgitation is then enough to seal the valve. This explanation again has been seriously misleading.

It would be a fundamental mistake to think that a certain reversed flow through a valve is essential to complete its closure, although in special cases a regurgitation may precede valve closure. Further, the emphasis on the role of the vortices tends to divert one's attention away from one of the primary functions of the adverse pressure gradient during deceleration of flow through a valve. The adverse pressure gradient not only decelerates the flow but also acts at the same time on the valve leaflets moving them toward closure, irrespective of whether vortices are present behind the leaflets or not.

---

*Present address: Dept. Physiologie, Universität Ulm

Aortic Valve

Bellhouse and Bellhouse [2] suggested that strong vortices are generated in the aortic sinuses during peak systolic ejection when, they assumed, the valve is fully open and the leaflets even project into the sinuses. Consequently, the sinuses were regarded as essential for a proper valve closure. In their model experiments, Bellhouse and Bellhouse [3] and Bellhouse and Talbot [5] used rigid sinuses and aorta. But there is no evidence that the aortic valve leaflets project into the sinuses in vivo. Padula et al. [11], using a direct cinematographic method, showed that, in a beating heart, the aortic valve opens fully very early in systole but for an extremely short time, after which the valve aperture becomes triangular. The anatomic specimens by Robel [15] suggest that the aortic valve aperture has to become triangular, as the valve commissures are dilated under the rising aortic pressure, after the leaflets cease to pull them radially inward. Aortic valve echograms taken recently by Laniado et al. [10] confirmed that the leaflets, after their maximum excursion early in systole, move back a certain distance very quickly before peak systole, i.e., when the aortic pressure and flow velocity are still rising. Therefore, even a normal aortic valve will act like a stenosis during peak systole. This might be a possible reason for the peak systolic flow disturbances in the ascending aorta reported by Seed and Wood [16]. But strong sinus vortices will not be generated in this situation. It appears that the aortic valve closure is accomplished solely by the adverse pressure gradient that comes into action after peak systole. Further, the adverse pressure gradient should be effective on the leaflets even if the sinuses are covered, leaving only small pockets behind the leaflets.

The above characteristics were confirmed by model studies performed using a fully flexible trileaflet valve developed by Reul and Ghista [13] and elastic aorta and sinuses set in a hydraulic analogue model of the circulatory system developed by Reul et al. [14]. General flow patterns in the vicinity of the valve were made visible by suspending amberlite particles in the model fluid, a 36% aqueous solution of glycerine. To detect backflow through the valve, if any, hydrogen bubbles were generated just downstream of the valve. Flow patterns were observed in a longitudinal section of the aortic root and valve. The valve movement was observed from the aortic side through the transparent aortic wall. Flow patterns and valve motion were recorded on a 16-mm movie film as well as on triggered photographs.

In order to determine the influence of the aortic sinuses on the valve closing behavior, two sets of observations were made: 1) with open sinuses and 2) with closed sinuses. Practically no difference in valve actions between the two cases was found. In neither of the two cases was there any regurgitation. The movement of the aortic valve and the flow situations in its vicinity at different stages of the cardiac cycle may be described in the following way with reference to the illustrations of Figure 1 (corresponding to the points "a — i" shown on the ventricular ejection velocity curve).

a: The leaflets are beginning to move, as the ventricular pressure is just exceeding the aortic pressure.
b: The leaflets have bulged forward while the valve is yet to open.

270

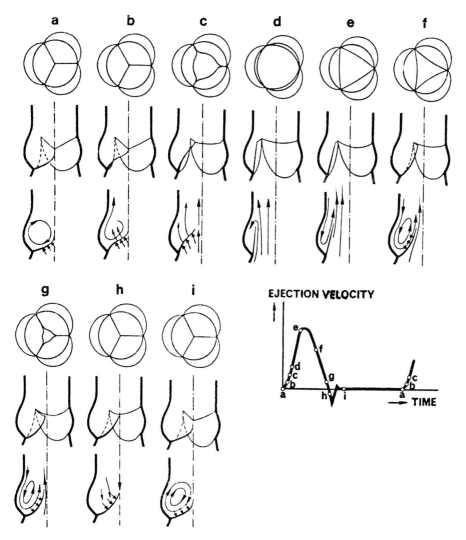

Fig. 1. Different stages of valve leaflet position and flow through the aortic valve during valve opening and valve closure.

c: The valve is partly open: and the leaflets are being displace laterally, causing a washout of the sinuses while the jet under formation is yet to pass the leaflets' edges.

d: The valve is almost fully open. Boundary layer blood is being diverted into the sinuses where the pressure is lower than at the jet, leading to a weak vortex motion in the sinuses.

e: The aortic jet is being ejected through a stenosis of nearly triangular aperture. Flow separation at the jet boundary and a local back flow near the aortic wall are very likely to follow.

f: The adverse pressure gradient strengthens the backflow near the wall and thus also the sinus vortices, and at the same time it acts on the leaflets moving them

271

toward closure and decelerates the jet that thus gets slower and narrower simultaneously.

g: The jet velocity and the valve aperture are greatly reduced.

h: The valve aperture is vanishing as leaflets and the blood are being displaced toward the ventricle causing a pseudoregurgitation (no backflow relative to the valve aperture).

i: The leaflets have reached their final, end systolic position. The aortic blood, after being suddenly stopped, slides on the slanting leaflet surfaces giving rise to strong, diastolic sinus vortices that rotate against the systolic ones.

The following conclusions are drawn. The aortic valve closure is primarily accomplished by the adverse pressure gradient that simultaneously decelerates the flow and brings the valve gradually toward closure. Sinus vortices are produced mainly after peak systole, during flow deceleration, and especially after valve closure, as secondary effects of the adverse pressure gradient. Neither the vortices nor the aortic sinuses appear to play any indispensable role in valve closure. The normal aortic valve closes without regurgitation.

Mitral Valve

The mitral valve, after opening early in diastole, undergoes a partial closure in mid-diastole after which it opens again due to atrial contraction prior to final closure. The mitral flow has a typical M shape with two peaks corresponding to the two openings of the valve, as shown by Laniado et al. [9]. During ventricular filling, vortices are very likely to be generated in the ventricle, as illustrated in Figure 2 whereby the valve leaflet positions and the ventricular shape are drawn after the echograms taken by Pohost et al. [12].

According to Bellhouse [1], the ventricular vortices raise the pressure at the back of the leaflets. Brockman [6] has shown that the atrioventricular pressure gradient is reversed as a result of ventricular filling. The mid-diastolic partial valve closure may be attributed to both the ventricular vortices and the mid-diastolic adverse pressure gradient, the latter also accounting for the deceleration. The actual valve closure we are concerned with, however, takes place after atrial contraction (Fig. 2, f-i).

As shown by Laniado et al. [8], the ventricular contraction starts when the mitral flow is near its second peak (Fig. 2, f) and the valve is almost fully open. This is in contrast to the opinion shared by Brockman [6] and Bellhouse and Bellhouse [4] that the mitral valve, in order to minimize regurgitation, has to be partially closed before the ventricle contracts. The subsequent strong deceleration of mitral flow (Fig. 2, f-h) is the result of the strong adverse pressure gradient due to the rapid rise of the ventricular pressure. During this deceleration, the pressure forces can also act on the valve leaflets to move them toward closure. As shown by Laniado et al. [8], the valve aperture practically vanishes when the velocity of flow through the valve comes down to zero so that no backflow through the valve is possible. The apparent backflow or pseudoregurgitation that follows (Fig. 2, h) is due to a displacement of valve leaflets along with the adjacent blood toward the atrium until the chordae tendineae suddenly stop them.

272

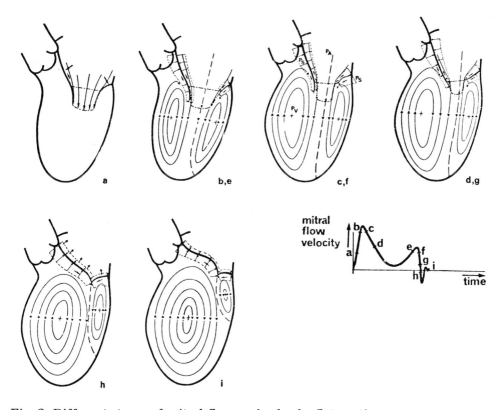

Fig. 2. Different stages of mitral flow and valve leaflet motion

The closure of the mitral valve is thus basically very similar to that of the aortic valve, the differences being that the mitral valve closes more quickly and that strong vortices are present behind the valve leaflets before and after the adverse pressure gradient comes into action. But it appears that the pressure gradient would be closing the valve efficiently even without the help of the vortices, as in the case of the aortic valve. This, however, remains to be verified experimentally.

Bellhouse and Bellhouse [3], in their model experiments, found considerable regurgitation when they started the ventricular contraction after the fluid in the ventricle came to a standstill. While eliminating the vortices, they also precluded flow deceleration by the rising ventricular pressure due to ventricular contraction. In our experiments which are still in progress, the vortices are going to be prevented from acting on the valve leaflets, without impairing the pulsatility of the mitral flow. As in a beating heart, the adverse pressure gradient produced by the ventricular contraction should be allowed to decelerate the flow and to act on the valve leaflets at the same time. The results of our experiments will provide a more definite evaluation of the role of the ventricular vortices in the valve closure mechanism.

273

References

1. Bellhouse, B.J.: Fluid mechanics of a model mitral valve and left ventricle. Cardiovasc. Res. 6, 199 (1972)
2. Bellhouse, B.J., Bellhouse, F.H.: Mechanism of closure of the aortic valve. Nature 217, 86 (1968)
3. Bellhouse, B.J., Bellhouse, F.H.: Fluid mechanics of model normal and stenosed aortic valves. Circ. Research 25, 693 (1969)
4. Bellhouse, B.J., Bellhouse, F.H.: Fluid mechanics of the mitral valve. Nature 224, 615 (1969)
5. Bellhouse, B.J., Talbot, L.: The fluid mechanics of the aortic valve. J. Fluid Mech. 35, 721 (1969)
6. Brockman, S.K.: Mechanism of the movements of the atrioventricular valves. Am. J. Cardiol. 17, 682 (1968)
7. Henderson, Y., Johnson, F.E.: Two modes of closure of the heart valves. Heart 4, 69 (1912)
8. Laniado, S., Yellin, E.L., Millner, H., Frater, R.W.M.: Temporal relation of the first heart sound to closure of the mitral valve. Circulation 47, 1006 (1973)
9. Laniado, S., Yellin, E.L., Kotler, M., Levy, L., Stadler, J., Terdiman, R.: A study of the dynamic relation between the mitral valve echogram and phasic mitral flow. Circulation 51, 104 (1975)
10. Laniado, S., Yellin, E.L., Terdiman, R., Meytes, J., Stadler, J.: Hemodynamic correlates of the normal aortic valve echogram. Circulation 54, 729 (1976)
11. Padula, R.T., Cowan, S.M. (Jr.), Camishion, R.C.: Photographic analysis of the active and passive components of cardiac valvular action. J. Thor. Cardiovasc. Surg. 56, 6 (1968)
12. Pohost, G.M., Dinsmore, R.E., Rubenstein, J.J., O'Keefe, D.D., Grantham, R.N., Scully, H.E., Bierholm, E.A., Fredriksen, J.W., Weisfeldt, M.L., Daggett, W.M.: The echogram of the anterior leaflet of the mitral valve. Circulation 51, 88 (1975)
13. Reul, H., Ghista, D.N.: Optimum prosthetic aortic leaflet valve: design criteria, prototype design and in vitro testing. Digest 11th ICEMB (Ottawa) 328 (1976)
14. Reul, H., Minamitani, H., Runge, J.: A hydraulic analog of the systemic and pulmonary circulation for testing artificial hearts. Proc. ESAO 2, 120 (1976)
15. Robel, S.B.: Structural mechanics of the aortic valve. In: Prosthetic Replacement of the Aortic Valve. Sauvage, L.R., Viggers, R.F., Berger, K., Robel, S.B., Sawyer, P.N., Wood, S.J. (eds.). Springfield (Illinois), Thomas, p.3 (1972)
16. Seed, W.A., Wood, N.B.: Velocity patterns in the aorta. Cardiovas. Res. 5, 319 (1971)

Early Mortality Due to Ventricular Fibrillation, and the Vulnerability of the Heart Following Acute Experimental Coronary Occlusion: Possible Mechanisms and Pharmacological Prophylaxis*

W. Meesmann, V. Wiegand, U. Menken, W. Komhard, and U. Rehwald

Institute of Pathophysiology, University Essen (GHS), Hufelandstraße 55
D-43 Essen 1, Fed. Rep. Germ.

Ventricular fibrillation (VF) is by far and away the most common cause of early mortality in patients with acute myocardial infarction [12, 13]. This also applies equally to acute experimental coronary occlusion [12, 13]. Early mortality within the first 24 h attains a maximum in the 1st h and then drops exponentially. The mean interval between the onset of symptoms and sudden death is reported as 21 min [12, 13]. In experimental cardiology, we distinguish between two characteristic phases of arrhythmias following acute one-step coronary ligation [9]: an initial early phase lasting 20-30 min immediately following ligation and a second phase of arrhythmias after an interval of 6-10 h with few extrasystoles; this second phase lasts for a period of 24-48 h. The present study is an investigation of the first phase of arrhythmias described by Harris [9].

Pantridge et al. [18,22]have also described ventricular premature beats (VPB) and sudden onset VF in this initial period in patients with myocardial infarction. A detailed analysis of the frequency and distribution of these VPB and VF is, of course, only possible on the basis of experiments.

Before we give a brief description of our infarction model in dogs, it must first be mentioned that, in contrast to man, the dog has a left coronary preponderance, the region supplied by the circumflex branch of the left coronary artery usually being considerably larger than that supplied by the left anterior descending branch. Moreover, in the dog, a distinction must also be made between animals with functionally effective intercoronary collaterals and those without. We established this situation in every dog, in postmortem examinations, employing a special method of selective coronary angiography. The extent of the retrograde filling of the vascular system of the acutely ligated coronary artery was determined by orthograde injection into the neighbouring coronary trunks [14].

Table 1 shows the results, obtained from studies in a total of 62 dogs, of the frequency of VF after acute occlusion of the circumflex or anterior descending branch of the left coronary artery, as a function of the coronary collaterals [14]. These results clearly reveal the prerequisites for an experimental animal study of the protective measures, including the protective effects of a drug, in particular against VF in the acute phase following coronary occlusion, viz, 1) ligation of the largest coronary branch (in the dog), the circumflex branch, and 2) exclusion of effective collaterals.

---

* Supported by the Landesamt f. Wissenschaft u. Forschung, Düsseldorf, FRG.

Table 1. Frequency of ventricular fibrillation after occlusion of the circumflex branch or the anterior descending branch of the left coronary artery in anesthetized dogs as a function of coronary collaterals

	Total n	Ventricular Fibrillation	
		n	%
ram. descendens			
with collaterals	7	0 *	0
without "	9	5	55,6
ram. circumflexus			
with collaterals	27	1 *	3,7
without "	19	19	100,0

(from Meesmann et al 1970) * = p < 0,001

On the other hand, the frequency and distribution of VPB in time can be better investigated on the basis of the ligation of the anterior descending branch, since here the percentage of surviving animals is greater, even in the absence of collaterals [14]. For the same reason, we also determined the electric ventricular fibrillation threshold (VFT) of the heart in animals with ligated descending branch. For this purpose, R wave triggered square wave pulse currents of 2-ms duration, delivered at 3-ms intervals, in one train lasting 140-ms, were applied during the vulnerable period of the cardiac cycle under oscilloscopic control. As stimulating electrodes, chlorided silver plates (diameter 7 mm) were sutured 3 cm outside the ischemic area directly onto the epicardium. The VFT was taken to be the current intensity, in mA, which just sufficed to produce VF. A few seconds after the start of VF, sinus rhythm was reestablished by defibrillation (DC countershock) employing plate electrodes of 3-cm diameter on the affixed pericard [15].

In a number of experimental series involving various conditions of anesthesia, it was revealed that the vulnerability of the heart after sudden coronary occlusion has a bimodal distribution in the initial phase of arrhythmia previously considered to be uniform in nature [13, 16]. This is shown in Figure 1 by the distribution of VPB and the mortality rate due to VF under different narcoses in 65 dogs. In addition, the course of the VFT following acute occlusion of the descending branch of a further group of 18 dogs is also recorded [15]. Two phases, in which VPB and VF occur frequently, can clearly be differentiated. In the early phase (termed Ia), an unequivocal coincidence in time of the maxima of the frequency of the VPB, the VF, and also the drop of the VFT is obtained. It is noteworthy that the VFT, which is determined only in normal sinus rhythm, manifests no drop in the second phase (termed Ib).
The presence of these two phases — as far as we know, first mentioned by Haase and Schiller [8] in 1969 and to date virtually ignored in the international litera-

276

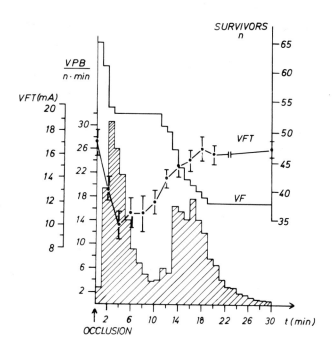

Fig. 1. Frequency of distribution in time of ventricular PB, mortality rate (VF), and fibrillation threshold (VFT) after acute ligation of the descending branch. The abscissa represents the time in minutes after acute occlusion (occlusion at time 0), the ordinate (VPB/n × min) the mean figure of the ventricular PB/min for each animal still living, the ventricular fibrillation threshold (VFT), and the survival rate (survivors)

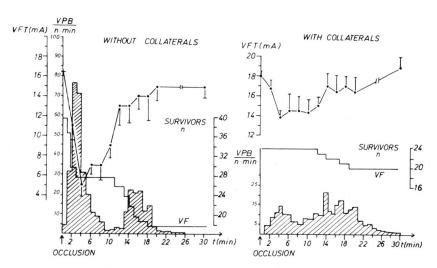

Fig. 2. Frequency and distribution in time of ventricular PB, mortality rate (VF), and fibrillation threshold (VFT) after acute ligation of the anterior descending branch (untreated animals). Ordinate and abscissa as in Figure 1. Animals are divided into those with and those without coronary collaterals

ture — becomes even more clearly recognizable when the animals are divided into those with and those without collaterals. This is shown in Figure 2. The ordinate and abscissa are unchanged, merely the scale for the VPB is smaller. In the case of the animals without coronary collaterals, a clearly recognized maximum of the frequency of VPB and VF is reached between the 2nd and the 6th min and coincides with the maximum of the VFT drop. Following this, VPB and VF are strongly reduced for several minutes — in many cases regular pauses are present — and finally, the Ib phase develops from the 12th min onward. Its ectopic maximum is not so high — rather somewhat broadened. In comparison, in the case of animals with collaterals, this differentiation is somewhat unsharper, although here too, a phase course that in principle is identical can be recognized. Only four of these animals have VF. The VFT drop is significantly smaller. In the great majority of cases, these arrhythmias are monotopic VPB. These phases Ia and Ib (Fig. 4, left) are even more marked and show an almost dramatic course during ligation of the circumflex branch [20]. The ordinates and the abscissae are again identical. All 19 animals in this group died of VF within 21 min. The onset and the maximum of the Ia phase are earlier than is the case with ligation of the anterior descending branch. Here, the pause prior to the onset of the Ib phase can clearly be recognized.

Noteworthy and almost pathognomonic for the Ia and Ib phases are the different transitions to VF in the ECGs. Figure 3 shows two typical courses for ligation of the descending branch. In the upper example (ECG, lead II), multiple individual or groups of VPB or ventricular tachycardias occur. They may suddenly remit or (as here) they may develop into ventricular flutter and then ventricular fibrillation (here 1 min and 49 s following ligation).

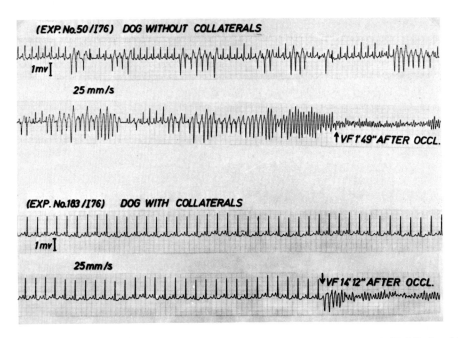

Fig. 3. Two examples of arrhythmia with development of VF (ECG, lead II) in the early (Ia) and late (Ib) phases after acute ligation of the anterior descending branch (untreated animals)

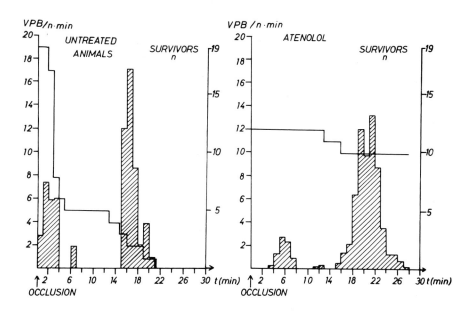

Fig. 4. Frequency and distribution in time of ventricular VPB and survival rate (VF) after acute ligation of the circumflex branch following oral administration of atenolol, in comparison with an untreated group (animals without collaterals). Ordinate and abscissa as in Figure 1

The situation is completely different in the case of an animal with collaterals, in which very often no Ia phase develops. Here, in the presence of a regular sinus rhythm, a VPB suddenly occurs in the Ib phase, a second VPB occurring in the vulnerable phase of the first. Following ventricular flutter of short duration, VF now rapidly develops (here 14 min and 12 s after ligation).

Numerous experimental and clinical findings now indicate the decisive importance of the sympathetic nervous system in this early phase of myocardial infarction [12, 13]. In this conjunction, it has not yet been established how a local activation of the sympathetic system triggers the arrhythmias and the VF, or at least plays a supporting role in their initiation. Thus, it seemed obvious to try to influence the arrhythmias by the use of β-blockers. The main idea behind this is that if the fateful early VF can be influenced effectively at all, then decisively by means of prophylactic measures, in this case antiarrhythmic drugs, which can and must be administered prophylactically to endangered patients. Clinically, this question is very difficult to investigate.

Experiments in animals [13], with acute ligation of coronary vessels following previous intravenous administration of β-blockers, have to date been carried out with propranolol, sotalol, and practolol and in our work group with practolol and atenolol [1, 21]. In particular, the following serious objections have to be made against these investigations: 1) nonconsideration of collaterals, 2) ligation of the anterior descending branch, and 3) the groups studied are too small. If, nevertheless, the animals with anterior descending branch and circumflex liga-

279

tions are collected together in respective groups, a marked positive survival effect of an acute β-blockade in coronary ligation is revealed [1, 13].

The objective of further studies was to investigate the effect of chronic oral pre-treatment of the animals with the pure β_1-blocker atenolol[1] on the survival rate following coronary occlusion and to establish whether there was any influence on the frequency and distribution in time of VPB. These points were to be studied at various dose levels. In each animal, acute high ligation of the circumflex branch was carried out under anesthesia with morphine-chloralose und urethane, and only animals with no functionally important collaterals were evaluated. The animals had an average weight of 22 kg. As a measure of the β-blockade obtained in each case, we determined the percentage inhibition of isoproterenol tachycardia following the administration of 1 mcg/kg isoproterenol. In addition, the plasma atenolol level at the moment of ligation was determined using Kaye's spectro-photofluometric method [13].

The results are summarized in Table 2 [13, 16]. All the animals in the control group died of VF. The three atenolol groups had all been given one daily oral dose of 10 or 2 mg/kg body weight atenolol over a period of 5 days. Although, 18 h after the last 10 mg dose, all the animals survived the Ia phase, they then all died of VF in the Ib phase. Apparently after this period of 18 h, the blood level of the drug and the extent of the β-blockade after chronic oral administra-

Table 2. Protective effect of prophylactic atenolol administration against early ventricular fibrillation after acute occlusion of the circumflex branch (animals without collaterals)

groups	oral daily dose/kg	interval: last dose - occlusion	number of dogs n	incidence of VF	plasma-concentration of atenolol [mcg/ml]	inhibition of isoprot.-induced tachycardia [1 mcg/kg i.v.]
control	———	———	19	19	———	———
atenolol A	10 mg for 5 days	18 h	5	5	0,15 ± 0,02	42 % *
atenolol B	10 mg for 5 days	6 h	6	1 *	0,82 ± 0,05	77 % *
atenolol C	2 mg for 5 days	6 h	6	1 *	0,34 ± 0,02	59 % *

$* = p < 0,001$

tion are inadequate for the Ib phase. Six hours after the last administration, however, both at 10 mg and 2 mg/kg body weight dose levels, only one animal of six died

---

[1] Tenormin (R), ICI Pharma, Plankstadt/Heidelberg, FRG.

of VF in each group, again both in the Ib phase (15 min, 5 s and 12 min, 30 s, respectively). These results are highly significant.

The temporal distribution of the VPB and the mortality rate of the atenolol groups B and C can be seen in Figure 4. On the left we have the control group and on the right the treated group. In the pretreated group, the Ia phase extends from the 3rd to the 8th min and clearly manifests fewer VPB than in the control group. Of the 12 atenolol animals (without collaterals), only 7 manifested VPB, of wich 1 animal, together with another without previous VPB, died of VF at the beginning of the Ib phase.

In earlier studies [13], we had already found the VFT to be elevated after atenolol administration in individual measurements, also during coronary ligation. Now, for the entire course of the VFT, after ligation of the descending branch following prior chronic oral administration of atenolol (dose level, atenolol group B), it was established that both the initial values and also all the values during ligation were significantly higher than those of the control group [13, 16].

The summarized results show that a chronic oral β-blockade can almost completely prevent VF and VPB after acute coronary ligation; this also applies in the case of ligation of the largest coronary branch in the dog and in hearts without collaterals. The doses and the blood level of atenolol and also the extent of the β-blockade corresponds to the values determined in man. The so-called first arrhythmic phase described by Harris can no longer — as formerly assumed — be considered a uniform phase. Rather, in this phase, the VPB and the VF are bimodally distributed and, in the typical case, can be differentiated from each other by an interval into an Ia and an Ib phase, which can both abruptly change to sinus rhythm, even in a stage of most marked arrhythmia. A particular feature proves to be the fact that a drop in the VFT can be established only in the Ia phase and that the Ia phase is considerably more sensitive to β-blockade than is the Ib phase. Finally, the development of VF, as far as it can be recognized in the ECG, seems to be so unequivocally different in each phase that this has also contributed to the opinion that the mechanisms of origination of the two phases are different.

The question as to the possible mechanisms also includes the question as to the mode of operation of the β-blocker in this early stage of infarction. With respect to the Ia phase, a reduced electric instability may be deduced from the reduced lowering of the VFT, i.e., there is probably also a reduced dispersion of the refractory periods of the action potentials in the central region of the infarction. Without β-blockade, a characteristic inhomogeneity of the cellular responses to stimulation rapidly develops. In contrast, in these extensive infarctions, we consider diminishment of the area of infarction resulting from a reduced oxygen consumption representing the balance of the hemodynamic changes of the β-blockade to be of little importance, especially at this early point in time. It is, however, certainly possible that a diminished myocardial oxygen consumption, in the center of the ischemic region, might delay the onset and the time course of the cellular sequelae of anoxia. This would be of significance, since in the early arrhythmic phase in the nontreated infarction the cellular processes are more strongly stimulated β-adrenergically. This is indicated by the values for cyclic

3' 5' adenosine monophosphate (cAMP), which are increased in the cells of the ischemic zone but not in normal cardiac muscle [11]. This prevents the necessary rapidity and the simultaneity of fatal anoxic events in a sufficiently large area of myocardium necessary to the development of VF. In an extreme case, the subsequent infarction might develop without ventricular fibrillation comparable to slow coronary occlusion or well-developed coronary collaterals. Here, there may be certain similarities to the recent investigations carried out by Reimer et al. [19] and Nayler [17] with respect to the protective effect of propranolol on the extent of the muscular ischemia and release of CPK.

The decisive antifibrillatory and also antiarrhythmic effect of a prophylactic β-blockade in these early phases following acute coronary occlusions seems to us, in agreement with the latest findings [1, 4, 13], rather to lie in its electrophysiologic effects and may be envisaged as follows: In consequence of the rapid onset ischemic anoxia, a partial depolarization of the cell membrane and K^+ efflux out of the cells of the ventricular myocardium occurs simultaneously with the increasing acidosis. Associated with this, there is an increasing inactivation of the fast Na^+ channel with depressed conduction. With complete inactivation of the fast inward flow of Na^+, however, the myocardial fiber does not completely lose its ability to propagate an impulse. Under certain conditions, the cell can "make use" of the slow current of Na^+ and Ca^{++} to produce action potentials — a process which was first named the "slow response" by Cranefield [5] in 1972.

It is known that in ischemic anoxia, a high extracellular concentration of K^+ develops very rapidly — as has been shown recently by the group led by Kessler [10] with ion-selective superficial electrodes in the liver. Initial experiments carried out jointly by us and the Dortmund group under Kessler indicate that under our experimental conditions also in the ischemic myocardium an extracellular concentration of K^+ of 15 mM and more is reached in only a few minutes [23]. At the same time, in the ischemic myocardium, locally increased amounts of noradrenalin are released. This is occasioned by cardiac sympathetic reflex mechanisms and direct effects of anoxia and elevated concentrations of extracellular K^+ on the local adrenergic neurones. In the presence of partial depolarization, and the thus elevated extracellular K^+ concentration, these catecholamines are able to activate the slow Na^+ and Ca^{++} channel and trigger a "slow response." This has been frequently demonstrated experimentally in specially prepared Purkinje fibers or papillary muscle [4]. Such action potentials manifest a very slow rise and are frequently associated with a slow conduction and unidirectional block.

If, as the response of the myocardial cell to excitation, a slow response occurs in a sufficiently large ischemic area in a closely limited period of time, before a total depolarization occurs, virtually optimal conditions for the development of a reentry are achieved (circus movement through excitable gap, reentry by unidirectional block, reexcitation at different repolarization) and VF can originate. After prophylactic administration of a β-blocker, as a result of the β-blockade, the catecholamines cannot activate the slow Na^+ and Ca^{++} channel, even in the presence of high concentrations of extracellular K^+. A slow response is either not triggered or only incompletely, i.e., inadequate to develop propagated action potentials. Thus, the preconditions for VF would not be satisfied. The extent to which the recently described presynaptic β_1-receptors of the adrenergic neuron [2, 3] are also present in the heart and whether they are inhibited by the selective β_1-blocker atenolol is uncertain. If this applies, then the local release of catecholamines would be reduced in this way.

At the present time, it is in these processes in the center of the infarction that we see the probable mechanism of the origin of the Ia phase. In contrast, it would seem improbable that the Ib phase also arises by means of similar mechanisms in the center of the infarction. From the investigations of the group led by Durrer [6. 7], we know that, in typical cases, the myocardial cells in the center of the infarction become nonexcitable after only 10-12 min. This virtually corresponds to the time of the interval between the Ia phase and Ib phase. Thus, it would seem obvious to look for the origin of the Ib phase in the marginal zone of the infarction rather than in its center. The type of VF that is usually of sudden onset, arising out of sinus rhythm after brief ventricular flutter in the presence of normal VFT, points rather to a circumscribed focus of partially depolarized fibers which in a multifarious manner, also in slow channel activation, become the "starting point" of the VF. Our results have shown to date only that, here too, a β-blockade can interrupt the chain of causality leading to VF.

References

1. Abendroth, R.-R., Meesmann, W., Stephan, K., Schley, G., Hübner, H.: Wirkung des β-Sympathikolytikums Atenolol auf die Arrhythmien, speziell das Kammerflimmern und die Flimmerschwelle des Herzens beim akuten experimentellen Koronarverschluß. Z. Kardiol. 66. 341 (1977)
2. Åblad, B., Carlsson, E., Dahlof, C., Ek, L.: Some aspects on the pharmacology of adrenergic β-receptor blockers. In: Pathophysiology and Management of Arterial Hypertension. Berglund, G., Hansson, L., Werkö, L. (ed.). Proc. Conf. Kopenhagen, Univ. Göteborg, pp. 152-166, 1975
3. Adler-Graschinsky, E., Langer, S.Z.: Possible role of a betaadrenoceptor in regulation of noradrenaline release by nerve stimulation through a positive feed-back mechanism. Br. J. Pharmacol. 53, 43 (1975)
4. Cranefield, P.F.: The Conduction of the Cardiac Impulse. New York: Mount Kisco 1975
5. Cranefield, P.F., Wit, A.L., Hoffman, B.F.: Conduction of the cardiac impulse. III. Characteristics of very slow conduction. J. Gen. Physiol. 59, 227 (1972)
6. Downar, E., Janse, M.J., Durrer, D.: The effect of acute coronary artery occlusion on subepicardial transmembrane potentials in the intact porcine heart. Circulation 56, 217 (1977)
7. Downar, E., Janse, M.J., Durrer, D.: The effect of "ischemic" blood on transmembrane potentials of normal porcine ventricular myocardium. Circulation 55, 455 (1977)
8. Haase, M., Schiller, U.: Zur zeitlichen Parallelität zwischen der Aktivität ektopischer Schrittmacher und dem Eintritt von Kammerflimmern nach Ligatur eines Hauptkoronarastes beim Hund. Acta Biol. Med. Ger. 23, 413 (1969)

9. Harris, A.S.: Delayed development of ventricular ectopic rhythms following experimental coronary occlusion. Circulation 1, 1318 (1950)

10. Höper, J., Kessler, M., Simon, W.: Measurements with ion-selective surface electrodes (pK, pNa, pCa, pH) during no-flow anoxia. In: Ion and Encyme Electrodes in Biology and Medicine. Kessler, M. et al., (eds.). München-Berlin-Wien: Urban & Schwarzenberg 1976, 331

11. Lubbe, W., Bricknell, O.L., Podzuweit, T., Opie, L.H.: Cyclic AMP as a determinant of vulnerability to ventricular fibrillation in the isolated rat heart. Cardiovasc. Res. 10, 697 (1976)

12. Meesmann, W., Stephan, K., Schley, G., Gülker, H.: Zur Problematik einer Differentialtherapie der Arrhythmien beim akuten Herzinfarkt. Dtsch. Med. Wochenschr. 100, 954 (1975)

13. Meesmann, W., Stephan, K., Abendroth, R.-R., Menken, U., Wiegand, V.: Frühe Arrhythmien, insbesondere Kammerflimmern, nach akutem experimentellen Koronarverschluß und Beta-Rezeptorenblocker. In: Betablockade 1977. Mäurer, W., Schönig, A., Dietz, R., Lichtlen, P. (eds.). Stuttgart: Thieme 1977, p. 244

14. Meesmann, W., Schulz, F.W., Schley, G., Adolphsen, P.: Überlebensquote nach akutem experimentellem Coronarverschluß in Abhängigkeit von Spontankollateralen des Herzens. Z. Ges. Exp. Med. 153, 246 (1970)

15. Meesmann, W., Gülker, H., Krämer, B., Stephan, K.: Time course of changes in ventricular fibrillation threshold in myocardial infarction: characteristics of acute and slow occlusion with respect to the collateral vessels of the heart. Cardiovasc, Res. 10, 466 (1976)

16. Menken, U., Wiegand, V., Meesmann, W., Stephan, K., Bucher, P.: Prophylaxe des Kammerflimmerns und verminderte Vulnerabilität des akut ischämischen Myokards durch chronische β-Blockade. Z. Kardiol. Suppl. 4, R 77 (1977)

17. Nayler, W.G.: Pharmacological protection of the hypoxic heart. 7th Europ. Con. Cardiol. Amsterdam (20.-25.6.1976) p. 687

18. Pantridge, J.F., Webb, S.W.: Autonomic disturbance at the onset of acute myocardial infarction. In: Kardiale Sympathikolyse als therapeutisches Prinzip. Lydtin, H., Meesmann, W. (eds.). Stuttgart: Thieme 1975, p. 136

19. Reimer, K.A., Rasmussen, M.M., Jennings, R.B.: On the nature of protection by propranolol against myocardial necrosis after temporary coronary occlusion in dogs. Am. J. Cardiol. 37, 520 (1976)

20. Schley, G., Meesmann, W., Schulz, F.W., Amann, L., Tüttemann, J., Wilde, A.: Untersuchungen über den Einfluß von Spontankollateralen des Herzens auf die Herzrhythmusstörungen nach experimentellem Koronarverschluß. Arch. Kreislaufforsch. 67, 305 (1972)

21. Stephan, K., Meesmann, W.: Beeinflussung der frühen Arrhythmien nach akutem Koronarverschluß durch β-Blockade mit Practolol. Z. Kardiol. 63, 603 (1974)

22. Webb, S.W., Adgey, A.A.J., Pantridge, J.F.: Autonomic disturbance at onset of acute myocardial infarction. Br. Med. J. 3, 89 (1972)

23. Wiegand, V., Güggi, M., Meesmann, W., Kessler, M., Greitschus, F.: Extracellular [K^+]e changes after acute coronary occlusion. Pflügers Arch. [Suppl.] 373, R17 (1978)

Direct Nervous Effects on Coronary Flow in Conscious Dogs[*]

E. Bassenge, J. Holtz, and W. v. Restorff

Physiologisches Institut der Universität, D - 8000 München 15, Pettenkoferstr. 12

Introduction

The role of the sympathetic coronary innervation under physiologic and pathophysiologic conditions has not been clarified. Both a- and β-adrenergic receptors have been demonstrated in the coronary bed [1, 2, 3, 5, 6, 12, 16], but their significance under physiologic conditions has remained obscure [11], mainly because of the difficulty in separating direct nervous influences on the coronary bed from indirect, metabolically induced effects. In this study, different approaches were used to demonstrate and quantitate direct sympathetic influences on the coronary bed. The results demonstrate that in the coronary bed of conscious dogs a surprisingly high sympathetic constrictive tone is effective which can be modulated by reflex.

Methods

1. Induction of Regional Sympathectomy in Left Canine Ventricles to Demonstrate Steady-State Effects of Sympathetic Coronary Control

Mongrel dogs were equipped with silastic catheters into the left atrium (for microsphere injection), into the aorta (determination of heart rate and arterial pressure), and into the pulmonary artery (for drug administration). 6-Hydroxydopamine causes degeneration of the adrenergic nerve endings and was applied to one defined section of the left ventricle through a microcatheter into the left circumflex coronary artery in appropriate dosages during temporary stop of perfusion by an implanted coronary occluder. This method is described in detail elsewhere [4]. Microspheres of 9 μm diameter with five different labels were used to measure myocardial blood flow and its distribution comparing the chemically sympathectomized and the normally innervated control section of the left ventricle in the resting conscious dog.

*Supported by Deutsche Forschungsgemeinschaft

2. Reflex Modulations of the Constrictive Coronary Control

Mongrel dogs with atrioventricular block (AV block) were used, and the heart rate was fixed using an external pacemaker. Electromagnetic flow probes were applied to estimate aortic and left circumflex coronary flow. Continuous measurement of myocardial oxygen extraction rate was used to differentiate direct and indirect effects of sympathetic nerves on coronary flow using reflexion oximetry of arterial and coronary venous blood [9]. Two pneumatic occlusion cuffs around the common carotid arteries were used to elicite a pressure response upon brief occlusion periods of the cuffs. An intracarotid microcatheter was used for the application of minute nicotine doses for the induction of a pulmonary hyperinflation reflex [13]. Mean values ± SD are given throughout the paper.

Results and Discussion

Under resting conditions, striking differences in myocardial perfusion rates between the sympathectomized sections and the normally innervated control sections of the left ventricle were observed. The results are demonstrated in Figure 1. In the center of regional chemical sympathectomy, myocardial blood flow amounted to 108 ± 16 ml/100 g · min in contrast to the normally innervated control area with a flow rate of 65 ± 15 ml/100 g · min. Upon administration of a-blocking agents, the flow rate in the innervated control area reached that of the sympathectomized section (Fig. 1).

These highly significant differences in perfusion rates can be related to direct effects of sympathetic innervation on the coronary vessels; hemodynamic parameters affecting myocardial blood flow, such as heart rate, coronary perfusion pressure, left ventricular pre- and afterload were identical for both the innervated and the denervated sections of the same ventricle. This pattern of flow distribution between the various sections of the left ventricle indicates a substantial a-adrenergic constrictive effect on the coronary system of resting unanesthetized animals. Differences in extravascular coronary resistance due to differences in the contractile state between the sympathectomized section and the innervated section could not have brought about this distribution pattern of myocardial blood flow; when β-adrenergic blockers were applied, no diminution in excess blood flow to the sympathectomized sections were observed [4]. Therefore, these experiments show a tonic vasoconstrictive influence on the coronary bed of a surprisingly high magnitude; in the absence of the a-adrenergically mediated coronary vasoconstriction, myocardial perfusion rates in the resting state are almost doubled.

These findings led us to the next series of experiments, in the course of which we tried to bring about phasic modifications of this a-adrenergic tone. This was mainly done in order to test the hypothesis of whether or not a-sympathetically induced coronary constrictions may explain PRINZMETALS functional variant angina [14, 15]. Recently, Mudge et al. [7] reported on steep increases in coronary resistance leading to angina during a cold pressor test in patients with ischemic

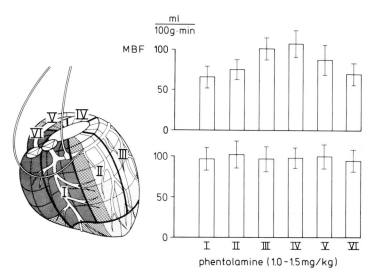

Fig. 1. Left ventricular blood flow in regional sympathectomy of the canine heart. Left: the schematic drawing represents the normally innervated dark control sections I and VI. The bright sections III and IV represent the center of chemical sympathectomy induced by 6-hydroxydopamine injections through a coronary microcatheter. Right, upper panel: distribution of myocardial blood flow (MBF) under resting conditions within the various sections of the regionally sympathectomized heart. Columns I to VI represent the flow rates within the respective sections of the schematic drawing. Data from 22 experiments in 12 dogs under resting control conditions. Heart rate: 95 ± 14 min^{-1}; mean arterial pressure: 101 ± 8 mm Hg. Lower panel: flow rates to identical ventricular sections after administration of 1.0-1.5 mg/kg phentolamine. The a-blocking agent induces identical flow rates to all ventricular sections. Data from 12 experiments in 12 dogs. Heart rate: 125 ± 32 min^{-1}; mean arterial pressure: 88 ± 10 mm Hg.

heart disease. These anginal attacks could be prevented by previous administration of a-blocking agents.

In order to mimic such an exaggerated coronary vasoconstriction, we stimulated the hypothalamic defense area at various points and observed the changes in several hemodynamic parameters of dogs, in which the heart rates were experimentally kept constant. We never observed any signs of coronary vasoconstriction; the electric stimulation of the hypothalamic defense area resulted in either no immediate response on the coronary resistance, or in a small dilation, which was apparently β-adrenergically mediated and led to a lowered O_2 extraction from the coronary blood [8].

Due to the impossibility of demonstrating such an enhanced constrictive influence on the coronary vessels, we tested whether and to what extent the coronary bed participates in a generalized pressor response induced by intracarotid hypotension, using a similar dog preparation in the next series of experiments. The results are shown in Figure 2. A sudden bilateral carotid occlusion resulted in a fall of the

287

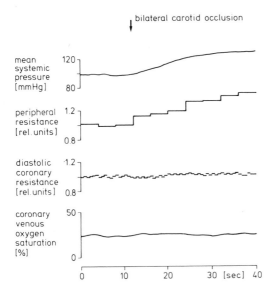

Fig. 2. Effect of bilateral carotid occlusion on total peripheral and coronary resistance. Redrawing of a typical experiment in a resting dog with fixed heart rate (AV block). Upon bilateral carotid occlusion at the arrow, a steady increase in total peripheral resistance is observed (calculations from aortic flow and mean systemic pressure in the thoracic aorta in 4-s intervals). No increase in diastolic coronary resistance was observed (beat to beat calculations from left circumflex coronary flow and aortic pressure). Coronary venous oxygen saturation remained constant. Ten identical experiments were carried out in four dogs with experimental AV block and the hearts paced at 90 min^{-1}

intracarotid blood pressure, which in turn triggered a typical pressor response. Mean systemic pressure steadily increased by 30 mm Hg over a period of 25 s. This increase mainly resulted from a substantial rise in total-peripheral resistance due to the sudden pressure drop at the carotid baroreceptors. However, from this generalized vasoconstriction, the coronary bed is completely excluded and did not even show a minute increase in resistance. This finding was substantiated by continuous recordings of arterial and coronary venous saturation. Following the bilateral carotid occlusion, myocardial oxygen extraction was virtually unaffected.

Similar experiments were carried out in three dogs, in which a mercury-filled occluder around the left circumflex coronary was used to produce an experimental coronary stenosis in order to mimic myocardial perfusion in patients suffering from coronary artery disease. The experimental coronary stenosis was quantified by its effect on postischemic reactive hyperemia (using a second occlusion cuff downstream to the mercury-filled occluder). Under the condition of a completely abolished coronary reserve (comparable to patients with severe coronary artery disease), various tests to induce general vasoconstriction and increase coronary resistance were applied: cold pressor test by immersion of the paw into ice water, dextran infusion at –1°C into the brachial artery and/or into the carotid artery, sudden pressure release at the carotid baroreceptors. None of these interventions resulted in an increase in coronary resistance (comparable to the observations by Mudge et al. [7] on patients with coronary artery disease). Hence, a modulation of the a-adrenergic constrictive influence on the coronary arteries towards an enhanced vasoconstriction or spasm could not be elicited by the interventions tested in our experiments.

However, the opposit effect, a sudden withdrawal of the a-adrenergic constrictive influence, leading to a steep, immediate rise in coronary flow and augmented coronary venous oxygen saturation, could be well demonstrated. This reflex-induced excess perfusion was observed during a pulmonary hyperinflation. The results of these experiments are shown in Figure 3. A hyperinflation, either a spontane-

Fig. 3. Coronary dilation induced by pulmonary hyperinflation. Original tracing from a conscious dog with fixed heart rate (AV block and ventricular pacing at 120 min^{-1}). Left panel: control condition at rest; middle panel: β-adrenergic blockade using propranolol; right panel: a-adrenergic blockade (in addition to the β-adrenergic blockade) using phentolamine. Chemoreceptor stimulation by intracarotid nicotine (arrows) results in a deep inspiration (see short periods of negative end-diastolic pressure in the left ventricular pressure recording). This

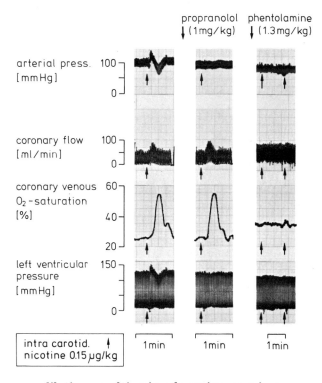

hyperinflation triggers a coronary dilation resulting in a large increase in coronary venous oxygen saturation. The changes in arterial and peak ventricular pressure following nicotine are minimized by β-adrenergic blockade, while the coronary dilation is unaffected. However, additional a-adrenergic blockade offsets the hyperinflation-induced coronary dilation (right panel)

ous deep breath or following the injection of 0.15 μg/kg nicotine into the carotid artery, resulted in a sudden steep rise in coronary flow and in coronary venous oxygen saturation from 24% saturation to 56% saturation. Application of a-blocking agents resulted in the complete disappearance of the hyperinflation-induced coronary excess perfusion.

In the same series of experiments, the transmural distribution of myocardial blood flow in the left ventricle was tested in two different states: [a] under resting conditions following 1.0 mg/kg propranolol and [b] during the maximum of hyperinflation-induced coronary dilation. The results are shown in Figure 4. During resting conditions under propranolol, myocardial blood flow was 65 ± 9 ml/100 g/min,

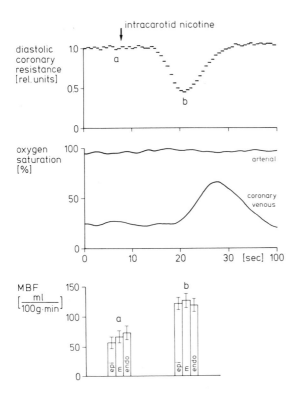

Fig. 4. Transmural distribution of myocardial blood flow (MBF) during hyperinflation-induced coronary dilation. Hyperinflation was induced by intracarotid nicotine (see Fig. 3) in eight experiments in eight dogs with fixed heart rate (AV block and ventricular pacing at 120 min^{-1}) under β-adrenergic blockade. Myocardial blood flow in different layers (epi = subepicardial; m = middle; endo = subendocardial) of left ventricle was measured by microspheres prior to nicotine injection [a], and during peak hyperinflation-induced coronary dilation [b]. Diastolic coronary resistance and arterial and coronary venous oxygen saturation are redrawn from one typical experiment.

favoring the subendocardial perfusion, which was found to be 32% higher than the subepicardial perfusion rate. At the maximum of hyperinflation-induced coronary dilation, the ventricular flow rate was doubled, amounting to 122 ± 11 ml/100 g/min and was similar in all ventricular layers. This demonstrates the existence of the a-constrictive influence throughout all layers of the left ventricular wall. The withdrawal of this a-constrictive influence on the coronary bed, results in an excess perfusion of 90%, a figure which compares very well to the excess perfusion obtained in the center of regional ventricular sympathectomy (+80%).

Similar experiments were carried out in three patients whose heart rates were kept constant by external ventricular pacing (unpublished experiments, K. Theisen, W. v. Restorff, and E. Bassenge). Using reflexion oximetry [9], coronary venous oxygen saturation was continuously monitored and amounted to 36%-45%. Upon a deep inspiration, the increase in coronary venous oxygen saturation never exceeded 5% saturation. Angiographically, there were very little or no signs of coronary artery disease, but the coronary reserve was not tested. It is not clear why these human probands did not show the amount of coronary excess perfusion which could be elicited by hyperinflation in the dog. One could speculate that the a-adrenergic constrictive control on the coronary bed in resting humans is less effective than in dogs (which in general exhibit coronary venous oxygen saturation levels [10] substantially below the ones reported for humans).

However, according to the findings in this study, the constrictive coronary tone in resting dogs is apparently very high, as indicated by the low coronary venous oxygen saturation. In contrast to humans, the coronary venous O_2 saturation declines even below 10% saturation in dogs during severe exercise, although an additional coronary dilatory capacity was still observed [10]. The high constrictive coronary tone could not be enhanced in our experiments. This might be explained by the fact that the interventions applied were not adequate to cause coronary vasoconstriction. The applied exposure to cold in dogs — in contrast to humans — does not result in any substantial increase in arterial pressure or peripheral resistance. Effects of baroreceptor reflexes on the coronary bed are relatively small; even with electric stimulation of the carotid sinus nerve in dogs, the sympathetic coronary tone is not offset, and coronary resistance decreases by less than 20% [12]. The hyperinflation reflex, however, is much more effective in offsetting the sympathetic coronary constrictive tone. This hyperinflation-induced excess perfusion of 90%, qualitatively and quantitatively confirms the conclusion derived from the studies on distribution of myocardial blood flow in regionally sympathectomized hearts: a surprisingly high coronary sympathetic constrictive tone in the resting dog. This tone might be beneficial for the efficiency of myocardial contraction, since at the onset of ventricular contraction, a part of the intramural blood volume is squeezed out of the myocardium, thus affecting rapid tension development. The sympathetic constrictive coronary tone reduces the intramural blood volume, and therefore increases the efficiency.

Summary

A defined regional ventricular sympathectomy was obtained by repeated intra-coronary injections of 6-hydroxydopamine in dogs. This regional sympathectomy resulted in an excess blood flow to the sympathectomized sections of 80%. a-blocking agents resulted in the disappearance of the different perfusion rates between the normally innervated and the sympathectomized sections, demonstrating a constrictive sympathetic tone on the coronary bed in the normally innervated control sections of these ventricles.
In another series of experiments in dogs without any pretreatment by 6-hydroxydopamine, modulations of this sympathetic coronary control were studied. An enhancement of the constrictive tone could not be elicited by electric stimulation of the hypothalamic defense area, baroreceptor reflex, or exposure to cold. However, a sudden withdrawal of the a-sympathetic constrictive tone resulting in coronary dilation could be elicited by a pulmonary hyperinflation, induced by chemoreceptor stimulation using intracarotid nicotine. During this coronary dilation, left ventricular myocardial blood flow increased by 90% and coronary venous oxygen saturation rose from 24% to 56%. This excess perfusion cannot be explained as metabolically induced and was completely offset by a-adrenergic blockade. Thus, a substantial sympathetic constrictive tone on the coronary bed was demonstrated and quantified using two basically different approaches.

References

1. Berne, R.M., DeGest, H., Levy, M.N.: Influence of the cardiac nerves on coronary resistance. Am. J. Physiol. 208, 763-769 (1965)
2. Doutheil, U., Ten Bruggencate, G., Kramer, K.: Koronarvasomotorik unter L-Noradrenalin und Isopropylnoradrenalin nach Blockierung der adrenergen β-Rezeptoren durch Nethalide. Pflügers Arch. 281, 181-190 (1964)
3. Feigl, E.O.: Sympathetic control of coronary circulation. Circ. Res. 20, 262-271 (1967)
4. Holtz, J., Mayer, E., Bassenge, E.: Demonstration of alpha-adrenergic coronary control in different layers of canine myocardium by regional myocardial sympathectomy. Pflügers Arch. 372, 187-194 (1977)
5. Klocke, E.J., Kaiser, G.A., Ross, J. (Jr.), Braunwald, E.: An intrinsic adrenergic vasodilator mechanism in the coronary vascular bed of the dog. Circ. Res. 16, 376-382 (1965)
6. McRaven, D.R., Merk, A.L., Abboud, F.M., Mayer, H.E.: Responses of coronary vessels to adrenergic stimuli. J. Clin. Invest. 50, 773-778 (1971)
7. Mudge, G.H., Grossman, W., Mills, R.M., Jr., Lesch, M., Braunwald, E.: Reflex increase in coronary vascular resistance in patients with ischemic heart disease. N. Engl. J. Med. 295, 1333-1337 (1976)
8. Restorff, W. von, Bassenge, E.: Evaluation of a neurogenic rapid coronary dilatation during an excitatory response in conscious dogs. Pflügers Arch. 367, 157-164 (1976)
9. Restorff, W. von, Bassenge, E.: Transient effects of norepinephrine on myocardial oxygen balance. Pflügers Arch. 370, 131-137 (1977)
10. Restorff, W. von, Holtz, J., Bassenge, E.: Exercise induced augmentation of myocardial oxygen extraction in spite of normal coronary dilatory capacity in dogs. Pflügers Arch. 372, 181-185 (1977)
11. Ross, G.: Adrenergic responses of the coronary vessels. Circ. Res. 39, 641-466 (1976)
12. Vatner, S.F., Franklin, D., Citters, R.L. van, Braunwald, E.: Effects of carotid sinus nerve stimulation on the coronary circulation of the conscious dog. Circ. Res. 27, 11-21 (1970)
13. Vatner, S.F., McRitchie, R.J.: Interaction of the chemoreflex and the pulmonary inflation reflex in the regulation of coronary circulation in conscious dogs. Circ. Res. 37, 664-673 (1975)
14. Yasue, H., Touyama, M., Shimamoto, M., Kato, H., Tanaka, S., Akiyama, F.: Role of autonomic nervous system in the pathogenesis of Prinzmetal's variant form of angina. Circulation 50, 534-539 (1974)
15. Yasue, H., Touyama, M., Kato, H., Tanaka, S., Akiyama, F.: Prinzmetal's variant form of angina as a manifestation of alpha-adrenergic receptor-mediated coronary artery spasm: documentation by coronary arteriography. Am. Heart J. 91, 148-155 (1976)
16. Zuberbuhler, R.C., Bohr, D.F.: Responses of coronary smooth muscle to catecholamines. Circ. Res. 16, 431-440 (1965)

Laudatio

Laudatio für Herrn Professor Dr. E. Wetterer

T. Kenner

Wir dürfen heute einem Arzt, Lehrer und Wissenschaftler unsere Reverenz erweisen, der in größter Bescheidenheit nie dem Erfolg nachgelaufen ist, und dessen Leistungen doch die moderne Kardiologie und Kreislaufforschung geprägt haben.

Für mich ist es eine ganz besonders große Ehre, dazu ausersehen worden zu sein, einige Worte über Herrn Wetterer, sein Leben und sein Werk, zu sagen.

Herr Wetterer wurde am 25. Jänner 1909 in Mannheim geboren. Gymnasium und Medizinstudium absolvierte er in Heidelberg. Nach der Promotion war Herr Wetterer als Medizinalpraktikant an der Medizinischen Klinik in Heidelberg tätig. Daher sind ihm klinische Probleme aus erster Hand bekannt. Er war jedoch nach seiner Promotion von den Vorzügen eines Physiologischen Instituts so überzeugt, daß er 1934 als Assistent zu Broemser nach München übersiedelte. Er wurde dadurch zum Mitglied der Frankschen Schule, sozusagen getauft durch die Arbeiten an der berühmten Broemserschen Wasserkunst, einem Modell des Arteriensystems an Hand dessen zu allererst die Frage der optimalen Abstimmung zwischen Herz und Arteriensystem vermutet worden war.

Nach der 1935 geschriebenen Dissertation über Versuche zur Kreislaufdynamik erfolgt bereits 1937 die Publikation der Erfindung des elektromagnetischen Strömungsmeßgerätes, des sogenannten Induktions-Tachographen.

Zur Beurteilung des Kreislaufzustandes ist einerseits die Messung des Blutdruckes, andererseits die Messung der Blutströmung notwendig. In den 30er Jahren war vor allem aufgrund der Leistungen Otto Franks und Philip Broemsers die Messung des pulsatilen Blutdrucks schon mit großer Genauigkeit möglich. Demgegenüber waren für die Messung der Blutströmung unzählige Methoden entworfen worden, die letztlich alle unbefriedigend waren, angefangen von der Ludwigschen Stromuhr über den Kriesschen Gastachographen bis zu Versuchen Broemsers mit einem Differentialmanometerprinzip.

Die große Leistung der Erfindung des elektromagnetischen Strömungsmeßgerätes besteht in der Idee der Anwendung eines bisher zu diesem Zweck nicht angewendeten Prinzips, der strömungsbedingten Induktion einer Spannung in einem Magnetfeld. Dieses Prinzip, das im Gegensatz zu früheren komplizierteren Methoden auch eine Eröffnung des Gefäßes überflüssig macht, eignet sich für die Strömungsmessung so hervorragend, daß die Methode auch heute noch zu den Standardmethoden der Strömungsmessung gezählt werden kann.

Wie es manchmal vorkommt, lag die Erfindung sozusagen in der Luft. Gleichzeitig mit Wetterer arbeitete in den USA Kolin unabhängig an der gleichen Erfindung. Kolins Beschreibung seiner Erfindung war, zunächst unbemerkt von Wetterer, 1936 erschienen. Die Entdeckung, daß die Priorität einem anderen gebühre, war nach der mühsamen Arbeit an der Perfektionierung der Methode für den jungen Wissenschaftler eine große Enttäuschung.

Bedingt durch den Krieg sind beide Herren erst lange Zeit später, durch das gemeinsame Interesse zusammengeführt, in freundschaftliche Verbindung getreten.

In den Jahren nach der Entwicklung der neuen Methode wurde diese von Wetterer zu einer Reihe von experimentellen Untersuchungen praktisch angewendet. Gemeinsam mit Deppe wurden die Ergebnisse der exakten Strömungsmessung mit den verschiedenen vorgeschlagenen Methoden der physikalischen Schlagvolumenbestimmung verglichen. Diese Messungen, die viel zu wenig bekannt geworden sind, zeigten die wesentlichen Fehlerquellen nicht-invasiver Methoden auf. Die heute wieder moderne Problematik nicht-invasiver Methoden war seit jeher ein Hauptanliegen der so oft als etwas weltfremd angesehenen "Pulsologen" der Frankschen Schule.

Auch für die experimentellen Studien, zu der als nächster akademischer Schritt geplanten Habilitation, wurden Messungen mit dem Induktionstachographen durchgeführt.

Die 1939 verfaßte Habilitationsschrift befaßte sich mit den "Beziehungen zwischen Stromstärke und Druck im natürlichen Kreislauf bei zeitlich variabler Elastizität des arteriellen Windkessels". Diese Arbeit lenkte die Aufmerksamkeit von der damals im Vordergrund stehenden Windkesselbetrachtung, auf die Wellendynamik des Arteriensystems.

1940 wurde Herr Wetterer zum Dozenten für Physiologie an der Universität München ernannt.

Wann immer heute in der Klinik oder im experimentellen Labor eine exakte Beurteilung eines verzerrungsfrei registrierten Blutdruckverlaufs im Herzen oder in einer Arterie notwendig ist, wird zur Registrierung ein Katheterspitzenmanometer verwendet. Kaum jemand, der heute ein solches Gerät um teures Geld kauft, weiß, daß Herr Wetterer bereits 1943 ein Katheterspitzenmanometer selbst gebaut, erprobt und publiziert hatte. Die besonderen Probleme beim Bau eines solchen Manometers bestehen in der Miniaturisierung des Manometers und in der Konstruktion der Kautschukmembran. Beide Probleme waren schon anfangs der 40er Jahre von Wetterer gelöst worden. Ein umfangreicher praktischer Einsatz des neuen Gerätes erfolgte erst später. Der erste Bau eines derartig miniaturisierten Manometers, das an der Spitze eines Herzkatheters Platz hat, war wegen der hierbei zu lösenden mechanischen und elektronischen Probleme kaum eine geringere Leistung als die Erfindung eines neuen Meßprinzips.

Neben seinen theoretischen und experimentellen Studien über hämodynamische Fragen und neben seinen Arbeiten an dem Miniaturmanometer, befaßte sich Herr Wetterer damals mit der Entwicklung und der technischen Verbesserung von biologisch anwendbaren Verstärkern. Im Jahre 1944 erschien eine Arbeit über Gleichspannungsverstärkung mittels Trägerfrequenz, eine Methode, die heute gang und gäbe ist, damals jedoch eine Neuheit darstellte.

Neben seinen Forschungsarbeiten hielt Herr Wetterer Vorlesungen über Physik für Zahnmediziner, eine Aufgabe der er mit einigen Unterbrechungen, mit viel Liebe bis zu seiner Berufung nach Erlangen nachkam.

Von den Ereignissen der Nachkriegszeit, die für Herrn Wetterer die Erfahrung der Arbeit in der medizinisch-technischen Industrie brachte, ist zu erwähnen, daß sein Lebensweg seit 1948 von Frau Erna begleitet wird.

Da es unmöglich ist, hier auf die Bedeutung der zahlreichen, in den folgenden Jahren erschienenen Arbeiten im einzelnen einzugehen, möchte ich im folgenden nur die wichtigsten, methodischen und theoretischen Studien von Herrn Wetterer erwähnen.

Von besonders weitreichender Bedeutung stellt sich jetzt die Entwicklung einer Methodik zur Beobachtung des diastolischen Abstromes aus dem gesamten Arteriensystem heraus, die gemeinsam mit Pieper durchgeführt wurde. In dieser Arbeit wurde das nichtlineare bzw. nicht proportionale Verhalten des gesamten peripheren Widerstandes quantitativ erfaßt und seine Beeinflussung durch verschiedene physiologische und pharmakologische Eingriffe untersucht. Diese Fragen sind im Zusammenhang mit der Theorie der Schlagvolumenformel, mit der Deutung der sogenannten Windkesselfunktion des Arteriensystems und hinsichtlich der Grundlage verschiedenster Kreislaufmodelle von größter Bedeutung. Weitere Studien aus den 50er Jahren betreffen Untersuchungen über Schlauchwellen und technische Arbeiten über die Anwendung von Transistoren als Kathodenwiderstände für elektrobiologische Zwecke.

Wie dies offenbar überall auf der Welt vorkommt, bei uns aber wohl besonders deutlich fühlbar, ist der Prophet im eigenen Land am wenigsten angesehen.

Als erste Anerkennung seiner Arbeiten erfolgte 1953 eine Einladung zu einer Vortragsreise in die USA. Eine Anerkennung in der Heimat erhielt Herr Wetterer erst 3 Jahre später durch die Einladung, ein Übersichtsreferat bei der Tagung der Deutschen Gesellschaft für Kreislaufforschung in Bad Nauheim 1956 zu halten. 1960 erhielt Herr Wetterer eine Einladung, einen Artikel für die Ergebnisse der Physiologie zu schreiben. In einem schwachen Moment hat er mich damals dazu ausersehen, als Mitautor daran teilzunehmen. Wie bekannt, ist aus dem geplanten Artikel durch laufende Perfektion, später eine umfangreiche Monographie geworden. 1961 wurde Herr Wetterer eingeladen, ein Hauptreferat über Blutströmungsmessung auf der „4th International Conference on Medicals Electronics" über elektromagnetische Strömungsmessung zu halten. 1963 erschien ein zusammenfassender Artikel über elektromagnetische Strömungsmessung aus seiner Hand im „Handbook of Physiology".

Ein Thema, das die Arbeiten in diesen Jahren nicht immer ganz angenehm und vorteilhaft begleitete, war der Frage gewidmet, ob sich die Wellenlänge der sogenannten stehenden Welle im Arteriensystem zu der Länge dieses Systems im Verhältnis 1:4 oder 1:2 verhalte. Dieses Problem, das im Zusammenhang mit der physikalischen Schlagvolumenmessung steht, und gewisse Fragen betreffend die Theorie der elastischen Dehnbarkeit der kleinen Gefäße, ergaben einen immer wieder aufflackernden Zwist mit dem Frankfurter Institut.

Die schriftstellerische Arbeit an dem großen, zunächst für die Ergebnisse der Physiologie geplanten Artikel, wurde sofort nach Beginn unterbrochen, um Versuche aufzubauen und durchzuführen. Die ersten gemeinsamen Überlegungen und Entwürfe hatten einen Mangel an experimentellen Überprüfungen der theoretisch geforderten und auch mathematisch unterbauten Vorstellungen über die Wellenausbreitung und die Wellenreflexion in den Arterien ergeben. Herr Wetterer und seine Familie wohnte damals unter dem Dach des Münchner Physiologischen Instituts, sodaß wir, ich darf mich hier einschließen, Tag und Nacht fast durchgehend arbeiteten, nur durch die Essenszeit und die Kaffeepausen unterbrochen, während der die Diskussionen auch nicht abbrachen. Danach entstanden die Versuchsaufbauten zur Demonstration des Effektes von Stoßstellen und der Wirkung der kontinuierlichen Zunahme des Wellenwiderstandes auf die Pulsformen. Es muß erwähnt werden, daß mindestens die Hälfte unserer experimentellen Erfolge als Verdienst der seelischen und körperlichen Betreuung durch Frau Wetterer anzusehen sind.

Seit 1965 ist Herr Wetterer Vorstand des II. Physiologischen Instituts der Universität Erlangen-Nürnberg und wurde gleich nach dem ersten Jahr seiner Übersiedlung zum Dekan der Medizinischen Fakultät gewählt. In der Zeit nach der Übersiedlung wurde die Monographie trotz mancher Schwierigkeiten fertiggestellt, sodaß sie 1968 erscheinen konnte.

Hier ist auch zu erwähnen, daß Herr Wetterer immer mit viel Liebe die offenbar unvermeidlichen psychologischen Schwierigkeiten des Personals und mancher Assistenten behoben bzw. mit der größten Geduld ertragen hat.

1966 wurde er mit dem wohlverdienten Arthur Weber-Preis ausgezeichnet. 1967 erschien, auch als Frucht seiner Lehrtätigkeit, der Beitrag „Bau und Funktion des Gefäßsystems" im kurzgefaßten Lehrbuch der Physiologie, das von Herrn Keidel herausgegeben wurde.

Ebenso exakt wie alle seine Arbeiten, ist auch die Vorlesung organisiert. Ich erinnere mich noch an die Zeit, wo wir mit der sogenannten Kanone bewaffnet, das ist ein langes Rohr, in dem die Wandtafeln vor Regen geschützt transportiert werden konnten, durch den Schloßpark zum Hauptgebäude in die Vorlesung marschierten. Von Herrn Wetterer geprüft zu werden, war bei allen Studenten beliebt, da es niemals passierte, daß er, der sehr genau und ausgiebig prüft, jemand ungerecht beurteilt hätte.

Das Werk Wetterers wird 1971 durch den Bau des Instituts in der Waldstraße physisch gekrönt. Eine neue Periode beginnt mit der Zusammenarbeit mit den Assistenten, die ihren Dank nun durch dieses Symposion ausdrücken.

Die Übersiedlung in das neugebaute Institut erfolgte Anfang 1972. Noch im gleichen Jahr findet in Erlangen unter dem Vorsitz Wetterers die Frühjahrstagung der Deutschen Physiologischen Gesellschaft statt.

Die wissenschaftliche Arbeit im neuen Institut bringt die Fortsetzung und Erfüllung früherer Pläne.

Die inhomogene Wellenleitung wird mittels eines Computermodells simuliert. Fragen der Entstehung der Pulsformen in verschiedenen Arterien werden durch Vergleich dieses Modells mit Messungen am Menschen und im Tierversuch geprüft. Ein altes schon in den Anfängen der 60er Jahre bearbeitetes Problem wird wieder aufgegriffen: die Problematik der Umfang-Druckbeziehung während der schnellen Pulsation der Arterien. Eine neue Methode der optischen Registrierung der Durchmesserpulsationen wird entwickelt. Die beobachteten Resultate geben neue Fragen, und aus der Diskussion folgen neue Ideen und Experimente. Die Frage der Nichtlinearität der Wandviskosität der Blutgefäße ist vorläufig eine der letzten Früchte dieser Arbeit.

1974 leitet Wetterer als Vorsitzender der Deutschen Gesellschaft für Kreislaufforschung deren traditionsreiche Jahrestagung in Bad Nauheim über das Thema „Das arterielle System".

Im Frühjahr 1977 wird Herrn Wetterer in Anbetracht seiner Verdienste um die physiologische Forschung und Lehre die Ehrenmitgliedschaft der Deutschen Physiologischen Gesellschaft verliehen.

Es muß erwähnt sein, daß manche Autoren von wissenschaftlichen Arbeiten und selbst von Lehrbüchern, die sich mit hämodynamischen Problemen befassen, offensichtlich die Leistungen Wetterers noch nicht verstanden haben. Die Folgen dieser Ignoranz sind Fehler der Interpretation, die leicht hätten vermieden werden können. Allzu offensichtliche und überraschende Unkenntnis bestraft sich sozusagen selbst.

Wetterers Institut steht allen jenen ständig offen, die mit Fragen, betreffend spezielle hämodynamische Probleme, beladen nach Erlangen kommen. Es kommt nicht selten vor, daß die von einem Besucher bei langen Diskussionen gewonnenen Einsichten, später ohne Nennung der wahren Quelle publiziert, in Sonderdruckform mit freundlicher Widmung in Erlangen auf den Chefschreibtisch flattern.

Nie hat Herr Wetterer offen über diese Wermutstropfen geklagt und nie hat er bei Tagungen oder anderen Zusammenkünften den betreffenden Kollegen ihre Handlungsweise spüren lassen.

Von all den Dingen, die wir von Herrn Wetterer gelernt haben oder hätten lernen sollen, ist wohl leider seine Bescheidenheit am wenigsten nachgeahmt und kopiert worden. In unserer schnellebigen und überheblichen Zeit, wird Bescheidenheit als Schwäche angesehen, ja sogar als Zeichen von Dummheit interpretiert. So manchem, der dieser Meinung war, ist allerdings bei Diskussionen mit Herrn Wetterer demonstriert worden, daß Bescheidenheit, gepaart mit profunder Kenntnis, in den meisten Lebenslagen weiterführt, als der Versuch, sich nur auf ein gutes Mundwerk zu verlassen.

Das Leben besteht nicht allein aus Wissenschaft und Arbeit. Herrn Wetterers besondere Neigung gilt neben der Wissenschaft dem Bergsteigen, der Musik und der Kunst der orientalischen Teppichknüpferei. Es ist schon viel über die enge Beziehung zwischen Wissenschaft und Kunst philosophiert worden. Ich glaube aber, das Geheimnis liegt darin, daß die wirklich großen Entdeckungen und Erfindungen nur dem gelingen, der abseits von allem Ehrgeiz das Schöne sucht. Darum sind auch die meisten großen Forscher und Ärzte gleichzeitig auch Musiker und Künstler und selbst, wenn sie die Kunst nicht aktiv ausüben, spiegelt sich in der Ausübung der Wissenschaft das Erfinderische des Künstlers wieder.

Ich vermute, daß für Herrn Wetterer die Verarbeitung des königlichen Themas im Musikalischen Opfer und in der Kunst der Fuge ähnlich begeisternd wirkt, wie das klar durchdachte Schaltschema eines Verstärkers oder die Anwendung der Reflexionsgesetze zur Deutung der Pulsformen.

Neben seiner Bescheidenheit, ist als wesentliches Kennzeichen seiner Persönlichkeit das Streben nach Perfektion zu erwähnen. Die wichtigsten seiner Arbeiten, Entdeckungen und Erfindungen haben nur deswegen eine schnelle Anerkennung und eine technische Nutzung nicht umgehend erhalten, weil die gewissenhafte Bearbeitung eine rasche Publikation der ersten Idee, ohne genaue Austestung, nicht zuließ und auch nicht erlaubte, den zweiten und dritten Schritt zu planen, bevor der erste abgeschlossen war.

Das elektronische Basteln ist für Herrn Wetterer gleichzeitig Hobby, Entspannung und wissenschaftliche Arbeit und ist immer in jener Perfektion gelungen, die vor ihm selbst die Arbeit rechtfertigt. Leider hat er daneben die aktive Ausführung der Musik aufgegeben, weil ihm hierfür jene von ihm selbst geforderte Perfektionierung neben dem Beruf nicht möglich erschien.

Wenn abends im Institut noch bis in die Nacht hinein Licht brennt, dann wird wohl im Chef-Labor eine neue Schaltung ausprobiert. Es ist für einen Physiologen eine ideale Fähigkeit, Geräte für die Experimente selbst bauen zu können, und es ist ein besonderes Glück, wenn Arbeit und Vergnügen praktisch übereinstimmen.

Herr Wetterer ist ein Lehrer, der Tag und Nacht zu Diskussionen und Experimenten bereit ist. Ich habe nie erlebt, daß er bei den durch mich verursachten zahlreichen Störungen jemals ungeduldig geworden wäre. Erst durch seine Diskussionen und seine konstruktive Kritik ist manche unreife Idee praktikabel geworden.

Das Haus Wetterer ist immer ein offenes Haus. Was immer auf der Welt an hämodynamischen Problemen untersucht wird, ist irgendwann bei Kaffee im Dachgeschoß des Münchner Physiologischen Instituts oder im Haus in Buckenhof diskutiert worden. Aber nicht nur Hämodynamik. Dies gilt nun auch für die Kunst des Teppichknüpfens, für Fragen der Interpretation der Bachschen Musik, und für Diskussion von literarischen Werken. Ich habe viele Geschichten erzählen gehört über die Zeit der Meister in München, die Erlebnisse in den Labors beim Begrübeln von Problemen und unerwarteten Resultaten, die Erlebnisse auf Bergtouren und Wanderungen, die teils wissenschaftliche und teils vergnügliche Ziele hatten.

Hier sind jene anwesend, die würdiger und kompetenter als ich hierüber erzählen könnten.

Ich möchte diese Laudatio nicht beenden, ohne auch Frau Wetterer mit einzubeziehen. Sie ist der Stützpunkt der Wissenschaft und hütet das stets bereite Refugium. Vieles wäre ohne sie nicht oder doch nur unvollständig gelungen. Ohne ihre Geduld, bei Tisch, bei Kaffee, bei Spaziergängen, das viele Fachsimpeln zu ertragen, wäre so manche Idee noch vor der Formulierung zugrundegegangen.

Ich glaube abschließend sagen zu dürfen, daß wir und unsere Studenten das Beispiel eines aufrechten, offenen und bescheidenen Mannes wie Wetterer und das Beispiel einer Frau, die immer für ihren Mann bereitsteht, bitter nötig brauchen.

Für dieses Beispiel zu danken, ist uns Ehre und Pflicht.

Subject Index

W. A. McAlpine
Heart and Coronary Arteries
An Anatomical Atlas for Clinical Diagnosis, Radiological Investigation, and Surgical Treatment
1975. 1098 figures mostly in color. XVI, 224 pages
Cloth DM 198,–; US $ 99.00
ISBN 3-540-06985-2
Distribution rights for Japan:
Igaku Shoin Ltd., Tokyo

W. Wenz
Abdominale Angiography
Unter Mitarbeit von G. van Kaick, D. Beduhn, F.-J. Roth
1972. 183 zum Teil farbige Abbildungen in 351 Einzeldatstellungen und 34 Zeichnungen. X, 225 Seiten
Gebunden DM 116,–; US $ 58.00
ISBN 3-540-05788-9
Vertriebsrechte für Japan:
Igaku Shoin Ltd. Tokyo
Auch in englischer Sprache lieferbar

H. M. Duvernoy
The Superficial Veins of the Human Brain
Veins of the Brain Stem and of the Base of the Brain.
1975. 71 figures (138 separate illustr.).
VI, 110 pages
Cloth DM 96,–; US $ 48.00
ISBN 3-540-06876-7
Distribution rights for Japan:
Nankado Co. Ltd., Tokyo

P. Meiisel, D. E. Apitzsch
Atlas der Nierenangiographie
Unter Mitarbeit von L. Laasonen, S. Tötterman, M. Valle
Mit einem Geleitwort von W. Frommhold
1978. 336 Abbildungen. IX, 201 Seiten
Gebunden DM 148,–; US $ 74.00
ISBN 3-540-08486-X

G. B. Bradac, R. Oberson
Arterial Cerebral Occlusive Disease
Angiography and Complementary examinations
1978. Approx. 137 figures.
Approx. 200 pages
ISBN 3-540-08898-9
Scheduled for publication Winter 1978
Prices are subject to change without notice

Angiography of the Human Brain Cortex
Atlas of Vasculat Patterns and Stereotactic Cortical Localization
By G. Szikla, G. Bouvier, T. Hori, V. Petrov
With collaboration of E. A. Cabanis, P. Farnarier, M. T. Iba-Zizen, Foreword by J. Talairach
1977. 22 figures, 199 plates. X, 273 pages
Cloth DM 340,–; US $ 170.00
ISBN 3-540-08285-9
Distribution rights for Japan:
Maruzen Co. Ltd., Tokyo

Prices are subject to change without notice
Preisänderungen vorbehalten

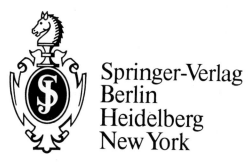

Springer-Verlag
Berlin
Heidelberg
New York

M. Bessis

Blood Smears Reinterpreted

Translated from the French by G. Brecher

1977. 342 figures, some in color. XV, 270 pages
Cloth DM 96,–; US $ 48.00
ISBN 3-540-07206-3

M. Bessis

Corpuscles

Atlas of Red Blood Cell Shapes
1974. 121 figures, 147 pages
Cloth DM 96,–; US $ 48.00
ISBN 3-540-06375-7
Distribution rights for Japan:
Maruzen Co. Ltd., Tokyo

M. Bessis

Living Blood Cells and their Ultrastructure

Translated by R. I. Weed

1973. 521 figures, 2 color plates. XXI, 767 pages
Cloth DM 168,–; US $ 84.00
ISBN 3-540-05981-4
Distribution rights for Japan:
Maruzen Co. Ltd., Tokyo

R. Djindjian, J.-J. Merland

Super-Selective Arteriography of the External Carotid Artery

With collaboration of J. Théron
Translated from the French by
I. F. Moseley
Preface by R. Houdart

1978. 1068 figures, 5 plates, some in color.
XVIII, 550 pages
Cloth DM 430,–; US $ 215.00
ISBN 3-540-08118-6

Handbuch der allgemeinen Pathologie

Herausgeber: H.-W. Altmann, F. Büchner, H. Cottier, E. Grundmann, G. Holle, E. Letterer, W. Masshoff, H. Meessen, F. Roulet, G. Seifert, G. Siebert

Band 3

Zwischensubstanzen, Gewebe, Organe

Teil 7

Mikrozirkulation/ Microcirculation

Von M. Boutet, U. Fuchs, P. Gaethgens, O. H. Gauer, F. Hammersen, D. L. Heene, I. Hüttner, K. Kirsch, J. Lang, H. G. Lasch, D. W. Lübbers, R. G. Mason, R. Poche, G. Rona, H. Schmid-Schönbein, D. E. Sharp
Redigiert von H. Meessen

1977. 256 Abbildungen. XXVI, 1138 Seiten (34 Seiten in Englisch)
Gebunden DM 560,–; US $ 280.00
ISBN 3-540-07750-2

Prices are subject to change without notice
Preisänderungen vorbehalten

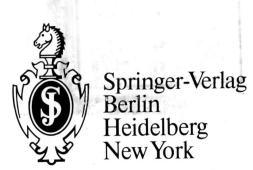

Springer-Verlag
Berlin
Heidelberg
New York